In his 1988 report on nutrition and health, Surgeon General C. Everett Koop said, "Of greatest concern is our excessive intake of dietary fat and its relationship to risk for chronic diseases such as coronary heart disease, some types of cancers, diabetes, high blood pressure, strokes and obesity."

The first recommendation in the Surgeon General's report is, "Reduce consumption of fat." Americans eat too much fat; 37% of all our calories are fat. Experts recommend that we reduce our fat intake by one-third.

The Food Marketing Institute in a recent survey found that the top nutritional concern of American consumers is the amount of fat in their food. Americans know that they eat more fat than is good for them. They want to do something about it.

Now it's easier to watch your fat intake—and protect your health—with the more than 10,000 handy alphabetical listings in *The Fat Counter*.

ANNETTE B. NATOW, PH.D., R.D., and JO-ANN HESLIN, M.S., R.D., are the authors of thirteen books on nutrition, including *The Cholesterol Counter*, *The Diabetes Carbohydrate and Calorie Counter*, *The Fat Attack Plan* and *The Pregnancy Nutrition Counter*. Both are former faculty members of Adelphi University and State University of New York, Downstate Medical Center. They are editors of *The Journal of Nutrition for the Elderly*, serve as editorial board members for *American Baby* and *Environmental Nutrition Newsletter*, and are frequent contributors to magazines and journals.

Look for *The Sodium Counter*
Coming from Pocket Books in July 1993

Books by Annette B. Natow and Jo-Ann Heslin

The Cholesterol Counter
The Diabetes Carbohydrate and Calorie Counter
The Fat Attack Plan
The Fat Counter
The Iron Counter
Megadoses
No-Nonsense Nutrition for Kids
The Pocket Encyclopedia of Nutrition
The Pregnancy Nutrition Counter
The Sodium Counter

Published by POCKET BOOKS

THE
·FAT·
COUNTER

SECOND EDITION
REVISED AND UPDATED

Annette B. Natow, Ph.D., R.D.,
and Jo-Ann Heslin, M.A., R.D.

POCKET BOOKS

New York   London   Toronto   Sydney   Tokyo   Singapore

An *Original* Publication of POCKET BOOKS

POCKET BOOKS, a division of Simon & Schuster Inc.
1230 Avenue of the Americas, New York, NY 10020

Copyright © 1989, 1993 by Annette Natow and Jo-Ann Heslin

All rights reserved, including the right to reproduce
this book or portions thereof in any form whatsoever.
For information address Pocket Books, 1230 Avenue
of the Americas, New York, NY 10020

ISBN: 0-671-69564-9

First Pocket Books printing February 1993

10 9 8 7 6 5 4 3

POCKET and colophon are registered trademarks of
Simon & Schuster Inc.

Cover design by Tom McKeveny

Printed in the U.S.A.

To our families who support us through every project: Harry, Allen, Irene, Susan, Meryl, Louis, Mark, George, Cindy, Steven, Joseph, Kristen, and Karen

ACKNOWLEDGMENTS

Without the tireless cooperation of Steven and Stephen *The Fat Counter* would never have been completed. A special thanks to our editor, Sally Peters, and our agent, Nancy Trichter.

Our thanks also go to all the food manufacturers who graciously shared their data.

SOURCES OF DATA

Values in this counter have been obtained from the Composition of Foods, United States Department of Agriculture, Agricultural Handbooks: No. 8-1, Dairy and Egg Products; No. 8-2, Spices and Herbs; No. 8-3, Baby Foods; No. 8-4, Fats and Oils; No. 8-5, Poultry Products; No. 8-6, Soups, Sauces and Gravies; No. 8-7, Sausages and Luncheon Meats; No. 8-8, Breakfast Cereals; No. 8-9, Fruits and Fruit Juices; No. 8-10, Pork Products; No. 8-11, Vegetables and Vegetable Products; No. 8–12, Nut and Seed Products; No. 8-13, Beef Products; No. 8–14, Beverages; No. 8-15, Finfish and Shellfish Products; No. 8-16, Legumes and Legume Products; No. 8-17, Lamb, Veal and Game Products; No. 8-19, Snacks and Sweets; No. 8-20, Cereal Grains and Pasta; No. 8-21, Fast Foods; Supplements 1989, 1990.

Nutritive Value of Foods, United States Department of Agriculture, Home and Garden Bulletin No. 72.

J. Davies and J. Dickerson, Nutrient Content of Food Portions. Cambridge, UK: The Royal Society of Chemistry, 1991.

G. A. Leveille, M. E. Zabik and K. J. Morgan, Nutrients in Foods. Cambridge, MA: The Nutrition Guild, 1983.

Souci, Fachmann and Kraut, Food Composition and Nutrition Tables. Stuttgart: Wissenschaftliche Verlagsgesellschaft MbH, 1989.

Information from food labels, manufacturers and processors. The values are based on research conducted prior to 1992. Manufacturers' ingredients are subject to change, so current values may vary from those listed in the book.

"Too much fat is a disadvantage . . . laying the foundation for troubles with the heart."

"Foods very high in fuel value, i.e., fats and dishes containing much fat, should be avoided."

MARY SWARTZ ROSE, PH.D.
Feeding the Family
The Macmillan Company, 1919

many of which result in death or disability.

INTRODUCTION

". . . the primary priority for dietary change is the recommendation to reduce intake of total fats."

C. EVERETT KOOP
Surgeon General's Report on Nutrition
and Health, 1988

The first recommendation in the Surgeon General's report is "Reduce consumption of fat." Americans eat too much fat; 37 percent of all our calories are fat. Experts believe that we should be eating much less. They recommend that we reduce our fat intake by one-third.

The Food Marketing Institute in a recent survey found that the top nutritional concern of American consumers is the amount of fat in their food. Americans know that they eat more fat than is good for them. They want to do something about it.

FAT FACTS

Too Much Is Not Safe

High fat diets are unhealthy. Almost three-fourths of the two million Americans who died last year died from diseases linked to our high fat diet.

Eating too much fat increases the risk for:

HEART ATTACK—Americans have more than one and a half million heart attacks each year with more than half a million deaths as a result.

STROKE—Americans have one half million strokes each year, many of which result in death or disability.

CANCER—Studies suggest that high fat intake increases risk for breast, colon and prostate cancer.

OVERWEIGHT—Diets high in fat lead to overweight more easily than do diets high in protein or carbohydrate. High fat diets make you fatter faster.

GALLBLADDER DISEASE—People with high fat diets who are overweight have a greater risk of gallbladder trouble.

OSTEOARTHRITIS—High fat diets cause overweight, putting more strain on the joints.

HEARING LOSS—Studies suggest that as people age, high fat and high cholesterol intakes coupled with high blood pressure can lead to hearing loss.

GOUT—A high fat diet aggravates gout.

DIABETES—High fat diets cause overweight, increasing the risk for diabetes and complicating treatment.

Most foods contain fat. Some have more, some less, few have none. Some fat can be easily seen—butter, margarine, salad oils and the fat on your steak or chop. Much of the fat you eat can't be seen. There's invisible fat in meat, milk, egg yolks, olives, walnuts, cakes, pies, cookies and candy. Whether you can see the fat or not, it adds up quickly.

FAT FACT #1: *Everyone should be eating less fat.* Americans eat too much fat. Almost 40 percent of all the calories we eat are from fat! Experts agree that we should be eating much less; 30 percent of our calories should come from fat.

FAT FACT #2: *Fat makes you fatter faster.* The fat we eat gets turned into body fat much easier than the other things we eat. Fat calories make us fatter than calories from protein, sugar or starch.

FAT FACT #3: *Fat comes in three forms*—saturated, polyunsaturated and monounsaturated.

The different kinds of fat in foods depend on the fatty acids they contain. Fats can be saturated, polyunsaturated or monounsaturated. Most foods contain all three of these fats. Some foods have more of one type than another. For example, beef has a lot more saturated fat, margarine a lot of polyunsaturated fat, and olive oil is high in monounsaturated fat.

Saturated Fat

How can you tell the difference between the three fats? If you left a stick of butter on the kitchen counter all day it would soften but it wouldn't melt. Butter is high in saturated fat. Saturated fat is solid at room temperature.

Research shows that eating a lot of saturated fats raises blood cholesterol levels. People with higher blood cholesterol levels are more likely to have a heart attack. Recently it has been found that not all saturated fats raise cholesterol. Even though that is true, foods we eat never contain only one type of saturated fat. All fats in foods are mixtures of fats. Foods often contain some saturated fats that raise cholesterol and other saturated fats that may not. That makes it difficult to translate these studies into food recommendations. *The safest recommendation: eat less total fat.*

FOODS HIGH IN SATURATED FATS

Whole milk
Cheese
Butter
Cream
Sour cream
Whipped cream
Half & Half
Ice cream
Beef
Pork
Lamb
Veal
Duck
Chicken
Fish
Hot dogs
Lunch meats
Sausage
Chocolate
Coconut
Coconut oil
Palm oil
Palm kernel oil

Polyunsaturated Fat

Corn oil left out on the kitchen counter will not get solid. It doesn't even get solid in the refrigerator. Polyunsaturated fats are liquid at room temperature. These fats may help lower cholesterol levels in the blood. Research suggests that too much polyunsaturated fat may not be good. High intake may cause gallbladder disease, depress the immune system and put you at greater risk for some cancers. *The safest recommendation: eat less total fat.*

FOODS HIGH IN POLYUNSATURATED FATS

Corn oil
Cottonseed oil
Sunflower oil
Safflower oil
Sesame oil
Soybean oil
Soft margarine
Salad dressing
Mayonnaise
Walnuts
Walnut oil
Wheat germ
Tuna
Salmon
Bluefish
Mackerel
Sablefish
Herring
Whitefish
Rainbow trout

Monounsaturated Fats

Olive oil left out on the kitchen counter never becomes solid. In the refrigerator olive oil gets cloudy as it becomes partly solid. Monounsaturated fat stays liquid at room temperature but becomes partly solid when chilled. You may have been hearing more about monounsaturated fats lately. Recent research shows these fats may help lower blood cholesterol. This sounds good but too much of any fat is not good for you. *The safest recommendation: eat less total fat.*

FOODS HIGH IN MONOUNSATURATED FAT

Canola oil
Olive oil
Peanut oil
Sesame oil
Soybean oil
Soybean oil margarine
Almonds
Cashews
Filberts (hazelnuts)
Macadamia nuts
Peanuts
Pignolia (pine nuts)
Pistachio nuts
Peanut butter
Chicken fat
Olives
Shortening made from vegetable fat

FINDING FAT IN FOODS

Doesn't everybody need some fat?

Yes, you do need a small amount of fat. Fat is part of every cell in your body. It is used to make hormones. Fat cushions bones and body organs. Fat insulates the body and helps maintain normal temperature. Food fats carry fat soluble vitamins, A, D, E and K. Fats stay in the stomach longer making you feel full so that you don't get hungry as soon.

Finding Food Fats

Most fruits and vegetables have little or no fat. There are a few exceptions, like avocados and olives (see page 10 and page 312).

Dried peas and beans are all pretty low in fat. Soybeans have a little more fat than other beans (see pages 442–43).

All nuts and seeds, including coconut and peanuts, have a lot of fat. All these are examples of hidden fat.

Grains like oats, rice, wheat, rye and barley contain little fat. Cereals, breads and pasta made from grains are usually low in fat. Exceptions are some granola-type cereals, cookies, pies, sweet rolls and cakes. You can tell how much fat is in a cookie by how soft it is. The softer the cookie, the more fat it has. Judge your cookies by breaking them in half; a cookie that bends instead of breaking is higher in fat. Place a croissant, muffin or danish on a napkin for a few minutes. If a grease ring forms, it's high in fat.

People think of animal foods like meat, milk, cheese, eggs, poultry and fish as good protein foods. While this is true, it is also true that all animal foods contain fat. In fact an ounce of lean meat has the same amount of calories from protein as from fat. In fatty meat like spare ribs, there may be twice as many calories from fat as from protein. Meats like bacon should really be thought of as fat not meat. The fat in one slice of bacon is equal to the fat in a pat of butter.

Choosing Low Fat Proteins

1. Choose skim or low fat milk and yogurt. Use skim milk cheese or reduced fat cheese. On occasions when you eat regular cheese, limit the portion.

2. Use low fat yogurt in place of sour cream.

3. Choose the leanest cuts of meat; remove all visible fat before cooking.

4. Choose ground beef that has as little fat as possible. Supermarkets label the ground beef with the percentage of fat; sometimes it is as low as 10 percent or less. Ground poultry is a good substitute for ground meat. It is usually lower in fat.

5. Roast, broil or grill meats on a rack so that fats drip

off during cooking. When making soups, stews or sauces, skim fat off the top.

6. Avoid turkey and turkey breasts that are "self basted." The basting usually adds more fat.

7. Poultry skin is high in fat. Remove it before eating.

8. All fish contains less fat than most cuts of meat. Very lean fish choices are: cod, scrod, flounder, halibut, pollock, sole and haddock. Shellfish like shrimp, lobster, scallops and crab are low in fat too.

9. Choose tuna canned in water. Tuna is a low fat fish, but when it is canned in oil it contains seven times more fat than when it is canned in water.

10. Choose poached, steamed or broiled fish instead of breaded, battered and fried.

Reading Labels

There's a lot of information on labels but sometimes it can be confusing. When you want to know more about a food, look at the list of ingredients. Packaged foods have ingredient listings. The first ingredient listed is the main one in the food. If it is fat, this is a high fat food. But even if fat is the second or third ingredient listed, the food is fairly high in fat.

Fats on labels can appear as any of the following:

> Animal fats (lard, suet, chicken fat)
> Butter
> Cocoa butter
> Cream
> Cheese
> Whole milk
> Diglycerides
> Fat

Hydrogenated fat
Hydrogenated oil
Margarine
Monoglycerides
Oil
Partially hydrogenated fat
Partially hydrogenated oil
Shortening
Vegetable fat
Vegetable oil

Choosing the Best Fats

Once in a while everyone feels like having some toast with butter or margarine. In most homes you find butter, margarine and some kind of cooking oil. Even low fat recipes may call for some oil or shortening. There are things you should remember to help you choose the best fats.

When selecting a margarine, choose one with a liquid oil as the first ingredient. Avoid margarines with tropical oils, such as palm oil and palm kernel oil. Soft tub margarines are often highest in polyunsaturates. For example, if liquid sunflower oil is the first ingredient, this would be a highly polyunsaturated oil. If the nutrition information panel lists 4 grams polyunsaturated oil and 2 grams fat per serving, twice as much polyunsaturated fat as saturated fat, this is a good ratio. Using moderate amounts of this or a similar margarine would be a good choice.

You may have also seen butter blends which are a combination of some butter and some margarine. Blends have less saturated fat than butter but more saturated fat than margarines.

A good, all purpose cooking oil is tasteless and fries without smoking. Corn, safflower, sunflower, soybean, cottonseed are all highly polyunsaturated oils. Peanut, olive, and canola oil are high in polyunsaturates and monounsaturates. All are good choices.

FINDING FAT CALORIES IN FOOD

Fat calories make you fatter faster. The food fat we eat is easily turned into body fat. You can limit fat calories by counting fat grams.

Nutrition labels can help you find out how much fat is in a food. Fat is listed in grams.

$$1 \text{ gram of fat} = 9 \text{ calories}$$

For example, 1 oz. of corn chips has 155 calories and 9 grams of fat.

$$9 \text{ grams of fat} \times 9 \text{ calories} = 81 \text{ fat calories}$$

More than one-half of the calories in corn chips come from fat.

Fat foods have a lot of calories. One teaspoon of fat has 45 calories. A teaspoon of protein, sugar or starch has only 20 calories.

Another example: 1 oz. of pretzels has 120 calories and 1 gram of fat.

$$1 \text{ gram of fat} \times 9 \text{ calories} = 9 \text{ fat calories}$$

Less than one-tenth of the calories in pretzels come from fat. Pretzels are a good snack choice. Less fat, less fat calories, less fattening for you.

There is an easy rule of thumb that will help you pick lower fat foods having fewer than 30 percent of their calories as fat. *Choose foods that contain no more than one gram of fat for every 30 calories.* For example: a raisin cookie has 70 calories and one gram of fat, less than one gram of fat in 30 calories. That would be a better choice than a chocolate chip cookie with 85 calories and 5 grams of fat, which has more than one gram of fat for 30 calories.

How Much Fat Should You Eat?

Americans eat too much fat. A few years ago, the average American got over 40 percent of his calories from fat. We eat a little less now. But still, we get a whopping 37 percent of our calories from fat. Experts agree we should be eating much less.

The American Heart Association, The American Cancer Society, The American Health Foundation and the Surgeon General all recommend lowering fat intake. Americans should eat no more than 30 percent of their food as fat each day.

That's a good suggestion. How do you do it? The question is how many grams of fat can you eat and still limit your fat to no more than 30 percent of your calories? It's easy to find out.

1. *Find out how many calories you eat each day.* If you maintain the same weight, you are probably eating:

   13 calories a pound, if you are not very active
   15 calories a pound, if you are moderately active
   17 calories a pound, if you are very active
   20 calories a pound, if you are extremely active

For example, if you weigh 145 pounds and are moderately active you need 2175 calories a day. (145 pounds × 15 calories = 2175 calories a day). Round that number to 2200 calories. You need 2200 calories a day to maintain your weight.

If you are overweight, estimate your desirable weight and multiply that by the appropriate number of calories per pound. For example if you would like to weigh 130 pounds and are not very active, estimate your calorie need as follows:

130 pounds × 13 calories a pound = 1690 calories

Round answer to 1700 calories.

2. *Find out how many of grams of fat you should be eating each day.* In Step 1 you found out how many calories you need each day. Find the number of calories you need each day on the list below. Next to it is the maximum grams of fat allowed for the day. For example, if you need 1800 calories a day, you should be eating no more than 60 grams of fat a day.

MAXIMUM GRAMS OF FAT ALLOWED

CALORIES	GRAMS OF FAT	CALORIES	GRAMS OF FAT
1200	40	2200	73
1300	43	2300	77
1400	47	2400	80
1500	50	2500	83
1600	53	2600	87
1700	57	2700	90
1800	60	2800	93
1900	63	2900	97
2000	67	3000	100
2100	70		

Now that you know how many grams of fat you should be eating each day, it's time to count up your fat.

COUNT UP YOUR FAT

We often eat on the run and pick foods high in fat. By the end of the day, we've eaten too much fat. You know you shouldn't be eating so much fat. You want to cut back. The fat counter will help you do it. For the first time it's simple to find out the amount of fat in all the foods you are eating.

Let's look at a typical day. Are the food choices familiar? Let's see how much fat this sample day has in it.

FAT COUNTING
A SAMPLE DAY OF POOR FOOD CHOICES

Breakfast	FAT GRAMS	CALORIES
Orange juice (½ cup)	0	56
French toast (1 slice)	7	155
Syrup (2 tbsp)	0	100
Sausage (2 links)	8	96
Coffee w/ Half & Half (2 tbsp)	4	40
Lunch		
Cheeseburger w/ bun	15	320
Catsup (1 tbsp)	0	15
French fries (10 strips)	4	111
Vanilla shake (10 oz)	8	314
Snack		
Doughnut	13	235
Coffee w/ Half & Half (2 tbsp)	4	40
Dinner		
Batter dipped fried chicken (2.9 oz)	11	218
Baked potato &	tr	145
Sour cream (2 tbsp)	6	52
Tossed salad &	0	10
French dressing (2 tbsp)	12	120
Apple pie (1 slice)	22	420
Tea &	0	0
Sugar (1 tsp)	0	16
TV Snack		
Rich vanilla ice cream (½ cup)	12	175
Total	**126**	**2638**

126 grams of fat × 9 calories = 1134 fat calories
Calories from fat divided by total calories = percent of calories from fat
1134 fat calories divided by 2638 total calories = 43% fat

This is too much fat for one day—43% of the day's calories came from fat. Now you can see how easy it is to eat too much fat.

FAT COUNTING
A SAMPLE DAY OF WISE FOOD CHOICES

Breakfast	FAT GRAMS	CALORIES
Orange juice (½ cup)	0	56
All Bran &	1	70
Lowfat milk (½ cup)	2	51
Toast (1 slice) &	0	55
Jelly (1 tbsp)	0	50
Coffee &	0	0
Lowfat milk (2 tbsp)	0	20
Lunch		
Hamburger w/ bun	12	275
Catsup (1 tbsp)	0	15
French fries (10 strips)	4	111
Cola	0	98
Snack		
Pear	1	98
Dinner		
Roasted chicken breast, no skin (½ breast)	3	142
Baked potato &	tr	145
Plain yogurt (2 tbsp)	1	18
Tossed salad &	0	10
Oil & vinegar dressing (2 tbsp)	14	140
Fruit cocktail (½ cup)	0	60
Tea &	0	0
Sugar (1 tsp)	0	16
TV Snack		
Vanilla ice milk (½ cup)	3	92
Total	**41**	**1522**

41 grams of fat × 9 calories = 369 calories
calories from fat divided by total calories = percent of fat calories
369 fat calories divided by 1522 total calories = 24% fat

Wise food choices! A much healthier intake of fat for the day. When you cut down on grams of fat, you cut down on calories too. In this sample day fat calories are only 24% of the total.

Now it's your turn to count your fat. Note everything you eat today, then look up the fat in each food you have eaten and see how much fat you ate today. While you're at it, jot down the calories, too!

FAT COUNTING:
A SAMPLE WORKSHEET FOOD AMOUNT

FOOD	PORTION	FAT GRAMS	CALORIES
Breakfast			
Snack			
Lunch			
Snack			
Dinner			
Snack			

**TOTAL
FAT GRAMS:** ____   **TOTAL
CALORIES:** ____

Grams of fat × 9 calories = total fat calories

(Your total) ____ grams of fat × 9 calories = your total fat
  calories for today

Calories from fat divided by total calories = percent of calories
  from fat

(Your total) ____ fat calories divided by ____ your total calories
  = percent of fat you ate today

Did you eat more than 30% fat today? If you did, you're eating too much fat. Turn back to page xxvi, "Maximum Grams of Fat Allowed."

Start right now to make lower fat food choices.

TEN STEPS TO LOWER YOUR FAT INTAKE

1. Choose skim or low fat milk, evaporated milk, yogurt and cheese. Look for the words: skim, 1% fat, 2% fat, 99% fat free, fat-free.

Beware: Cheeses labeled "made with partially skimmed milk" may contain almost as much fat as regular cheese.

2. Choose lean meats trimmed of all visible fat; poultry without skin. Look for ground meat and poultry containing 10% or less fat (90% fat free) or the new low-fat ground beef that contains fiber fillers like oat bran and carrageenan.

Beware: Meat, poultry and fish contain invisible fat. Limit portion size to 4 oz., about the size of the palm of your hand.

3. Choose lean fish like cod, scrod, haddock and halibut. When using fatty fish like salmon, bluefish or mackerel, remove the skin and all visible fat.

4. Roast, broil, grill, bake or poach meat, poultry and fish so no extra fat is added. During cooking fat drips off, discard it.

Beware: When you add bread crumbs to ground meat for meat loaf or hamburgers, the crumbs act like a blotter, soaking up fat instead of allowing it to drip off.

5. Use jelly or jam as a spread on toast and bread instead of butter, margarine or cream cheese; good taste and no fat.

6. Sour cream as a topping for baked potatoes is a lower fat choice than butter. Plain, lowfat yogurt is even better. Use butter flavor sprinkles.

7. Use lowfat milk in tea or coffee instead of half and half, cream or nondairy creamers (whiteners). More flavor and less fat.

8. Dress your salad with lemon juice or herb flavored vinegar, or no-fat dressings instead of regular oil-based salad dressing or mayonnaise.

9. Sweet rolls, donuts and Danish pastries are high fat snacks. Try cinnamon raisin bread for a low fat sweet treat.

10. Use cooking spray to grease pans and sauté foods.

These suggestions are just a beginning. To reduce the total amount of fat you eat you have to learn how to recognize fat when you see it and even when you don't see it. It's not always easy. *The Fat Counter* will help.

PROJECT LEAN
LOW-FAT EATING FOR AMERICA NOW

Project Lean, initiated by the Henry J. Kaiser Family Foundation in 1987, is a national public awareness campaign to promote low-fat eating. The campaign is now being sponsored by the National Center for Nutrition and Dietetics (NCND), the public education initiative of the American Dietetic Association and its Foundation. The Center was selected as the national organization to carry on this project because of its consumer-based goals and its position as an established authority on nutrition topics. Project Lean is directed to consumers as well as food industries and government agencies that influence what people eat.

Project Lean has three main objectives:

1. Reduce dietary fat intake from present levels to 30% of total calories, by teaching consumers the skills necessary to identify, buy, request or prepare low-fat meals and snacks.

2. Increase availability of low-fat foods in supermarkets, restaurants, and cafeterias in worksites and schools.

3. Increase collaboration among national and community organizations committed to reducing dietary fat.

WHEN IS A FAT NOT A FAT?

In spite of the fact that high fat foods make us fat and are not healthy, we love fatty foods. Fried foods, cakes, pies, cookies, butter and ice cream are often listed as favorites.

Scientists working with food manufacturers are busily

developing fat substitutes that will help make our favorite high fat foods lower in calories and healthier for us.

Fat substitutes contain fewer calories than fat and are used to replace all or part of the fat in processed foods. N-OIL, OATRIM, STELLAR, LITESSE, SLENDID and AVICEL are made from carbohydrates. You will see them listed as ingredients in frozen desserts, baked goods, puddings, salad dressings and sauces.

SIMPLESSE, ULTRA-BAKE, ULTRA-FREEZE are made from milk, egg or corn protein. They are used in frozen desserts, baked goods, butter, sour cream and margarine. DUR-LO and VERI-LO are fat-based fat replacers that have the same calorie value as fat, but they can be used in lesser amounts so the fat and calorie content is reduced. They can replace all or part of the fat in cake mixes and cookies. CAPRENIN, made from fat that is only partially absorbed, thus providing fewer calories, is used in candy. Other fat-based fat substitutes OLESTRA, TATCA, DDM and EPG are awaiting FDA approval and may be available in processed foods in the near future.

Even though these new fat substitutes sound exciting, it may be a while before we can take advantage of all of them. Even then we'll still have to watch our fat intake because these new fat substitutes will replace only part of the fat in our foods.

USING YOUR FAT COUNTER

This book lists the fat and calorie content of over 10,000 foods. For the first time, information about fat values is at your fingertips. Now you will find it easy to follow a low fat diet.

Before *The Fat Counter* it was impossible to compare so many foods at one time. When you want to pick a low fat cookie, look up the cookie category, page 140. Fresh foods like meat, chicken, fish and cheese do not usually have a label. The same goes for take-out items like potato salad, coleslaw, ice cream, or foods bought at the bakery. How can you tell how much fat there is in a burger or taco that you enjoy at the local fast food restaurant? *The Fat Counter* lists them all!

The Fat Counter is divided into two main sections.

Part I: Brand Name and Generic Foods lists foods alphabetically. For each group, you will find brand name foods listed first in alphabetical order, followed by an alphabetical listing of generic foods. Large categories are divided into subcategories—canned, fresh, frozen, ready-to-use—to make it easier to find what you are looking for.

If you want to know how much fat is in the hamburger you are having for lunch: look under HAMBURGER where you will find all kinds of hamburgers listed, or if you are making a homemade hamburger, look under ROLL where you will find the hamburger roll listed alphabetically and under BEEF where you will find a listing for a cooked chopped beef patty. For foods like FRENCH TOAST, HONEY or SALAD DRESSING, simply look for the specific food alphabetically in the complete listing. For example, FRENCH TOAST is found on page 207, listed alphabetically between FRENCH FRIES and FROG'S LEGS. Two slices have 14 grams of fat.

If you are eating at home, simply look up the individual foods you are eating and total the fat for the meal. For example, your dinner may consist of:

	FAT (GRAMS)
Rib Lamb Chops, broiled	50
Broccoli Cuts in Cheese Sauce (Green Giant)	3
Minute Rice Drumstick (General Foods)	4
French Cheese Cake (Sara Lee)	16
Glass of White Wine	0
TOTAL FAT FOR THE MEAL =	73 g

Most food categories will have a take-out subcategory. Items found in the take-out subcategory will help you estimate the fat and calories in similar restaurant or take-out menu items. For example, if you order spaghetti and meatballs, look under PASTA DINNERS, beginning on page 328.

Most foods are listed alphabetically. But, in some cases, foods are grouped by category. For example, all pasta dishes, like spaghetti and meat balls, lasagne and fettucini are found under the category PASTA DINNERS.

Other group categories include:

DINNERS (page 180): includes all frozen dinners by brand name

ICE CREAM AND FROZEN DESSERT (page 237): includes all dairy and non-dairy ice cream and frozen novelties

LIQUOR/LIQUEUR (page 266): includes all alcoholic beverages except wine or beer

LUNCHEON MEATS/COLD CUTS (page 268): includes all sandwich meats except chicken, ham and turkey

MEXICAN FOOD (page 282): includes all Mexican-type foods

NUTRITIONAL SUPPLEMENTS (page 304): includes all meal replacers, diet bars and diet drinks

ORIENTAL FOOD (page 315): includes all Oriental-type foods

Part II: Restaurant, Take-out and Fast Food Chains contains an alphabetical listing of 35 popular chains. Fast foods like BURGER KING, DOMINO'S PIZZA, TACO BELL and WENDY'S are listed alphabetically under the chain's name. For example, the fat values for McDONALD'S begins on page 536 under M.

We have tried to include all foods for which fat values are known. There will be some foods, however, that are not listed in *The Fat Counter* because the fat values are not available for that particular food.

When you can't locate your favorite brand, look at other similar foods. You will probably find a brand food, a generic product or a home recipe that is like your favorite food. For example, you may find that your favorite brand of vanilla yogurt is not listed. Look at the different vanilla yogurts listed on page 497. From these entries you can quickly determine that vanilla yogurt has from 0 to 4 grams of fat in a serving. You can then assume that your favorite brand has a comparable amount.

With *The Fat Counter* as your guide, you will never again wonder how much fat is in food. You will always be able to tell if a food is high in fat, moderate in fat or low in fat. Your goal is to pick low fat foods each time you eat.

DEFINITIONS

as prep (as prepared): refers to food that has been prepared according to package directions

cooked: refers to food cooked without the addition of fat (oil, butter, margarine, etc.); steaming, poaching, broiling and dry roasting are examples of this type of preparation

generic: describes a food without a brand name

home recipe: describes homemade dishes; those included can be used as a guide to the fat and calorie values of similar products you may prepare or take-out food you buy ready-to-eat

lean & fat: describes meat with some fat on its edges that is not cut away before cooking or poultry prepared with skin and fat as purchased

lean only: lean portion, trimmed of all visible fat

shelf stable or shelf ready: refers to prepared products found on the supermarket shelf that are ready to be heated and do not require refrigeration.

take-out: describes prepared dishes that you purchase ready-to-eat; those included serve as a guide to the fat and calorie values of similar products you may purchase.

trace (tr): value use when a food contains less than one calorie or less than one gram of fat.

ABBREVIATIONS

avg	=	average	reg	=	regular
diam	=	diameter	sm	=	small
frzn	=	frozen	sq	=	square
g	=	gram	tbsp	=	tablespoon
lb	=	pound	tr	=	trace
lg	=	large	tsp	=	teaspoon
med	=	medium	w/	=	with
mg	=	milligram	w/o	=	without
oz	=	ounce	"	=	inch
pkg	=	package	<	=	less than
pkt	=	packet			
pt	=	pint			
prep	=	prepared			

EQUIVALENT MEASURES

1 tablespoon	=	3 teaspoons
4 tablespoons	=	¼ cup
8 tablespoons	=	½ cup
12 tablespoons	=	¾ cup
16 tablespoons	=	1 cup
1000 milligrams	=	1 gram
28 grams	=	1 ounce

LIQUID MEASUREMENTS

2 tablespoons	=	1 ounce
¼ cup	=	2 ounces
½ cup	=	4 ounces
¾ cup	=	6 ounces
1 cup	=	8 ounces
2 cups	=	1 pint
4 cups	=	1 quart

DRY MEASUREMENTS

16 ounces	=	1 pound
12 ounces	=	¾ pound
8 ounces	=	½ pound
4 ounces	=	¼ pound

NOTES

All cooking methods are without added fat unless indicated.

You can assume that all generic cooked foods are prepared without added fat unless indicated.

Discrepancies in figures from the first edition of *The Fat Counter* are due to rounding, product reformulation and reevaluation.

ALL FAT VALUES OF FOODS ARE GIVEN IN GRAMS (g)

PART I
Brand Name and Generic Foods

FOOD	PORTION	CALORIES	FAT

ABALONE
fried	3 oz	161	6

ACEROLA
acerola	1 fruit	2	tr
juice	1 cup	51	1

ADZUKI BEANS

CANNED
sweetened	1 cup	702	tr

DRIED
Arrowhead	2 oz	190	1
cooked	1 cup	294	tr
raw	1 cup	649	1

READY-TO-USE
yokan, sliced	3.25 oz	112	tr

AKEE
fresh	3.5 oz	223	20

ALE
(see BEER AND ALE)

ALFALFA
Arrowhead Alfalfa Seeds	1 cup	40	1
sprouts	1 cup	40	tr
sprouts	1 tbsp	1	tr

ALLIGATOR
tail, cooked	3.5 oz	143	3

ALLSPICE
ground	1 tsp	5	tr

FOOD	PORTION	CALORIES	FAT
ALMONDS			
Almond Butter (Erewhon)	1 tbsp	90	8
Almonds (Planters)	1 oz	170	15
Blanched Slivered Almonds (Dole)	1 oz	170	14
Blanched Whole Almonds (Dole)	1 oz	170	14
Chopped Natural Almonds (Dole)	1 oz	170	14
Honey Roasted (Planters)	1 oz	170	13
Sliced (Planters)	1 oz	170	15
Sliced Natural Almonds (Dole)	1 oz	170	14
Slivered (Planters)	1 oz	170	15
Whole Natural Almonds (Dole)	1 oz	170	14
almond butter, honey & cinnamon	1 tbsp	96	8
almond butter w/ salt	1 tbsp	101	9
almond butter w/o salt	1 tbsp	101	10
almond meal	1 oz	116	5
almond paste	1 oz	127	8
dried, blanched	1 oz	166	15
dried, unblanched	1 oz	167	15
dry roasted, unblanched	1 oz	167	15
dry roasted, unblanched, salted	1 oz	167	15
oil roasted, blanched	1 oz	174	16
oil roasted, blanched, salted	1 oz	174	16
oil roasted, unblanched	1 oz	176	16
toasted, unblanched	1 oz	167	14
AMARANTH			
Amaranth Cereal w/ Bananas (Health Valley)	½ cup	110	2
Amaranth Crunch w/ Raisins (Health Valley)	¼ cup	110	3

FOOD	PORTION	CALORIES	FAT
Amaranth Flakes 100% Organic (Health Valley)	½ cup	90	tr
Amaranth Seeds (Arrowhead)	2 oz	200	3
Fast Menu Amaranth w/ Garden Vegetables (Health Valley)	7.5 oz	140	3
cooked	½ cup	59	tr
uncooked	½ cup	366	6

ANASAZI BEANS

DRIED			
Arrowhead	2 oz	200	1

ANCHOVY

CANNED			
in oil	5	42	2
in oil	1 can (1.6 oz)	95	4
FRESH			
raw	3 oz	62	4

ANGLERFISH

raw	3.5 oz	72	1

ANISE

seed	1 tsp	7	tr

ANTELOPE

roasted	3 oz	127	2

APPLE

CANNED			
Apple Sauce			
(Mott's)	4 oz	88	0
(Mott's)	6 oz	132	0

FOOD	PORTION	CALORIES	FAT
Apple Sauce *(cont.)*			
100% Gravenstein Sweetened (S&W)	½ cup	90	0
100% Gravenstein Unsweetened (S&W)	½ cup	55	0
Cherry Fruit Pak (Mott's)	3.75 oz	65	0
Chunky (Mott's)	4 oz	57	0
Chunky (Mott's)	6 oz	86	0
Cinnamon (Mott's)	4 oz	72	0
Cinnamon (Seneca)	½ cup	90	0
Cinnamon (Tree Top)	½ cup	80	0
Cinnamon (White House)	4 oz	100	0
Diet (S&W)	½ cup	55	0
Natural (Mott's)	4 oz	44	0
Natural (Mott's)	6 oz	66	0
Natural (Seneca)	½ cup	50	0
Natural (Tree Top)	½ cup	60	0
Natural Packed w/ Apple Juice (White House)	4 oz	60	0
Original (Tree Top)	½ cup	80	0
Peach Fruit Pak (Mott's)	3.75 oz	70	0
Pineapple Fruit Pak (Mott's)	3.75 oz	79	0
Regular (Seneca)	½ cup	90	0
Regular or Chunky (White House)	4 oz	80	0
Strawberry Fruit Pak (Mott's)	3.75 oz	70	0
Sweetened (S&W)	½ cup	55	0
Unsweetened (S&W)	½ cup	25	2
Unsweetened (White House)	4 oz	50	0
sweetened	½ cup	97	tr
sweetened	1 cup	136	1
unsweetened	½ cup	53	tr

FOOD	PORTION	CALORIES	FAT
Escalloped Apples (White House)	4 oz	120	0
Fried Apples (Luck's)	8 oz	190	0
Sliced Apples (White House)	4 oz	55	0
Spiced Apple Rings (White House)	1 ring	25	0
DRIED			
Apples (Mariani)	¼ cup	150	0
cooked w/ sugar	½ cup	116	tr
cooked w/o sugar	½ cup	172	tr
rings	10	155	tr
FRESH			
Dole	1	80	1
apple	1	81	tr
w/o skin, sliced	1 cup	62	tr
w/o skin, sliced & cooked	1 cup	91	tr
w/o skin, sliced & microwaved	1 cup	96	tr
FROZEN			
Apple Fritters (Mrs. Paul's)	2	270	9
sliced, w/o sugar	½ cup	41	tr
JUICE			
Juice & More	8 oz	120	0
Juice Works	6 oz	100	0
Kern's Cinnamon Apple Nectar	6 oz	110	0
Libby's Apple Nectar	6 oz	100	0
Mott's	6 oz	88	0
Mott's	8.5 oz	124	0
Mott's	10 oz	148	0
Mott's Natural Style	6 oz	88	0
Ocean Spray	6 oz	90	0
S&W 100% Unsweetened	6 oz	85	0
Seneca	6 oz	90	0

8   APRICOTS

FOOD	PORTION	CALORIES	FAT
Seneca, frzn, as prep	6 oz	90	0
Seneca Natural, frzn, as prep	6 oz	90	0
Sippin' Pak 100% Pure	8.45 oz	110	0
Sipps Apple	8.45 oz	130	0
Tree Top	6 oz	90	0
Tree Top, frzn, as prep	6 oz	90	0
Tree Top Cider	6 oz	90	0
Tree Top Cider, frzn, as prep	6 oz	90	0
Tree Top Sparkling Juice	6 oz	90	0
Tree Top Unfiltered	6 oz	90	0
Tree Top Unfiltered, frzn, as prep	6 oz	90	0
Tree Top w/ Vitamin C	6 oz	90	0
White House	6 oz	90	0
apple	1 cup	116	tr
frzn, as prep	1 cup	111	tr
frzn, not prep	6 oz	349	1

APRICOTS

CANNED
	PORTION	CALORIES	FAT
Halves, Diet (S&W)	½ cup	35	0
Halves Unpeeled in Heavy Syrup (S&W)	½ cup	110	0
Halves Unsweetened (S&W)	½ cup	35	0
Whole Peeled, Diet (S&W)	½ cup	28	0
Whole Peeled in Heavy Syrup (S&W)	½ cup	100	0
heavy syrup w/ skin	3 halves	70	tr
juice pack w/ skin	3 halves	40	tr
light syrup w/ skin	3 halves	54	tr
water pack w/ skin	3 halves	22	tr
water pack w/o skin	4 halves	20	tr

FOOD	PORTION	CALORIES	FAT
DRIED			
Apricots (Mariani)	¼ cup	140	0
halves	10	83	tr
halves, cooked w/o sugar	½ cup	106	tr
FRESH			
apricots	3	51	tr
FROZEN			
sweetened	½ cup	119	tr
JUICE			
Kern's Nectar	6 oz	100	0
Libby's Nectar	6 oz	110	0
S&W Nectar	6 oz	35	0
nectar	1 cup	141	tr

ARROWHEAD

FOOD	PORTION	CALORIES	FAT
fresh, boiled	1 med (⅓ oz)	9	tr

ARROWROOT

FOOD	PORTION	CALORIES	FAT
flour	1 cup	457	tr

ARTICHOKE

FOOD	PORTION	CALORIES	FAT
CANNED			
Hearts Marinated (S&W)	½ cup	225	26
FRESH			
Dole	1 lg	23	tr
boiled	1 med (4 oz)	60	tr
hearts, cooked	½ cup	42	tr
jerusalem, raw, sliced	½ cup	57	tr
FROZEN			
Artichoke Hearts (Birds Eye)	½ cup	32	tr
cooked	1 pkg (9 oz)	108	1

FOOD	PORTION	CALORIES	FAT

ARUGULA

raw	½ cup	2	tr

ASPARAGUS

CANNED

Cut Spears (Owatonna)	½ cup	20	0
Points Water Pack (S&W)	½ cup	17	0
Spears Colossal Fancy (S&W)	½ cup	20	0
Spears Fancy (S&W)	½ cup	18	0
spears	½ cup	24	1

FRESH

Dole	5 spears	18	0
cooked	½ cup	22	tr
cooked	4 spears	14	tr
raw	½ cup	16	tr
raw	4 spears	14	tr

FROZEN

Cut (Birds Eye)	½ cup	23	tr
Harvest French Cuts (Green Giant)	½ cup	25	0
Spears (Birds Eye)	½ cup	24	tr
cooked	4 spears	17	tr
cooked	1 pkg (10 oz)	82	1

AVOCADO

FRESH

Avocado (California Avocados)	½	153	14
Avocado, mashed (California Avocados)	1 cup	407	36
avocado	1	324	31
puree	1 cup	370	35

FOOD	PORTION	CALORIES	FAT

BACON
(*see also* BACON SUBSTITUTES)

FOOD	PORTION	CALORIES	FAT
Armour Lower Salt, cooked	1 strip	38	3
Armour Star, cooked	1 strip	38	3
Nathan's Beef Bacon, cooked	3 slices	100	7
Oscar Mayer, cooked	1 strip (6 g)	35	3
Oscar Mayer Center Cut, cooked	1 strip (4.6 g)	24	2
Oscar Mayer Lower Salt, cooked	1 strip (6.1 g)	33	3
breakfast strips, beef, cooked	3 strips (34 g)	153	12
breakfast strips, cooked	3 strips (34 g)	156	12
cooked	3 strips	109	9
gammon, lean & fat, grilled	4.2 oz	274	15
grilled	2 slices (1.7 oz)	86	4

BACON SUBSTITUTES

FOOD	PORTION	CALORIES	FAT
Bacon Bits (Oscar Mayer)	¼ oz	21	1
Breakfast Strips Lean 'N Tasty Beef, cooked (Oscar Mayer)	1 strip (12 g)	46	4
Breakfast Strips Lean 'N Tasty Pork, cooked (Oscar Mayer)	1 strip (12 g)	54	5
Strips, frzn (Morningstar Farms)	3.5 oz	333	25
bacon substitute	1 strip	25	2

BAGEL

FRESH

FOOD	PORTION	CALORIES	FAT
egg	1 (3.5″ diam)	200	2
plain	1 (3.5″ diam)	200	2

FROZEN

FOOD	PORTION	CALORIES	FAT
Bagel Sandwich Ham & Cheese (Weight Watchers)	1 (3 oz)	210	6
Cinnamon Raisin (Sara Lee)	1 (3 oz)	240	2

FOOD	PORTION	CALORIES	FAT
Cinnamon 'N Raisin (Lender's)	1	200	1
Egg (Lender's)	1	150	1
Egg (Sara Lee)	1 (3 oz)	250	2
Ham, Cheese on a Bagel (Great Starts)	3 oz	240	8
Oat Bran (Sara Lee)	1 (3 oz)	220	1
Onion (Lender's)	1	160	1
Onion (Sara Lee)	1 (3 oz)	230	1
Plain (Lender's)	1	150	1
Plain (Sara Lee)	1 (3 oz)	230	1
Poppy Seed (Sara Lee)	1 (3 oz)	230	1
Sesame Seed (Sara Lee)	1 (3 oz)	240	2

BAKING POWDER

Calumet	1 tsp	3	tr
Clabber Girl	1 tsp	0	0
Davis	1 tsp	6	0
baking powder	1 tsp	5	0
low sodium	1 tsp	5	0

BAKING SODA

Arm & Hammer	1 tsp	0	0

BALSAM PEAR

leafy tips, cooked	½ cup	10	tr
leafy tips, raw	½ cup	7	tr
pods, cooked	½ cup	12	tr

BAMBOO SHOOTS

CANNED
| Empress Sliced | 2 oz | 14 | 0 |

FOOD	PORTION	CALORIES	FAT
La Choy	¼ cup	6	tr
sliced	1 cup	25	1
FRESH			
cooked	½ cup	15	tr
raw	½ cup	21	tr

BANANA

DRIED			
powder	1 tbsp	21	tr
FRESH			
Chiquita	1 (3.5 oz)	110	0
Dole	1	120	1
banana	1	105	tr
mashed	1 cup	207	1
JUICE			
Libby's Nectar	6 oz	110	0

BARLEY

Arrowhead Barley	2 oz	200	1
Arrowhead Barley Flakes	2 oz	200	1
Quaker Medium Pearled	¼ cup	172	1
Quaker Quick Pearled	¼ cup	172	1
Scotch Medium Pearled	¼ cup	172	1
Scotch Quick Pearled	¼ cup	172	1
pearled, cooked	½ cup	97	tr
pearled, uncooked	½ cup	352	1

BASIL

fresh, chopped	2 tbsp	1	tr
ground	1 tsp	4	tr
leaves, fresh	5	1	tr

FOOD	PORTION	CALORIES	FAT

BASS

FRESH
sea, cooked	3 oz	105	2
striped, baked	3 oz	105	3

BAY LEAF

crumbled	1 tsp	2	tr

BEAN SPROUTS

CANNED
La Choy	⅔ cup	8	tr

BEANS
(see also individual names)

CANNED
Baked Beans (Brick Oven)	½ cup	160	2
Baked Beans (Van Camp's)	1 cup	260	2
Barbeque Baked Beans (B&M)	⅞ cup	310	6
Barbecue Beans (Campbell)	½ can (7⅞ oz)	210	4
Barbecue Beans Texas Style (S&W)	½ cup	135	1
Beanee Weenee (Van Camp's)	1 cup	326	7
Big John's Beans 'n Fixin's (Hunt's)	4 oz	170	6
Boston Baked (Health Valley)	7.5 oz	190	tr
Boston Baked No Salt Added (Health Valley)	7.5 oz	190	tr
Brown Sugar Beans (Van Camp's)	1 cup	290	5
Chili (Gebhardt)	4 oz	115	1
Cut Green & Shelled Beans Seasoned w/ Pork (Luck's)	7.25 oz	200	6
Deluxe Baked Beans (Van Camp's)	1 cup	320	4
Fast Menu Honey Baked Organic Beans w/ Tofu Weiner (Health Valley)	7.5 oz	150	4

FOOD	PORTION	CALORIES	FAT
Four Bean Salad (Hanover)	½ cup	80	0
Green Beans & Wax Beans (S&W)	½ cup	20	0
Home Style Beans (Campbell)	½ can (8 oz)	220	4
Honey Baked Beans (B&M)	⅞ cup	280	2
Hot Chili Beans (Campbell)	½ can (7.75 oz)	180	4
Maple Sugar Beans (S&W)	½ cup	150	1
Mexican Style Chili Beans (Van Camp's)	1 cup	210	2
Mixed Bean Salad Marinated (S&W)	½ cup	90	1
Mixed Beans Seasoned w/ Pork (Luck's)	7.25 oz	200	5
Old Fashioned Beans in Molasses & Brown Sugar Sauce (Campbell)	½ can (8 oz)	230	3
Pork & Beans (Hunt's)	4 oz	135	1
Pork & Beans (Van Camp's)	1 cup	216	2
Pork & Beans in Tomato Sauce (Campbell)	½ can (8 oz)	200	3
Pork & Beans in Tomato Sauce (Green Giant)	½ cup	90	1
Pork & Molasses (Libby)	½ cup	140	2
Pork & Tomato Sauce (Libby)	½ cup	140	2
Pork & Tomato Sauce (Seneca)	½ cup	140	2
Pork 'N Beans (S&W)	½ cup	130	2
Ranch Style (Ranch Style)	7.5 oz	200	4
Refried (Gebhardt)	4 oz	100	2
Refried (Rosarita)	4 oz	100	2
Refried Beans & Green Chili (Little Pancho)	½ cup	80	0
Refried Jalapeno (Gebhardt)	4 oz	115	2
Refried Spicy (Rosarita)	4 oz	100	2
Refried Vegetarian (Rosarita)	4 oz	100	2
Refried w/ Bacon (Rosarita)	4 oz	110	2

FOOD	PORTION	CALORIES	FAT
Refried w/ Green Chilies (Rosarita)	4 oz	90	2
Refried w/ Nacho Cheese (Rosarita)	4 oz	110	2
Refried w/ Onions (Rosarita)	4 oz	110	2
Smokey Ranch Beans (S&W)	½ cup	130	2
Three Bean Salad (Green Giant)	½ cup	70	tr
Tomato Baked Beans (B&M)	⅞ cup	270	3
Vegetarian (Libby)	½ cup	130	1
Vegetarian (Seneca)	½ cup	130	1
Vegetarian Baked Beans (B&M)	⅞ cup	250	2
Vegetarian Beans (Campbell)	½ can (7.75 oz)	170	1
Vegetarian Beans w/ Miso (Health Valley)	7.5 oz	180	1
Vegetarian Style (Van Camp's)	1 cup	206	1
baked beans, plain	½ cup	118	1
baked beans, vegetarian	½ cup	118	1
baked beans w/ beef	½ cup	161	5
baked beans w/ franks	½ cup	182	8
baked beans w/ pork	½ cup	133	2
baked beans w/ pork & sweet sauce	½ cup	140	2
baked beans w/ pork & tomato sauce	½ cup	123	1
refried beans	½ cup	134	1
FROZEN			
Romano Bean Medley (Hanover)	½ cup	25	0
TAKE-OUT			
baked beans	½ cup	190	6
barbecue beans	3.5 oz	120	tr
four bean salad	3.5 oz	100	tr
refried beans	½ cup	43	2
three bean salad	¾ cup	230	11

FOOD	PORTION	CALORIES	FAT

BEAR

| simmered | 3 oz | 220 | 11 |

BEAVER

| roasted | 3 oz | 140 | 6 |
| simmered | 3 oz | 141 | 5 |

BEECHNUTS

| dried | 1 oz | 164 | 14 |

BEEF

(*see also* BEEF DISHES, DINNER, HAMBURGER, HOT DOG, LUNCHEON
MEAT/COLD CUTS, VEAL)

Beef is graded according to its marbling, the little flecks of fat in the muscle.
Beef graded "Prime" has the highest percentage of fat, followed by
"Choice" with less fat and "Select" with the least fat.

CANNED

| corned beef | 1 oz | 71 | 4 |
| corned beef | 1 slice (21 g) | 53 | 3 |

FRESH

Note that values for cooked beef may differ slightly from values for raw
beef. When meat is cooked some moisture and fat are lost, changing the
nutritional value slightly. As a rule of thumb it can be assumed that a 4-
ounce raw portion will equal a 3-ounce cooked portion of meat.

Chuck Roast, raw (Dakota Lean)	3 oz	80	2
Eye Round, raw (Dakota Lean)	3 oz	80	2
Filet (Double J)	3.5 oz	130	4
Flank Steak, raw (Dakota Lean)	3 oz	80	1
Ground, raw (Dakota Lean)	3 oz	88	2
NY Strip (Double J)	3.5 oz	133	4
Outside Round, raw (Dakota Lean)	3 oz	80	1
Rib Eye (Double J)	3.5 oz	134	5

FOOD	PORTION	CALORIES	FAT
Ribeye, raw (Dakota Lean)	3 oz	90	2
Sirloin Tip, raw (Dakota Lean)	3 oz	90	3
Strip Loin, raw (Dakota Lean)	3 oz	90	2
Tenderloin, raw (Dakota Lean)	3 oz	70	1
Top Butt (Double J)	3.5 oz	136	5
Top Round, raw (Dakota Lean)	3 oz	80	1
bottom round, lean & fat			
trim 0", Choice, roasted	3 oz	172	8
trim 0", Select, braised	3 oz	171	6
trim 0", Select, roasted	3 oz	150	24
trim ¼", Choice, braised	3 oz	241	15
trim ¼", Choice, roasted	3 oz	221	14
trim ¼", Select, braised	3 oz	220	13
trim ¼", Select, roasted	3 oz	199	11
brisket, lean & fat			
flat half, trim 0", braised	3 oz	183	8
flat half, trim ¼", braised	3 oz	309	24
point half, trim 0", braised	3 oz	304	24
point half, trim ¼", braised	3 oz	343	29
whole, trim 0", braised	3 oz	247	17
whole, trim ¼", braised	3 oz	327	27
chuck arm pot roast, lean & fat, trim 0", braised	3 oz	238	14
chuck arm pot roast, lean & fat, trim ¼", braised	3 oz	282	20
chuck blade roast, lean & fat, trim 0", braised	3 oz	284	21
chuck blade roast, lean & fat, trim ¼", braised	3 oz	293	22
corned beef brisket, cooked	3 oz	213	16
eye of round, lean & fat			
trim 0", Choice, roasted	3 oz	153	5

FOOD	PORTION	CALORIES	FAT
trim 0", Select, roasted	3 oz	137	4
trim ¼", Choice, roasted	3 oz	205	12
trim ¼", Select, roasted	3 oz	184	10
flank, lean & fat, trim 0", braised	3 oz	224	14
flank, lean & fat, trim 0", broiled	3 oz	192	11
ground			
extra lean, broiled medium	3 oz	217	14
extra lean, broiled well done	3 oz	225	14
extra lean, fried medium	3 oz	216	14
extra lean, fried well done	3 oz	224	14
lean, broiled medium	3 oz	231	16
lean, broiled well done	3 oz	238	15
low-fat w/ carrageenan, raw	4 oz	160	7
regular, broiled medium	3 oz	246	18
regular, broiled well done	3 oz	248	17
porterhouse steak, lean & fat, trim ¼", Choice, broiled	3 oz	260	19
porterhouse steak, lean & fat, trim ¼", Choice, broiled	3 oz	260	19
porterhouse steak, lean only, trim ¼", Choice, broiled	3 oz	185	9
rib, lean & fat			
large end, trim 0", roasted	3 oz	300	24
large end, trim ¼", broiled	3 oz	295	24
large end, trim ¼", roasted	3 oz	310	25
small end, trim 0", broiled	3 oz	252	18
small end, trim ¼", broiled	3 oz	285	22
small end, trim ¼", roasted	3 oz	295	24
whole, trim ¼", Choice, broiled	3 oz	306	25
whole, trim ¼", Choice, roasted	3 oz	320	27
whole, trim ¼", Prime, roasted	3 oz	348	30

FOOD	PORTION	CALORIES	FAT
rib, lean & fat *(cont.)*			
whole, trim ¼", Select, broiled	3 oz	274	21
whole, trim ¼", Select, roasted	3 oz	286	23
rib eye small end, lean & fat, trim 0", Choice, broiled	3 oz	261	19
shank crosscut, lean & fat, trim ¼", Choice, simmered	3 oz	224	12
short loin top loin			
lean & fat, trim 0", Choice, broiled	1 steak (5.4 oz)	353	19
lean & fat, trim 0", Choice, broiled	3 oz	193	10
lean & fat, trim 0", Select, broiled	1 steak (5.4 oz)	309	14
lean & fat, trim ¼", Choice, broiled	1 steak (6.3 oz)	536	38
lean & fat, trim ¼", Choice, broiled	3 oz	253	18
lean & fat, trim ¼", Prime, broiled	1 steak (6.3 oz)	582	43
lean & fat, trim ¼", Select, broiled	1 steak (6.3 oz)	473	31
lean only, trim 0", Choice, broiled	1 steak (5.2 oz)	311	14
lean only, trim ¼", Choice, broiled	1 steak (5.2 oz)	314	15
shortribs, lean & fat, Choice, braised	3 oz	400	36
t-bone steak, lean & fat, trim ¼", Choice, broiled	3 oz	253	18
t-bone steak, lean only, trim ¼", Choice, broiled	3 oz	182	9
tenderloin			
lean & fat, trim 0", Choice, broiled	3 oz	208	12
lean & fat, trim 0", Select, broiled	3 oz	194	11
lean & fat, trim ¼", Choice, broiled	3 oz	259	19
lean & fat, trim ¼", Choice, roasted	3 oz	288	22
lean & fat, trim ¼", Prime, broiled	3 oz	270	20
lean & fat, trim ¼", Select, roasted	3 oz	275	21
lean only, trim 0", Select, broiled	3 oz	170	7
lean only, trim ¼", Choice, broiled	3 oz	188	10
lean only, trim ¼", Select, broiled	3 oz	169	7

FOOD	PORTION	CALORIES	FAT
tip round, lean & fat			
trim 0", Choice, roasted	3 oz	170	8
trim 0", Select, roasted	3 oz	158	6
trim ¼", Choice, roasted	3 oz	210	13
trim ¼", Prime, roasted	3 oz	233	15
trim ¼", Select, roasted	3 oz	191	10
top round, lean & fat			
trim 0", Choice, braised	3 oz	184	6
trim 0", Select, braised	3 oz	170	5
trim ¼", Choice, braised	3 oz	221	11
trim ¼", Choice, broiled	3 oz	190	9
trim ¼", Choice, fried	3 oz	235	13
trim ¼", Prime, broiled	3 oz	195	9
trim ¼", Select, braised	3 oz	199	8
trim ¼", Select, broiled	3 oz	175	7
top sirloin, lean & fat			
trim 0", Choice, broiled	3 oz	194	10
trim 0", Select, broiled	3 oz	166	6
trim ¼", Choice, broiled	3 oz	228	14
trim ¼", Choice, fried	3 oz	277	19
trim ¼", Select, broiled	3 oz	208	12
tripe, raw	4 oz	111	4
FROZEN			
patties, broiled medium	3 oz	240	17
READY-TO-USE			
Weight Watchers Oven Roasted Cured Deli Thin	5 slices (⅓ oz)	10	tr

BEEF DISHES
(see also DINNER)

CANNED			
Beef Stew (Chef Boyardee)	7 oz	220	13

FOOD	PORTION	CALORIES	FAT
Beef Stew (Healthy Choice)	½ can (7.5 oz)	140	2
Beef Stew (Wolf Brand)	1 cup	179	8
Manwich Extra Thick & Chunky	1 sandwich	330	13
Manwich Mexican	1 sandwich	310	13
Meat Ball Stew (Chef Boyardee)	8 oz	330	21
Sloppy Joe (Manwich)	1 sandwich	310	13
FROZEN			
Banquet Entree			
Beef Patties & Mushroom Gravy	7 oz	350	26
Meatloaf w/ Tomato Sauce	7 oz	350	22
Salisbury Steak & Gravy	7 oz	300	21
Banquet Family Entree			
Beef Stew	7 oz	140	5
Gravy & Salisbury Steak	7 oz	260	19
Gravy & Sliced Steak	7 oz	140	5
Mushroom Gravy & Charbroiled Beef Patties	7 oz	260	18
Noodles & Beef w/ Gravy	7 oz	180	6
Onion Gravy & Beef Patties	7 oz	260	19
Veal Parmagian Patties	7 oz	320	16
Chefwich Beef w/ Barbecue Sauce	1	340	10
Dining Light Salisbury Steak	9 oz	200	8
Dining Light Sauce & Swedish Meatballs	9 oz	280	10
Healthy Choice Beef Pepper Steak	9.5 oz	250	4
Le Menu Entree LightStyle Swedish LightStyle Meatballs	8 oz	260	8
Ovenstuffs Beef/Cheddar Deli Melt	1 (4.75 oz)	390	22
MIX			
Manwich Seasoning Mix	1 sandwich	320	13

FOOD	PORTION	CALORIES	FAT
SHELF STABLE			
Beef Stew (Healthy Choice)	7.5 oz cup	140	2
TAKE-OUT			
bubble & squeak	5 oz	186	13
cornish pasty	1 (8 oz)	847	52
kebab, indian	1 (5.4 oz)	553	40
kheena	6.7 oz	781	71
koftas	5	280	22
roast beef sandwich, plain	1	346	14
roast beef sandwich w/ cheese	1	402	18
roast beef submarine sandwich w/ tomato, lettuce, mayonnaise	1	411	13
samosa	2 (4 oz)	652	62
shepherd's pie	6 oz	196	10
steak & kidney pie w/ top crust	1 slice (5 oz)	400	26
steak sandwich w/ tomato, lettuce, salt, mayonnaise	1	459	14
stew	6 oz	208	13
stew w/ vegetables	1 cup	220	11
stroganoff	¾ cup	260	19
swiss steak	4.6 oz	214	9
toad in the hole	1 (4.7 oz)	383	29

BEEFALO

roasted	3 oz	160	5

BEER AND ALE
(see also MALT)

Amstel Light	12 oz	95	0
Anheuser Busch Natural Light	12 oz	110	0
Bud Light	12 oz	108	0

FOOD	PORTION	CALORIES	FAT
Coors Light	12 oz	105	0
Hamm's	12 oz	137	0
Michelob Light	12 oz	134	0
Miller Lite	12 oz	96	0
Molson Light	12 oz	109	0
Old Milwaukee	12 oz	145	0
Old Milwaukee Light	12 oz	122	0
Olympia	12 oz	143	0
Pabst	12 oz	143	0
Piels Light	12 oz	136	0
Schaefer	12 oz	138	0
Schaefer Light	12 oz	111	0
Schlitz	12 oz	145	0
Schlitz Light	12 oz	99	0
Schmidts Light	12 oz	96	0
Signature	12 oz	150	0
Stroh	12 oz	142	0
Stroh Light	12 oz	115	0
ale brown	10 oz	77	0
ale pale	10 oz	88	0
beer light	12 oz	100	0
beer regular	12 oz	146	0
lager	10 oz	80	0
stout	10 oz	102	0
NONALCOHOLIC			
Guiness Kaliber	12 oz	43	0
Hamm's	12 oz	55	0
Pabst	12 oz	55	0
Spirit	12 oz	80	0

FOOD	PORTION	CALORIES	FAT

BEETS

CANNED

FOOD	PORTION	CALORIES	FAT
Beets Pickled w/ Onions (Libby)	½ cup	80	0
Beets Pickled w/ Onions (Seneca)	½ cup	80	0
Cut (Libby)	½ cup	35	0
Cut (Seneca)	½ cup	35	0
Diced (Libby)	½ cup	35	0
Diced (Seneca)	½ cup	35	0
Diced Tender (S&W)	½ cup	40	0
Harvard (Libby)	½ cup	80	0
Harvard (Seneca)	½ cup	80	0
Julienne French Style (S&W)	½ cup	40	0
Pickled (Libby)	½ cup	35	0
Pickled (Seneca)	½ cup	35	0
Pickled Whole Extra Small (S&W)	½ cup	70	0
Pickled w/ Red Wine Vinegar Sliced (S&W)	½ cup	70	0
Sliced (Libby)	½ cup	35	0
Sliced (Seneca)	½ cup	35	0
Sliced Small Premium (S&W)	½ cup	40	0
Sliced Water Pack (S&W)	½ cup	35	0
Whole (Libby)	½ cup	35	0
Whole (Seneca)	½ cup	35	0
Whole Small (S&W)	½ cup	40	0
harvard	½ cup	89	tr
pickled	½ cup	75	tr
sliced	½ cup	27	tr

FRESH

FOOD	PORTION	CALORIES	FAT
beet greens, cooked	½ cup	20	tr
beet greens, raw	½ cup	4	tr

FOOD	PORTION	CALORIES	FAT
beet greens, raw, chopped	½ cup	4	tr
beets, cooked	½ cup	26	tr
beets, raw, sliced	½ cup	30	tr
JUICE			
beet juice	3.5 oz	36	0

BEVERAGES

(*see* BEER AND ALE, COFFEE, DRINK MIXERS, FRUIT DRINKS, MALT, MINERAL/BOTTLED WATER, LIQUOR/LIQUEUR, SODA, TEA/HERBAL TEA, WINE, WINE COOLERS)

BISCUIT

biscuit	1 (1 oz)	100	5
FROZEN			
Egg, Canadian Bacon & Cheese (Great Starts)	5.2 oz	420	22
Sausage (Great Starts)	4.7 oz	410	22
Sausage Biscuit (Weight Watchers)	3 oz	220	11
HOME RECIPE			
oatcakes	2 (4 oz)	115	5
MIX			
Biscuit Mix (Arrowhead)	2 oz	100	1
Buttermilk Biscuit Mix, not prep (Health Valley)	1 oz	100	1
biscuit	1 (1 oz)	95	3
REFRIGERATED			
1869 Brand Baking Powder	1	100	5
1869 Brand Butter Tastin'	1	100	5
1869 Brand Buttermilk	1	100	5
Ballard Ovenready	1	50	1
Ballard Ovenready Buttermilk	1	50	1
Big Country Southern Style	1	100	4

FOOD	PORTION	CALORIES	FAT
Hungry Jack			
Butter Tastin' Flaky	1	90	4
Buttermilk Flaky	1	90	4
Buttermilk Fluffy	1	90	4
Extra Rich Buttermilk	1	50	1
Flaky	1	80	4
Honey Tastin' Flaky	1	90	4
Pillsbury			
Big Premium Heat N' Eat	2	280	15
Big Country Butter Tastin'	1	100	4
Big Country Buttermilk	1	100	4
Butter	1	50	1
Buttermilk	1	50	1
Country	1	50	1
Deluxe Heat N' Eat Buttermilk	2	170	5
Good 'N Buttery Fluffy	1	90	5
Hearty Grains Multi-Grain	1	80	2
Hearty Grains Oatmeal Raisin	1	90	2
Tender Layer Buttermilk	1	50	1
biscuit	1 (¾ oz)	65	2
TAKE-OUT			
plain	1	276	34
w/ egg	1	315	20
w/ egg & bacon	1	457	31
w/ egg & sausage	1	582	39
w/ egg & steak	1	474	28
w/ egg, cheese & bacon	1	477	31
w/ ham	1	387	18
w/ sausage	1	485	32
w/ steak	1	456	26

FOOD	PORTION	CALORIES	FAT

BISON
roasted	3 oz	122	2

BLACK BEANS

CANNED
Fast Menu Organic Black Beans w/ Tofu Weiners (Health Valley)	7.5 oz	150	1
Fast Menu Western Black Beans w/ Garden Vegetable (Health Valley)	7.5 oz	160	5

DRIED
Arrowhead Turtle	2 oz	190	1
cooked	1 cup	227	1
raw	1 cup	661	3

BLACKBERRIES
canned, in heavy syrup	½ cup	118	tr
fresh blackberries	½ cup	37	tr
frozen, unsweetened	1 cup	97	1

BLACKEYE PEAS

CANNED
Blackeyes w/ Jalapeno (Ranch Style)	7.5 oz	180	2
Jalapeno (Trappey's)	½ cup	90	1
Ranch Style	7.5 oz	170	2
Seasoned w/ Pork (Luck's)	7.25 oz	200	6
Trappey's	½ cup	90	1
w/ pork	½ cup	199	4

DRIED
Hurst Brand	1 cup	233	1
cooked	1 cup	198	1
uncooked	1 cup	562	2

FOOD	PORTION	CALORIES	FAT

BLINTZE

TAKE-OUT
cheese | 2 | 186 | 6

BLUEBERRIES

CANNED
Blueberries in Heavy Syrup (S&W) | ½ cup | 111 | 0
in heavy syrup | 1 cup | 225 | 1

FRESH
blueberries | 1 cup | 82 | 1

FROZEN
unsweetened | 1 cup | 78 | 1

BLUEFIN

fillet, baked | 4.1 oz | 186 | 6

BLUEFISH

fresh, baked | 3 oz | 135 | 5

BOAR

wild, roasted | 3 oz | 136 | 4

BOK CHOY

Dole, shredded | ½ cup | 5 | tr

BORAGE

FRESH
cooked, chopped | 3.5 oz | 25 | 1
raw, chopped | ½ cup | 9 | tr

FOOD	PORTION	CALORIES	FAT

BOYSENBERRIES

FOOD	PORTION	CALORIES	FAT
canned, in heavy syrup	1 cup	226	tr
frozen, unsweetened	1 cup	66	tr
JUICE			
Smucker's	8 oz	120	0
Smucker's Sparkler	10 oz	130	tr

BRAINS

FOOD	PORTION	CALORIES	FAT
beef, pan-fried	3 oz	167	13
beef, simmered	3 oz	136	11
lamb, braised	3 oz	124	9
lamb, fried	3 oz	232	19
pork, braised	3 oz	117	8
veal, braised	3 oz	115	8
veal, fried	3 oz	181	14

BRAN

FOOD	PORTION	CALORIES	FAT
Fast Menu Oat Bran Pilaf w/ Garden Vegetables (Health Valley)	7.5 oz	210	7
Oat Bran (Arrowhead)	1 oz	110	1
Oat Bran (Mother's)	⅓ cup	92	2
Quaker Unprocessed Bran	2 tbsp	8	tr
Super Bran (H-O)	⅓ cup	110	2
Toasted Wheat Bran (Kretschmer)	⅓ cup	57	2
Wheat Bran (Arrowhead)	2 oz	50	2
corn	⅓ cup	56	tr
oat, cooked	½ cup	44	tr
oat, dry	½ cup	116	3
rice, dry	⅓ cup	88	6
wheat, dry	½ cup	65	1

FOOD	PORTION	CALORIES	FAT

BRAZIL NUTS

dried, unblanched	1 oz	186	19

BREAD

(*see also* BAGEL, BISCUIT, BREADSTICK, CROISSANT, ENGLISH MUFFIN, MUFFIN, ROLL, SCONE)

CANNED

Brown Bread (B&M)	½ slice	80	tr
Brown Bread Raisins (B&M)	½ slice	80	tr
Brown Bread New England Recipe (S&W)	2 slices	76	0
boston brown	1 slice	95	1

HOME RECIPE

datenut	½" slice	92	3
hush puppies	5 (2.7 oz)	256	12
pita, whole wheat	1 (6" diam)	247	1
whole wheat	1 slice	71	tr

MIX

Corn Bread (Ballard)	⅛ of bread	140	3
Corn Bread (Dromedary)	1 piece (2 oz)	130	3
Cornbread Blue Cornmeal (Zia Foods)	1 piece (1.2 oz)	110	6

READY-TO-EAT

9 Grain & Nut (Matthew's)	1 slice	80	3
Bran'nola Country Oat (Arnold)	1 slice	90	2
Bran'nola Dark Wheat (Arnold)	1 slice	80	1
Bran'nola Hearty Wheat (Arnold)	1 slice	90	2
Bran'nola Nutty Grains (Arnold)	1 slice	90	1
Bran'nola Original (Arnold)	1 slice	70	1
Butter Crust (Freihofer's)	1 slice	70	1
Canadian Oat (Freihofer's)	1 slice	80	1

FOOD	PORTION	CALORIES	FAT
Cinnamon (Matthew's)	1 slice	70	1
Cinnamon (Pepperidge Farm)	1 slice	90	3
Cinnamon Oatmeal (Oatmeal Goodness)	1 slice	90	2
Cinnamon Raisin (Weight Watchers)	1 slice	60	tr
Club Pullman (Freihofer's)	1 slice	70	1
Country White (Pepperidge Farm)	2 slices	190	2
Cracked Wheat (Pepperidge Farm)	1 slice	70	1
Cracked Wheat (Roman Meal)	1 slice	66	tr
Crunchy Oat 1½ lb Loaf (Pepperidge Farm)	2 slices	190	4
Date Walnut (Pepperidge Farm)	1 slice	90	3
Dijon Rye (Pepperidge Farm)	1 slice	50	1
Dijon Rye Thick Sliced (Pepperidge Farm)	1 slice	70	1
Family Pumpernickel (Pepperidge Farm)	1 slice	80	1
Family Rye (Pepperidge Farm)	3 oz	80	1
Family Wheat (Pepperidge Farm)	1 slice	70	1
Family Wheat (Wonder)	1 slice	70	1
French Style Fully Baked (Pepperidge Farm)	2 oz	150	2
Garlic (Arnold)	1 slice	80	3
Golden (Matthew's)	1 slice	70	1
Harvest Recipe 100% Whole Wheat (Roman Meal)	1 slice	66	tr
Hearty Slice 7 Grain (Pepperidge Farm)	2 slices	180	2
Hi-Fibre (Monks' Bread)	1 slice	50	1
Honey Bran (Pepperidge Farm)	1 slice	90	1
Honey Wheat Berry (Roman Meal)	1 slice	66	1
Honey Wheatberry Light (Roman Meal)	1 slice	40	tr

FOOD	PORTION	CALORIES	FAT
Honeybran Light (Roman Meal)	1 slice	40	tr
Italian Brown & Serve (Pepperidge Farm)	1 oz	80	1
Italian Francisco (Arnold)	1 slice	70	1
Italian Francisco Thick Sliced (Arnold)	1 slice	70	1
Italian Light (Arnold)	1 slice	40	tr
Italian No Seeds (Freihofer's)	1 slice	70	1
Italian Seeded (Freihofer's)	1 slice	70	1
Italian Sliced (Pepperidge Farm)	1 slice	70	1
Large Family White Thin Slice (Pepperidge Farm)	1 slice	70	1
Light Diet (Freihofer's)	1 slice	40	0
Light Italian (Wonder)	1 slice	40	0
Light Oatmeal (Pepperidge Farm)	1 slice	45	0
Light Sourdough (Wonder)	1 slice	40	0
Light Vienna (Pepperidge Farm)	1 slice	45	0
Light Wheat (Pepperidge Farm)	1 slice	45	0
Light Wheat (Wonder)	1 slice	40	0
Malsovit	1 slice	66	1
Malsovit Raisin	1 slice	77	1
Multi-Grain (Weight Watchers)	1 slice	40	tr
Oat (Roman Meal)	1 slice	71	1
Oat Bran (Matthew's)	1 slice	65	0
Oat Bran (Weight Watchers)	1 slice	40	tr
Oat, Milk & Honey (Arnold)	1 slice	60	1
Oatmeal (Pepperidge Farm)	1 slice	70	1
Oatmeal 1½ lb Loaf (Pepperidge Farm)	1 slice	90	1
Oatmeal & Sunflower Seeds (Oatmeal Goodness)	1 slice	90	2
Oatmeal & Bran (Oatmeal Goodness)	1 slice	90	2

FOOD	PORTION	CALORIES	FAT
Oatmeal Light (Arnold)	1 slice	40	tr
Oatmeal Very Thin Sliced (Pepperidge Farm)	1 slice	40	1
Old Fashion (Freihofer's)	1 slice	70	1
Party Pumpernickel (Pepperidge Farm)	4 slices	60	1
Party Rye (Pepperidge Farm)	4 slices	60	1
Pita, White Regular Size (Sahara Bread)	1 pocket (2 oz)	160	1
Pita, White Large Size (Sahara Bread)	1 pocket (3 oz)	240	2
Pita, White Mini Loaf (Sahara Bread)	1 pocket (1 oz)	80	1
Pita, Whole Wheat (Matthew's)	1 pocket	210	2
Pita, Whole Wheat Mini Loaf (Sahara Bread)	1 pocket (1 oz)	80	1
Pita, Whole Wheat Regular Size (Sahara Bread)	1 pocket (2 oz)	150	2
Pumpernickel (Arnold)	1 slice	80	1
Pumpernickel, Levy's (Arnold)	1 slice	80	1
Raisin (Monks' Bread)	1 slice	70	2
Raisin Orange (Arnold)	1 slice	70	1
Raisin Sun Maid (Arnold)	1 slice	70	1
Raisin Tea Loaf (Arnold)	1 slice	70	1
Raisin w/ Cinnamon (Pepperidge Farm)	1 slice	90	2
Rite Diet (Freihofer's)	2 slices	90	1
Rite Diet Wheat (Freihofer's)	2 slices	90	1
Round Top (Roman Meal)	1 slice	67	tr
Rye (Weight Watchers)	1 slice	40	tr
Rye, Dill Seeded (Arnold)	1 slice	80	1
Rye, Jewish Seeded (Arnold)	1 slice	80	1
Rye, Jewish Unseeded (Arnold)	1 slice	80	1

FOOD	PORTION	CALORIES	FAT
Rye, Levy's Real Jewish Seeded (Arnold)	1 slice	80	1
Rye, Levy's Real Jewish Unseeded (Arnold)	1 slice	80	1
Rye, Melba Thin (Arnold)	1 slice	40	tr
Rye, Stub Pullman (Freihofer's)	1 slice	70	1
Sandwich (Roman Meal)	1 slice	55	tr
Sandwich White (Pepperidge Farm)	2 slices	130	2
Seedless Family Rye (Pepperidge Farm)	1 slice	80	1
Sesame Wheat (Pepperidge Farm)	2 slices	190	3
Seven Grain (Roman Meal)	1 slice	68	tr
Seven Grain Light (Roman Meal)	1 slice	40	tr
Sodium Free (Matthew's)	1 slice	70	2
Soft Rye (Pepperidge Farm)	1 slice	70	1
Soft Rye, Dill & Onion (Freihofer's)	1 slice	70	1
Soft Rye No Seeds (Freihofer's)	1 slice	70	1
Soft Rye Pumpernickel (Freihofer's)	1 slice	70	1
Soft Rye Seeded (Freihofer's)	1 slice	70	1
Split Top Wheat (Freihofer's)	1 slice	70	1
Split Top White (Freihofer's)	1 slice	70	1
Sprouted Wheat (Pepperidge Farm)	1 slice	70	2
Sun Grain (Roman Meal)	1 slice	68	1
Sunbeam King (Freihofer's)	1 slice	70	1
Sunflower & Bran (Monks' Bread)	1 slice	70	1
The Original (Freihofer's)	1 slice	70	1
Toasting White (Pepperidge Farm)	1 slice	90	1
Twin French (Pepperidge Farm)	1 oz	80	1
Vienna Thick Sliced (Pepperidge Farm)	1 slice	70	1
Wheat (Freihofer's)	1½ slices	70	1

FOOD	PORTION	CALORIES	FAT
Wheat (Weight Watchers)	1 slice	40	tr
Wheat 1½ lb Loaf (Pepperidge Farm)	1 slice	90	2
Wheat Berry, Honey (Arnold)	1 slice	80	2
Wheat Brick Oven (Arnold)	1 slice of 32 oz loaf	90	2
Wheat Brick Oven (Arnold)	1 slice of 16 oz loaf	60	2
Wheat Brick Oven (Arnold)	1 slice of 8 oz loaf	60	2
Wheat Cottage (America's Own)	1 slice	70	1
Wheat Golden Light (Arnold)	1 slice	40	tr
Wheat Less (Arnold)	1 slice	40	tr
Wheat Light (Roman Meal)	1 slice	40	tr
Wheat Oatmeal (Oatmeal Goodness)	1 slice	90	2
Wheat Small (Freihofer's)	1½ slices	70	1
Wheat Stone Ground 100% Whole (Arnold)	1 slice	50	1
Wheat Stub Pullman (Freihofer's)	1 slice	70	1
Wheat Very Thin (Arnold)	1 slice	40	1
Wheat Very Thin Sliced (Pepperidge Farm)	1 slice	35	0
White (Freihofer's)	1 slice	70	1
White (Monks' Bread)	1 slice	60	1
White (Roman Meal)	1 slice	71	tr
White (Weight Watchers)	1 slice	40	tr
White (Wonder)	1 slice	70	1
White ½ Pullman (Freihofer's)	1 slice	70	1
White 7/16 Stub Pullman (Freihofer's)	1½ slices	70	1
White Brick Oven (Arnold)	1 slice of 8 oz loaf	60	1
White Brick Oven (Arnold)	1 slice of 16 oz loaf	60	1

FOOD	PORTION	CALORIES	FAT
White Brick Oven (Arnold)	1 slice of 32 oz loaf	90	1
White Cottage (America's Own)	1 slice	70	1
White Country (Arnold)	1 slice	100	2
White Less (Arnold)	1 slice	40	tr
White Light (Roman Meal)	1 slice	40	tr
White, Milk & Honey (Arnold)	1 slice	60	1
White Thin Slice (Pepperidge Farm)	1 slice	80	2
White Very Thin (Arnold)	1 slice	40	1
White Very Thin Sliced (Pepperidge Farm)	1 slice	40	0
Whole Wheat (Matthew's)	1 slice	70	1
Whole Wheat 100% (Freihofer's)	1 slice	75	1
Whole Wheat 100% Stone Ground (Monks' Bread)	1 slice	70	1
Whole Wheat 100% Stoneground (Wonder)	1 slice	80	1
Whole Wheat Thin Slice (Pepperidge Farm)	1 slice	60	1
Whole White Special Recipe (Stroehmann)	1 slice	70	1
Whole White Special Recipe Kids (Stroehmann)	1 slice	60	tr
cracked wheat	1 slice	65	1
cracked wheat, toasted	1 slice	65	1
french	1 slice (1.2 oz)	100	1
french	1 loaf (1 lb)	454	18
italian	1 loaf (1 lb)	454	4
italian	1 slice (1 oz)	85	tr
oatmeal	1 slice	65	1
pita	1 (2 oz)	165	1
pumpernickel	1 slice	80	1

FOOD	PORTION	CALORIES	FAT
raisin	1 slice	65	1
rye	1 slice	65	1
vienna	1 slice (.9 oz)	70	1
wheat	1 slice	65	1
white	1 slice	65	1
white, cubed	1 cup	80	1
whole wheat	1 slice	70	1
REFRIGERATED			
Crusty French Loaf (Pillsbury)	1	60	tr
Hearty Grains Country Oatmeal Twists (Pillsbury)	1	80	2
Hearty Grains Cracked Wheat Twists (Pillsbury)	1	80	2
Pipin' Hot Wheat Loaf (Pillsbury)	1	70	2
Pipin' Hot White Loaf (Pillsbury)	1	70	2
TAKE-OUT			
chapatis, as prep w/ fat	1 (2.5 oz)	230	9
chapatis, as prep w/o fat	1 (2.5 oz)	141	1
cornbread	2" × 2" (1.4 oz)	107	2
cornstick	1 (1.3 oz)	101	4
naan	1 (6 oz)	571	21
papadums, fried	2 (1.5 oz)	81	4
paratha	1 (4.4 oz)	403	18

BREAD COATING

Breading Frying Mix (Golden Dipt)	1 oz	90	0
Chicken Frying Mix (Golden Dipt)	1 oz	90	0
Mrs. Dash Crispy Coating Mix	½ oz	63	1
Onion Ring Mix (Golden Dipt)	1 oz	100	0
Oven Fry Extra Crispy Recipe for Chicken (General Foods)	¼ pkg (1 oz)	111	2

FOOD	PORTION	CALORIES	FAT
Oven Fry Extra Crispy Recipe for Pork (General Foods)	¼ pkg (1 oz)	115	2
Oven Fry Light Crispy Homestyle Recipe (General Foods)	¼ pkg (1 oz)	107	3
Shake 'N Bake			
Country Mild Recipe	¼ pkg (½ oz)	65	3
Italian Herb Recipe	¼ pkg (½ oz)	75	1
Original Barbecue Recipe for Chicken	¼ pkg (½ oz)	90	2
Original Barbecue Recipe for Pork	¼ pkg (½ oz)	75	2
Original Recipe for Chicken	¼ pkg (½ oz)	75	2
Original Recipe for Fish	¼ pkg (½ oz)	74	1
Original Recipe for Pork	¼ pkg (½ oz)	80	1

BREADCRUMBS

FOOD	PORTION	CALORIES	FAT
Contadina Seasoned	1 rounded tbsp	35	tr
Contadina Seasoned	1 cup	426	4
Friday's Seasoned	1 oz	56	tr
Organic Whole Wheat Bread Crumbs, Italian Style (Jaclyn's)	½ oz	28	1
Organic Whole Wheat Bread Crumbs, Plain (Jaclyn's)	½ oz	28	1
dry	1 cup	390	5
fresh	1 cup	120	2

BREADFRUIT

FOOD	PORTION	CALORIES	FAT
breadfruit	3.5 oz	109	tr
fresh	¼ small	99	tr
seeds, cooked	1 oz	48	1
seeds, raw	1 oz	54	2
seeds, roasted	1 oz	59	tr

FOOD	PORTION	CALORIES	FAT

BREADNUT SEEDS

FOOD	PORTION	CALORIES	FAT
dried	1 oz	104	tr

BREADSTICKS

FOOD	PORTION	CALORIES	FAT
Cheese (Angonoa)	1 oz	110	2
Cheese (Lance)	2	20	1
Dunking Sticks (Lance)	1⅜ oz	190	10
Garlic (Angonoa)	1 oz	120	2
Garlic (Keebler)	2	30	tr
Garlic (Lance)	2	30	1
Italian (Angonoa)	1 oz	120	2
Low Sodium (Angonoa)	1 oz	120	4
Mini Cheese (Angonoa)	1 oz	110	2
Mini Pizza (Angonoa)	1 oz	120	2
Mini Sesame (Angonoa)	1 oz	120	4
Mini Whole Wheat (Angonoa)	1 oz	120	4
Onion (Angonoa)	1 oz	120	3
Onion (Keebler)	2	30	tr
Onion (Stella D'Oro)	1	38	1
Plain (Keebler)	2	30	tr
Plain (Stella D'Oro)	1	41	1
Plain (Lance)	2	30	1
Plain Dietetic (Stella D'Oro)	1	43	1
Sesame (Keebler)	2	30	1
Sesame (Lance)	2	30	1
Sesame (Stella D'Oro)	1	50	2
Sesame Royale (Angonoa)	1 oz	120	4
Soft Bread Sticks (Pillsbury)	1	100	2
onion poppyseed (home recipe)	1	64	1

FOOD	PORTION	CALORIES	FAT

BREAKFAST BAR
(*see also* BREAKFAST DRINKS, NUTRITIONAL SUPPLEMENTS)

FOOD	PORTION	CALORIES	FAT
Apple (Nutri-Grain)	1 (1.3 oz)	150	5
Blueberry (Nutri-Grain)	1 (1.3 oz)	150	5
Chocolate Chip (Carnation)	1 (1.44 oz)	200	11
Chocolate Crunch (Carnation)	1 (1.34 oz)	190	10
Peanut Butter Crunch (Carnation)	1 (1.35 oz)	190	11
Peanut Butter w/ Chocolate Chips (Carnation)	1 (1.39 oz)	200	11
Raspberry (Nutri-Grain)	1 (1.3 oz)	150	5
Strawberry (Nutri-Grain)	1 (1.3 oz)	150	5

BREAKFAST DRINKS
(*see also* BREAKFAST BAR, NUTRITIONAL SUPPLEMENTS)

FOOD	PORTION	CALORIES	FAT
Chocolate Instant Breakfast (Carnation)	1 pkg (1.25 oz)	130	tr
Chocolate Instant Breakfast, as prep w/ skim milk (Carnation)	1 pkg + 8 oz milk	220	1
Chocolate Instant Breakfast, as prep w/ whole milk (Carnation)	1 pkg + 8 oz milk	280	8
Chocolate Instant Breakfast, as prep w/ whole milk (Pillsbury)	1 pkg + 8 oz milk	290	9
Chocolate Instant Breakfast No Sugar Added (Carnation)	1 pkg (.69 oz)	70	1
Chocolate Instant Breakfast No Sugar Added, as prep w/ skim milk (Carnation)	1 pkg + 8 oz milk	160	2
Chocolate Malt Instant Breakfast (Carnation)	1 pkg (1.24 oz)	130	1
Chocolate Malt Instant Breakfast, as prep w/ skim milk (Carnation)	1 pkg + 8 oz milk	220	2
Chocolate Malt Instant Breakfast, as prep w/ whole milk (Carnation)	1 pkg + 8 oz milk	280	9

FOOD	PORTION	CALORIES	FAT
Chocolate Malt Instant Breakfast, as prep w/ whole milk (Pillsbury)	1 pkg + 8 oz milk	290	9
Chocolate Malt Instant Breakfast No Sugar Added (Carnation)	1 pkg (.71 oz)	70	1
Chocolate Malt Instant Breakfast No Sugar Added, as prep w/ skim milk (Carnation)	1 pkg + 8 oz milk	160	2
Coffee Instant Breakfast (Carnation)	1 pkg (1.26 oz)	130	tr
Coffee Instant Breakfast, as prep w/ skim milk (Carnation)	1 pkg + 8 oz milk	220	1
Coffee Instant Breakfast, as prep w/ whole milk (Carnation)	1 pkg + 8 oz milk	280	8
Eggnog Instant Breakfast (Carnation)	1 pkg (1.2 oz)	130	tr
Eggnog Instant Breakfast, as prep w/ skim milk (Carnation)	1 pkg + 8 oz milk	220	1
Eggnog Instant Breakfast, as prep w/ whole milk (Carnation)	1 pkg + 8 oz milk	280	8
Strawberry Instant Breakfast (Carnation)	1 pkg (1.25 oz)	130	tr
Strawberry Instant Breakfast, as prep w/ skim milk (Carnation)	1 pkg + 8 oz milk	220	1
Strawberry Instant Breakfast, as prep w/ whole milk (Carnation)	1 pkg + 8 oz milk	280	8
Strawberry Instant Breakfast, as prep w/ whole milk (Pillsbury)	1 pkg + 8 oz milk	290	9
Strawberry Instant Breakfast No Sugar Added (Carnation)	1 pkg (.68 oz)	70	0
Strawberry Instant Breakfast No Sugar Added, as prep w/ skim milk (Carnation)	1 pkg + 8 oz milk	160	1
Vanilla Instant Breakfast (Carnation)	1 pkg (1.23 oz)	130	tr
Vanilla Instant Breakfast, as prep w/ whole milk (Pillsbury)	1 pkg + 8 oz milk	300	9
Vanilla Instant Breakfast, as prep w/ skim milk (Carnation)	1 pkg + 8 oz milk	220	1

FOOD	PORTION	CALORIES	FAT
Vanilla Instant Breakfast, as prep w/ whole milk (Carnation)	1 pkg + 8 oz milk	280	8
Vanilla Instant Breakfast No Sugar Added (Carnation)	1 pkg (.67 oz)	70	0
Vanilla Instant Breakfast No Sugar Added, as prep w/ skim milk (Carnation)	1 pkg + 8 oz milk	160	1
orange drink, powder	3 rounded tsp	93	0
orange drink powder, as prep w/ water	6 oz	86	0

BROAD BEANS

CANNED broad beans	1 cup	183	1
DRIED cooked	1 cup	186	1
raw	1 cup	511	2
FRESH cooked	3.5 oz	56	tr

BROCCOLI

Dole	1 med spear	40	1
chopped, cooked	½ cup	22	tr
raw, chopped	½ cup	12	tr
FROZEN Baby Spears (Birds Eye)	⅔ cup	29	tr
Broccoli w/ Cheese in Pastry (Pepperidge Farm)	1	230	16
Broccoli w/ Cheese Sauce (Birds Eye)	½ cup	115	6
Broccoli w/ Creamy Italian Cheese Sauce (Birds Eye)	½ cup	90	6

FOOD	PORTION	CALORIES	FAT
Chopped (Birds Eye)	⅔ cup	26	tr
Cut (Hanover)	½ cup	25	0
Cuts (Birds Eye)	⅔ cup	25	tr
Cuts (Green Giant)	½ cup	12	0
Florets (Birds Eye)	⅔ cup	26	tr
Florets (Hanover)	½ cup	30	0
Harvest Fresh Cut (Green Giant)	½ cup	16	0
Harvest Fresh Spears (Green Giant)	½ cup	20	0
In Butter Sauce (Green Giant)	½ cup	40	2
In Cheese Sauce (Green Giant)	½ cup	60	2
Mini Spears (Green Giant Select)	4–5 spears	18	0
One Serve Cuts in Butter Sauce (Green Giant)	1 pkg	45	2
One Serve Cuts in Cheese Sauce (Green Giant)	1 pkg	70	3
Spears (Birds Eye)	⅔ cup	26	tr
Valley Combinations Broccoli Fanfare (Green Giant)	½ cup	80	2
chopped, cooked	½ cup	25	tr
spears, cooked	10 oz pkg	69	tr
spears, cooked	½ cup	25	tr

BROWNIE

FOOD	PORTION	CALORIES	FAT
Brownie Ala Mode (Weight Watchers)	1	180	4
Chocolate Brownie (Weight Watchers)	1 (1.25 oz)	100	3
Mint Frosted (Weight Watchers)	1 (1.23 oz)	100	5
Monterey Hot Fudge Chocolate Chunk Brownie (Pepperidge Farm)	1	480	26
Newport Hot Fudge Brownie (Pepperidge Farm)	1	400	20

FOOD	PORTION	CALORIES	FAT
HOME RECIPE			
w/ nuts	1 (.8 oz)	95	6
MIX			
Chewy Recipe Fudge Brownie Mix (Duncan Hines)	1	130	5
Deluxe Family-Size Fudge Brownie, as prep (Pillsbury)	2	150	7
Deluxe Fudge Brownie, as prep (Pillsbury)	2	150	6
Deluxe Fudge Brownie w/ Walnuts, as prep (Pillsbury)	2	150	8
Estee Brownie Mix, as prep	1	50	2
Fudge Brownie Microwave, as prep (Pillsbury)	1	190	9
Gourmet Truffle Brownie Mix (Duncan Hines)	1	280	13
Gourmet Turtle Brownie Mix (Duncan Hines)	1	240	10
Gourmet Vienna White Brownie Mix (Duncan Hines)	1	240	12
Milk Chocolate Brownie Mix (Duncan Hines)	1	160	7
Original Fudge Brownie Mix (Duncan Hines)	1	160	7
Peanut Butter Chocolate Brownie Mix (Duncan Hines)	1	150	8
The Ultimate Carmel Fudge Chunk Brownie, as prep (Pillsbury)	2	170	7
The Ultimate Chunky Triple Fudge Brownie, as prep (Pillsbury)	2	170	7
The Ultimate Double Fudge Brownie, as prep (Pillsbury)	2	160	6
The Ultimate Rockey Road Fudge Brownie, as prep (Pillsbury)	2	170	8

FOOD	PORTION	CALORIES	FAT
READY-TO-EAT			
Charlotte Fudgey Brownie (Pepperidge Farm)	1	220	11
Fudge Walnut (Tastykake)	1	373	10
Lance Brownie	1 pkg (1.75 oz)	200	6
Little Debbie	1 pkg (2 oz)	230	8
Tahoe Milk Chocolate Pecan (Pepperidge Farm)	1	210	10
Westport Fudgey Brownies w/ Walnuts (Pepperidge Farm)	1	220	11
w/ nuts	1 (1 oz)	100	4
w/o nuts	1 (2 oz)	243	10

BRUSSELS SPROUTS

FOOD	PORTION	CALORIES	FAT
FRESH			
Dole	½ cup	19	tr
cooked	½ cup	30	tr
cooked	1 sprout	8	tr
raw	½ cup	19	tr
raw	1 sprout	8	tr
FROZEN			
Birds Eye	½ cup	37	tr
Hanover	½ cup	40	0
Green Giant	½ cup	7	0
Baby Brussels Sprouts w/Cheese Sauce (Birds Eye)	½ cup	113	6
In Butter Sauce (Green Giant)	½ cup	40	1
cooked	½ cup	33	tr

BUCKWHEAT

FOOD	PORTION	CALORIES	FAT
Buckwheat Groats Brown (Arrowhead)	2 oz	190	1

FOOD	PORTION	CALORIES	FAT
Buckwheat Groats White (Arrowhead)	2 oz	190	1
flour, whole groat	1 cup	402	4
groats, roasted, cooked	½ cup	91	tr
groats, roasted, uncooked	½ cup	283	2

BUFFALO
water, roasted	3 oz	111	2

BULGUR
cooked	½ cup	76	tr
uncooked	½ cup	239	tr

BURBOT (FISH)
fresh, baked	3 oz	98	1

BURDOCK ROOT
cooked	1 cup	110	tr
raw	1 cup	85	tr

BUTTER
(see also BUTTER BLENDS, BUTTER SUBSTITUTES, MARGARINE)

REGULAR			
Cabot	1 tsp	35	4
Cabot Unsalted	1 tsp	35	4
Hotel Bar	1 tsp	35	4
Land O'Lakes	1 tsp	35	4
Land O'Lakes Unsalted	1 tsp	35	4
butter	1 pat	36	4
butter	4 oz	813	92
butter oil	1 cup	1795	204

FOOD	PORTION	CALORIES	FAT
butter oil	1 tbsp	112	13
clarified butter	3.5 oz	876	99
WHIPPED			
Land O'Lakes	1 tsp	25	3
Land O'Lakes Unsalted	1 tsp	24	3
butter	4 oz	542	61
butter	1 pat	27	3

BUTTER BEANS

	PORTION	CALORIES	FAT
CANNED			
Butter Beans (Hanover)	½ cup	80	0
Butter Beans (Van Camp's)	1 cup	162	1
Butter Beans in Sauce (Hanover)	½ cup	100	0
Butter Beans Tender Cooked (S&W)	½ cup	100	0
Large White (Trappey's)	½ cup	80	1
Speckled Butter Beans Seasoned w/ Pork (Luck's)	7.5 oz	230	8

BUTTER BLENDS
(*see also* BUTTER, BUTTER SUBSTITUTES, MARGARINE)

	PORTION	CALORIES	FAT
REGULAR			
Blue Bonnet Better Blend	1 tbsp	90	11
Blue Bonnet Better Blend Unsalted	1 tbsp	90	11
Country Morning Blend	1 tsp	35	4
Country Morning Blend Unsalted	1 tsp	35	4
butter blend	1 stick	811	91
SOFT			
Blue Bonnet Better Blend	1 tbsp	90	11
Country Morning Blend	1 tsp	30	3
Country Morning Blend Light Tub	1 tsp	20	3
Country Morning Blend Unsalted	1 tsp	30	3

FOOD	PORTION	CALORIES	FAT
Downey's Cinnamon Honey-Butter	1 tbsp	52	1
Downey's Original Honey-Butter	1 tbsp	52	1
Le Slim Cow (St. Hubert)	1 tbsp	40	4
Touch of Butter Stick	1 tbsp	90	10
Touch of Butter Tub	1 tbsp	50	6

BUTTER SUBSTITUTES
(see also BUTTER BLENDS, MARGARINE)

Butter Buds	⅛ oz	12	0
Butter Buds Sprinkles	½ tsp	4	0
Molly McButter	½ tsp	3	tr
Molly McButter w/ Bacon	½ tsp	4	tr
Molly McButter w/ Cheese	½ tsp	4	tr
Molly McButter w/ Sour Cream	½ tsp	4	tr

BUTTERBUR

canned fuki, chopped	1 cup	3	tr
fresh fuki, raw	1 cup	13	tr

BUTTERFISH

baked	3 oz	159	9
fillet, baked	1 oz	47	3

BUTTERNUTS

dried	1 oz	174	16

CABBAGE

FRESH

Dole	1/12 med head	18	0
Dole Napa, shredded	½ cup	6	tr
chinese pak-choi raw, shredded	½ cup	5	tr

FOOD	PORTION	CALORIES	FAT
chinese pak-choi, shredded, cooked	½ cup	10	tr
chinese pe-tsai raw, shredded	1 cup	12	tr
chinese pe-tsai, shredded, cooked	1 cup	16	tr
green, raw, shredded	1 head (2 lbs)	215	2
green, raw, shredded	½ cup	8	tr
green, shredded, cooked	½ cup	16	tr
red, raw, shredded	½ cup	10	tr
red, shredded, cooked	½ cup	16	tr
savoy, raw, shredded	½ cup	10	tr
savoy, shredded, cooked	½ cup	18	tr
HOME RECIPE			
coleslaw w/ dressing	¾ cup	147	11
TAKE-OUT			
coleslaw w/ dressing	½ cup	42	2
stuffed cabbage	1 (6 oz)	373	22
sweet & sour red cabbage	4 oz	61	3
vinegar & oil coleslaw	3.5 oz	150	9

CAKE

(see also BROWNIE, COOKIES, DANISH PASTRY, DOUGHNUT, PIE)

FOOD	PORTION	CALORIES	FAT
FROSTING/ICING			
Cake & Cookie Decorator, all colors except chocolate (Pillsbury)	1 tbsp	70	2
Cake & Cookie Decorator, Chocolate (Pillsbury)	1 tbsp	60	2
Caramel Pecan Frosting Supreme (Pillsbury)	for ¹⁄₁₂ cake	160	8
Chocolate Chip Frosting Supreme (Pillsbury)	for ¹⁄₁₂ cake	150	5
Chocolate Creamy Frosting (Duncan Hines)	¹⁄₁₂ pkg	160	7
Chocolate Fudge (Pillsbury)	for ⅛ cake	110	5

FOOD	PORTION	CALORIES	FAT
Chocolate Fudge Frosting Supreme (Pillsbury)	for 1/12 cake	150	6
Chocolate Fudge Funfetti (Pillsbury)	1/12 can	140	6
Chocolate Mint Frosting Supreme (Pillsbury)	for 1/12 cake	150	7
Coconut Almond Frosting Mix, as prep (Pillsbury)	for 1/12 cake	160	10
Coconut Almond Frosting Supreme (Pillsbury)	for 1/12 cake	150	9
Coconut Pecan Frosting Mix, as prep (Pillsbury)	for 1/12 cake	150	7
Coconut Pecan Frosting Supreme (Pillsbury)	for 1/12 cake	160	10
Cream Cheese Frosting Supreme (Pillsbury)	for 1/12 cake	160	6
Dark Dutch Fudge Creamy Frosting (Duncan Hines)	1/12 pkg	160	7
Double Dutch Frosting Supreme (Pillsbury)	for 1/12 cake	140	6
Fluffy White Frosting Mix (Pillsbury)	for 1/12 cake	60	0
Frost It Hot Chocolate (Pillsbury)	for 1/8 cake	50	0
Frost It Hot Fluffy White (Pillsbury)	for 1/8 cake	50	0
Frosting Mix (Estee)	1.5 tsp	50	1
Lemon Frosting Supreme (Pillsbury)	for 1/12 cake	160	6
Milk Chocolate Creamy Frosting (Duncan Hines)	1/12 pkg	160	7
Milk Chocolate Frosting Supreme (Pillsbury)	for 1/12 cake	150	6
Mocha Frosting Supreme (Pillsbury)	for 1/12 cake	150	6
Sour Cream Vanilla Frosting Supreme (Pillsbury)	for 1/12 cake	160	6
Strawberry Frosting Supreme (Pillsbury)	for 1/12 cake	160	6
Vanilla (Pillsbury)	for 1/8 cake	120	5

FOOD	PORTION	CALORIES	FAT
Vanilla Creamy Frosting (Duncan Hines)	⅟₁₂ pkg	160	7
Vanilla Frosting Supreme (Pillsbury)	for ⅟₁₂ cake	160	6
Vanilla Funfetti Pink (Pillsbury)	⅟₁₂ can	150	6
Vanilla Funfetti White (Pillsbury)	⅟₁₂ can	150	6
FROZEN			
Amhurst Apple Crumb Coffee Cake (Pepperidge Farm)	1	220	11
Apple Crisp (Weight Watchers)	1 (3.5 oz)	190	5
Apple Crisp Cake Light (Sara Lee)	1 (3 oz)	150	2
Apple 'N Spice Bake Dessert Lights (Pepperidge Farm)	1 piece (4.25 oz)	170	2
Apple Streusel Pie Free & Light (Sara Lee)	1 slice (2.9 oz)	170	2
Apple Turnover (Pepperidge Farm)	1	300	17
Banana Single Layer Iced Cake (Sara Lee)	1 slice (1.7 oz)	170	6
Berkshire Apple Crisp (Pepperidge Farm)	1	250	8
Better Than Cheesecake Blueberry (Tofutti)	2 oz	160	10
Better Than Cheesecake Chocolate Brownie (Tofutti)	2 oz	160	10
Better Than Cheesecake Classic (Tofutti)	2 oz	160	10
Black Forest Cake Light (Sara Lee)	1 (3.6 oz)	170	5
Black Forest Two Layer Cake (Sara Lee)	1 slice (2.5 oz)	190	8
Blueberry Turnovers (Pepperidge Farm)	1	310	19
Boston Cream Supreme (Pepperidge Farm)	1 piece (2⅞ oz)	290	14
Brownie Cheesecake (Weight Watchers)	1 (3.5 oz)	200	5

FOOD	PORTION	CALORIES	FAT
Butter Pound (Pepperidge Farm)	1 slice (1 oz)	130	7
Carrott Classic (Pepperidge Farm)	1 cake	260	16
Carrot Light (Sara Lee)	1 (2.5 oz)	170	4
Carrot Single Layer Iced Cake (Sara Lee)	1 slice (2.4 oz)	250	13
Carrot w/ Cream Cheese Icing (Pepperidge Farm)	1 slice (1.5 oz)	150	9
Charleston Peach Melba Shortcake (Pepperidge Farm)	1	220	5
Cheese Sweet Roll (Weight Watchers)	1 (2.25 oz)	180	4
Cheeries & Cream Cake (Weight Watchers)	1 (3 oz)	150	2
Cherries Supreme Dessert Lights (Pepperidge Farm)	1 piece (3.25 oz)	170	11
Cherry Streusel Pie Free & Light (Sara Lee)	1 slice (3.6 oz)	160	2
Cherry Turnover (Pepperidge Farm)	1	310	19
Chocolate Cake (Weight Watchers)	1 (2.5 oz)	180	5
Chocolate Cake Free & Light (Sara Lee)	1 slice (1.7 oz)	110	0
Chocolate Eclair (Weight Watchers)	1 (2.1 oz)	120	4
Chocolate Fudge Large Layer (Pepperidge Farm)	1 slice (1⅝ oz)	180	10
Chocolate Fudge Strip Large Layer (Pepperidge Farm)	1 piece (1⅝ oz)	170	9
Chocolate Mousse Cake Dessert Lights (Pepperidge Farm)	1 piece (2.5 oz)	190	9
Chocolate Supreme (Pepperidge Farm)	1 piece (2⅞ oz)	300	16
Cholestrol Free Pound (Pepperidge Farm)	1 slice (1 oz)	110	6
Cinnamon Roll (Pepperidge Farm)	1 (2.25 oz)	220	14
Cinnamon Rolls (Weight Watchers)	1 (2.1 oz)	180	5

FOOD	PORTION	CALORIES	FAT
Coconut Classic (Pepperidge Farm)	1 cake	230	11
Coconut Large Layer (Pepperidge Farm)	1 slice (1⅝ oz)	180	8
Coffee Cake All Butter Butter Streusel (Sara Lee)	1 slice (1.4 oz)	160	7
Coffee Cake All Butter Cheese (Sara Lee)	1 slice (2 oz)	210	11
Coffee Cake All Butter Pecan (Sara Lee)	1 slice (1.4 oz)	160	8
Coffee Cake w/ Cinnamon Streusel (Weight Watchers)	2.25 oz	160	4
Devil's Food Large Layer (Pepperidge Farm)	1 slice (1⅝ oz)	180	9
Double Chocolate Cake Light (Sara Lee)	1 (2.5 oz)	150	5
Double Chocolate Classic (Pepperidge Farm)	1 cake	250	13
Double Chocolate Three Layer Cake (Sara Lee)	1 slice (2.2 oz)	220	11
Double Fudge (Weight Watchers)	1 piece (2.75 oz)	190	4
Elfin Loaves Apple Cinnamon	1	180	4
Elfin Loaves Banana	1	190	7
Elfin Loaves Blueberry	1	170	4
Elfin Loaves Carrot	1	210	10
French Cheesecake (Sara Lee)	1 slice (2.9 oz)	250	16
French Cheesecake Light (Sara Lee)	1 (3.2 oz)	150	4
Fruit Squares Apple (Pepperidge Farm)	1	220	12
Fruit Squares Cherry (Pepperidge Farm)	1	230	12
Fudge Golden Classic (Pepperidge Farm)	1 cake	260	14

FOOD	PORTION	CALORIES	FAT
German Chocolate Classic (Pepperidge Farm)	1 cake	250	13
German Chocolate Large Layer (Pepperidge Farm)	1 slice (1⅝ oz)	180	10
Golden Large Layer (Pepperidge Farm)	1 slice (1⅝ oz)	180	9
Lemon Cake Supreme Dessert Lights (Pepperidge Farm)	1 piece (2.75 oz)	170	5
Lemon Coconut Classic Cake (Pepperidge Farm)	3 oz	280	13
Lemon Coconut Supreme (Pepperidge Farm)	1 piece (3 oz)	280	13
Lemon Cream Cake Light (Sara Lee)	1 (3.2 oz)	180	6
Lemon Cream Supreme (Pepperidge Farm)	1 piece (1⅝ oz)	170	9
Manhattan Strawberry Cheesecake (Pepperidge Farm)	1	300	9
Original Cheesecake Cherry (Sara Lee)	1 slice (3.2 oz)	243	8
Original Cheesecake Plain (Sara Lee)	1 slice (2.8 oz)	230	11
Original Cheesecake Strawberry (Sara Lee)	1 slice (3.2 oz)	222	8
Peach Melba Supreme (Pepperidge Farm)	1 (3⅛ oz)	270	7
Peach Parfait Dessert Lights (Pepperidge Farm)	1 piece (4.25 oz)	150	5
Peach Turnover (Pepperidge Farm)	1	310	18
Pineapple Cream Supreme (Pepperidge Farm)	1 piece (2 oz)	190	7
Pound Cake All Butter Family Size (Sara Lee)	1 slice (1 oz)	130	7
Pound Cake All Butter Original (Sara Lee)	1 slice (1 oz)	130	7
Pound Cake Cholesterol Free (Pepperidge Farm)	1 slice (1 oz)	110	6

FOOD	PORTION	CALORIES	FAT
Pound Cake Free & Light (Sara Lee)	1 slice (1 oz)	70	0
Raspberry Turnovers (Pepperidge Farm)	1	310	17
Raspberry Vanilla Swirl Dessert Lights (Pepperidge Farm)	1 piece (3.25 oz)	160	5
Strawberry Cheesecake (Weight Watchers)	1 piece (3.9 oz)	180	4
Strawberry Cream Supreme (Pepperidge Farm)	1 piece (2 oz)	190	7
Strawberry French Cheesecake Light (Sara Lee)	1 (3.5 oz)	150	2
Strawberry Shortcake Dessert Lights (Pepperidge Farm)	1 piece (3 oz)	170	5
Strawberry Shortcake Two Layer Cake (Sara Lee)	1 slice (2.5 oz)	190	8
Strawberry Strip Large Layer (Pepperidge Farm)	1 piece (1.5 oz)	160	8
Strawberry Yogurt Dessert Free & Light (Sara Lee)	1 slice (2.2 oz)	120	1
Vanilla Fudge Swirl Classic (Pepperidge Farm)	1 cake	250	11
Vanilla Large Layer (Pepperidge Farm)	1 slice (1⅝ oz)	190	8
eclair w/ chocolate icing & custard filling, frzn	1	205	10
HOME RECIPE			
carrot w/ cream cheese icing	1 cake (10" diam tube)	6175	328
carrot w/ cream cheese icing	1/16 cake	385	21
fruitcake, dark	1 cake (7½" × 2¼")	5185	228
fruitcake, dark	1 slice	165	7
pound	1 loaf (8½" × 3½")	1935	94
pound cake	1 slice (1 oz)	120	5

FOOD	PORTION	CALORIES	FAT
sheet cake w/ white frosting	1 cake (9″ sq)	4020	129
sheet cake w/ white frosting	⅑ cake	445	14
sheet cake w/o frosting	⅑ cake	315	12
sheet cake w/o frosting	1 cake (9″ sq)	2830	108

MIX

FOOD	PORTION	CALORIES	FAT
Angel Food			
Chocolate (General Mills)	1/12 cake	150	0
Confetti (General Mills)	1/12 cake	160	0
Lemon Custard (General Mills)	1/12 cake	150	0
Strawberry (General Mills)	1/12 cake	150	0
Traditional (General Mills)	1/12 cake	130	0
White (General Mills)	1/12 cake	150	0
Apple Cinnamon Coffee Cake (Pillsbury)	⅛ cake	240	7
Banana (Pillsbury Plus)	1/12 cake	250	11
Banana Quick Bread (Pillsbury)	1/12 loaf	170	6
Bisquick (General Mills)	2 oz	230	7
Black Forest Cherry Bundt (Pillsbury)	1/16 cake	240	9
Blueberry Nut Quick Bread (Pillsbury)	1/12 loaf	150	4
Butter Recipe as prep (Pillsbury Plus)	1/12 cake	260	12
Butter Recipe Fudge (Duncan Hines)	1/12 cake	270	13
Butter Recipe Golden (Duncan Hines)	1/12 cake	270	13
Carrot (Dromedary)	1/12 cake	232	15
Carrot (Estee)	1/10 cake	100	2
Carrot Spice (Pillsbury Plus)	1/12 cake	260	11
Cheesecake No Bake Dessert (Jell-O)	⅛ cake	281	13
Cherry Nut Quick Bread (Pillsbury)	1/12 loaf	180	5

FOOD	PORTION	CALORIES	FAT
Chocolate (Estee)	⅒ cake	100	2
Chocolate Cake Microwave (Pillsbury)	⅛ cake	210	12
Chocolate Cake w/ Chocolate Frosting (Pillsbury)	⅛ cake	300	17
Chocolate Cake w/ Vanilla Frosting (Pillsbury)	⅛ cake	300	17
Chocolate Chip (Pillsbury Plus)	⅟₁₂ cake	270	14
Chocolate Lite Cake & Frosting Mix (Batter Lite)	⅑ cake	110	2
Cinnamon Streusel Swirl (Pillsbury)	⅟₁₆ cake	260	11
Cobbler Apple Crumb (Dromedary)	⅛ cake	237	6
Cobbler Cherry Crumb (Dromedary)	⅛ cake	231	6
Coffee Cake Easy Mix (Aunt Jemima)	⅛ cake	160	5
Corn Bread Easy Mix (Aunt Jemima)	⅙ cake	210	7
Cranberry Quick Bread (Pillsbury)	⅟₁₂ loaf	160	4
Dark Dutch Fudge (Duncan Hines)	⅟₁₂ cake	280	15
Date Nut (Dromedary)	⅟₁₂ cake	183	8
Date Nut Roll (Dromedary)	⅟₁₂ loaf	80	2
Date Quick Bread (Pillsbury)	⅟₁₂ loaf	160	2
Devil's Food (Duncan Hines)	⅟₁₂ cake	280	15
Devil's Food (Pillsbury Plus)	⅟₁₂ cake	270	14
Double Chocolate Supreme Microwave (Pillsbury)	⅛ cake	330	19
Double Lemon Supreme Microwave (Pillsbury)	⅛ cake	300	15
French Vanilla (Duncan Hines)	⅟₁₂ cake	260	11
Fudge Marble (Duncan Hines)	⅟₁₂ cake	260	11
Fudge Marble (Pillsbury Plus)	⅟₁₂ cake	270	12
German Chocolate (Pillsbury Plus)	⅟₁₂ cake	250	11
Gingerbread (Dromedary)	1 piece (2″ × 2″)	100	2

FOOD	PORTION	CALORIES	FAT
Gingerbread (Pillsbury)	3" sq	190	4
Lemon (Estee)	1/10 cake	100	2
Lemon (Pillsbury Plus)	1/12 cake	250	11
Lemon Cake Microwave (Pillsbury)	1/8 cake	220	13
Lemon Cake w/ Lemon Frosting (Pillsbury)	1/8 cake	300	17
Lemon Streusel Swirl (Pillsbury)	1/16 cake	270	11
Lemon Supreme (Duncan Hines)	1/12 cake	260	11
Nut Quick Bread (Pillsbury)	1/12 loaf	170	6
Pineapple Cream Bundt (Pillsbury)	1/16 cake	260	10
Pineapple Supreme (Duncan Hines)	1/12 cake	260	11
Pound (Estee)	1/10 cake	100	2
Pound Cake (Dromedary)	1/2" slice	150	6
Spice (Duncan Hines)	1/12 cake	260	11
Strawberry (Pillsbury Plus)	1/12 cake	260	11
Strawberry Supreme (Duncan Hines)	1/12 cake	260	11
Streusel Swirl Cinnamon Microwave (Pillsbury)	1/8 cake	240	11
Swiss Chocolate (Duncan Hines)	1/12 cake	280	15
Tunnel of Fudge Bundt (Pillsbury)	1/16 cake	270	12
Tunnel of Fudge Bundt Microwave (Pillsbury)	1/8 cake	290	17
Tunnel of Lemon Bundt (Pillsbury)	1/16 cake	270	9
White (Duncan Hines)	1/12 cake	250	10
White (Pillsbury Plus)	1/12 cake	240	10
White (Estee)	1/10 cake	100	2
White Lite Cake & Frosting Mix (Batter Lite)	1/8 cake	110	2
Yellow (Duncan Hines)	1/12 cake	260	11
Yellow (Pillsbury Plus)	1/12 cake	260	12
Yellow Cake Microwave (Pillsbury)	1/8 cake	220	13

FOOD	PORTION	CALORIES	FAT
Yellow Cake w/ Chocolate Frosting (Pillsbury)	⅛ cake	300	17
angelfood	¹⁄₁₂ cake	125	tr
angelfood	1 cake (9¾" diam)	1510	2
crumb coffeecake	1 cake (7¾" × 5⅝")	1385	41
crumb coffeecake	⅙ cake	230	7
devil's food cupcake w/ chocolate frosting	1	120	4
devil's food w/ chocolate frosting	1 cake (9" sq)	3755	136
devil's food w/ chocolate frosting	¹⁄₁₆ cake	235	8
gingerbread	1 cake (8" sq)	1575	39
gingerbread	⅛ cake	175	4
yellow w/ chocolate frosting	1 cake (9" diam)	3735	125
yellow w/ chocolate frosting	¹⁄₁₆ cake	235	8
READY-TO-USE			
Cheesecake La Creame (Formagg)			
Amaretto Almond	2 oz	115	6
Pineapple	2 oz	115	6
Plain	2 oz	115	6
Strawberry	2 oz	115	6
bakewell tart	1 slice (3 oz)	410	27
battenburg cake	1 slice (2 oz)	204	10
cheesecake	1 cake (9" diam)	3350	213
cheesecake	¹⁄₁₂ cake	280	18
crumpets, toasted	2 (4 oz)	119	1
eccles cake	1 slice (2 oz)	285	16
eclair	1 (1.4 oz)	149	10
madeira cake	1 slice (1 oz)	98	4

FOOD	PORTION	CALORIES	FAT
pound cake	1 slice (1 oz)	110	12
pound cake	1 cake (8½" × 3½")	1935	94
treacle tart	1 slice (2.5 oz)	258	10
vanilla slice	1 slice (2.5 oz)	248	13
white w/ white frosting	1/16 cake	260	9
white w/ white frosting	1 cake (9" sq)	4170	148
yellow w/ chocolate frosting	1 cake (9" diam)	3895	175
yellow w/ chocolate frosting	1/16 cake	245	11
REFRIGERATED			
Apple Turnovers (Pillsbury)	1	170	8
Baby Watson Cheesecake	1 pkg (4 oz)	420	31
Cherry Turnovers (Pillsbury)	1	170	8
Coffee Cake Cinnamon Swirl (Pillsbury)	1/8 cake	180	9
Coffee Cake Pecan Streusel (Pillsbury)	1/8 cake	180	9
Pastry Pockets (Pillsbury)	1	240	13
SNACK			
All Butter Pound Cake (Sara Lee)	1	200	11
Apple Delights (Little Debbie)	1 pkg (1.25 oz)	160	8
Apple Light & Fruity (Drake's)	1 (1.2 oz)	90	1
Apple Pie (Drake's)	1 (2 oz)	210	10
Apple Spice (Little Debbie)	1 pkg (2.2 oz)	300	17
Banana Slices (Little Debbie)	1 pkg (3 oz)	380	17
Banana Twins (Little Debbie)	1 pkg (2.2 oz)	280	13
Be My Valentine (Little Debbie)	1 pkg (2.2 oz)	290	15
Blueberry Light & Fruity (Drake's)	1 (1.2 oz)	90	1
Blueberry Pie (Drake's)	1 (2 oz)	210	10
Cherry Cordials (Little Debbie)	1 pkg (1.3 oz)	180	9

FOOD	PORTION	CALORIES	FAT
Cherry Pie (Drake's)	1 (2 oz)	220	10
Choc-O-Jel (Little Debbie)	1 pkg (1.16 oz)	170	10
Choco-Cakes (Little Debbie)	1 pkg (2.17 oz)	270	13
Chocolate Chip (Little Debbie)	1 pkg (2.4 oz)	310	16
Chocolate Cupcake (Tastykake)	1	113	3
Chocolate Fudge Cake (Sara Lee)	1	190	10
Chocolate Slices (Little Debbie)	1 pkg (3 oz)	360	17
Chocolate Twins (Little Debbie)	1 pkg (2.2 oz)	260	13
Christmas Tree Cakes (Little Debbie)	1 pkg (1.5 oz)	200	9
Cinnamon Raisin Light & Fruity (Drake's)	1 (1.2 oz)	90	1
Classic Cheesecake (Sara Lee)	1	200	14
Coconut (Little Debbie)	1 pkg (2.17 oz)	310	18
Coconut Crunch (Little Debbie)	1 pkg (2 oz)	340	24
Coconut Rounds (Little Debbie)	1 pkg (1.13 oz)	160	10
Coffee Cake			
(Drake's)	1 (1.1 oz)	140	6
(Little Debbie)	1 pkg (2 oz)	220	6
Apple Cinnamon (Sara Lee)	1	290	13
Butter Streusel (Sara Lee)	1	230	12
Chocolate Crumb (Drake's)	1 (2.5 oz)	245	9
Cinnamon Crumb (Drake's)	½12 cake (1.3 oz)	150	6
Pecan (Sara Lee)	1	280	16
Small (Drake's)	1 (2 oz)	220	9
Cream Filled Butter Cream Cupcake (Tastykake)	1	125	3
Cream Filled Chocolate Cupcake (Tastykake)	1	130	4
Creamies Banana Treat (Tastykake)	1	138	3
Creamies Chocolate (Tastykake)	1	174	7
Creamies Vanilla (Tastykake)	1	182	8

FOOD	PORTION	CALORIES	FAT
Deluxe Carrot Cake (Sara Lee)	1	180	7
Devil Cremes (Little Debbie)	1 pkg (1.3 oz)	170	7
Devil Dog (Drake's)	1 (1.5 oz)	160	6
Devil Slices (Little Debbie)	1 pkg (3 oz)	320	9
Devil Squares (Little Debbie)	1 pkg (2.2 oz)	300	17
Easter Bunny Cakes (Little Debbie)	1 pkg (2.5 oz)	320	14
Easter Puffs (Little Debbie)	1 pkg (1.25 oz)	150	4
Fancy Cakes (Little Debbie)	1 pkg (2.4 oz)	310	15
Fig Cake (Lance)	2⅛ oz	210	3
Figaroos (Little Debbie)	1 pkg (1.5 oz)	160	4
Fudge Crispy (Little Debbie)	1 pkg (2.08 oz)	330	20
Fudge Rounds (Little Debbie)	1 pkg (1.19 oz)	150	5
Funny Bones (Drake's)	1 (1.25 oz)	150	8
Golden Cremes (Little Debbie)	1 pkg (1.47 oz)	160	5
Holiday Cakes Chocolate (Little Debbie)	1 pkg (2.4 oz)	330	19
Holiday Cakes Vanilla (Little Debbie)	1 pkg (2.5 oz)	350	21
Honeybuns Glazed (Tastykake)	1	330	13
Honeybuns Iced (Tastykake)	1	342	12
Jelly Rolls (Little Debbie)	1 pkg (2.17 oz)	240	9
Juniors Chocolate (Tastykake)	1	364	8
Juniors Coconut (Tastykake)	1	317	4
Juniors Koffee Kake (Tastykake)	1	317	12
Kandy Kakes Chocolate (Tastykake)	1	99	4
Kandy Kakes Peanut Butter (Tastykake)	1	103	5
Koffe Kake Cream Filled (Tastykake)	1	143	6
Krimpets (TastyKake) Butterscotch	1	118	2
Cream Filled Chocolate	1	142	4
Cream Filled Vanilla	1	139	4

FOOD	PORTION	CALORIES	FAT
Krimpets *(cont.)*			
Jelly	1	96	tr
Lemon Pie (Drake's)	1 (2 oz)	210	11
Lemon Stix (Little Debbie)	1 pkg (1.5 oz)	220	11
Marshmallow Supremes (Little Debbie)	1 pkg (1.25 oz)	150	5
Mint Sprints (Little Debbie)	1 pkg (1.5 oz)	240	15
Nutty Bar (Little Debbie)	1 pkg (2 oz)	320	19
PB Krunch (Tastykake)	1	292	13
Pecan Twins (Little Debbie)	1 pkg (2 oz)	220	9
Pop-Tarts			
Apple Cinnamon	1	210	6
Blueberry	1	210	6
Brown Sugar Cinnamon	1	210	8
Cherry	1	210	6
Chocolate Graham	1	210	6
Frosted Brown Sugar Cinnamon	1	210	7
Frosted Cherry	1	210	5
Frosted Chocolate Fudge	1	200	5
Frosted Chocolate Vanilla Creme	1	200	5
Frosted Grape	1	200	5
Frosted Raspberry	1	220	5
Frosted Strawberry	1	200	5
Strawberry	1	210	6
Pound Cake (Drake's)	1/10 cake	110	5
Pumpkin Delights (Little Debbie)	1 pkg (1.13 oz)	140	6
Ring Ding (Drake's)	1 (1.5 oz)	180	10
Ring Ding Mint (Drake's)	1 (1.5 oz)	190	11
Snack Cake Chocolate (Little Debbie)	1 pkg (2.5 oz)	340	20
Snack Cake Vanilla (Little Debbie)	1 pkg (2.6 oz)	360	21
Star Crunch (Little Debbie)	1 pkg (1.08 oz)	150	7

FOOD	PORTION	CALORIES	FAT
Sunny Doodle (Drake's)	1 (1 oz)	100	3
Swiss Cake Roll (Little Debbie)	1 pkg (2.17 oz)	270	12
Swiss Rolls (Tastykake)	1	130	6
Tasty Twists (Tastykake)	1 pkg	211	8
Tempty (Tastykake)	1	94	2
Toaster Tart (Pepperidge Farm)			
Apple Cinnamon	1	170	7
Cheese	1	190	10
Strawberry	1	190	7
Toastettes (Nabisco)			
Apple	1	190	5
Blueberry	1	190	5
Cherry	1	190	5
Frosted Apple	1	190	5
Frosted Blueberry	1	190	0
Frosted Brown Sugar Cinnamon	1	190	5
Frosted Cherry	1	190	5
Frosted Fruit Punch	1	190	5
Frosted Fudge	1	200	5
Frosted Strawberry	1	190	5
Strawberry	1	190	5
Vanilla Cremes (Little Debbie)	1 pkg (1.3 oz)	160	7
Vanilla Cups (Tastykake)	1	116	3
Yankee Doodle (Drake's)	1 (1 oz)	100	4
Yodel's (Drake's)	1 (1 oz)	150	9
devil's food w/ creme filling	1 (1 oz)	105	4
sponge w/ creme filling	1 (1.5 oz)	155	5
toaster pastries	1 (1.9 oz)	210	6
TAKE-OUT			
baklava	1 oz	126	9

FOOD	PORTION	CALORIES	FAT
strudel	1 piece (4.1 oz)	272	8
trifle w/ cream	6 oz	291	16

CANADIAN BACON

FOOD	PORTION	CALORIES	FAT
Oscar Mayer	1 slice (28 g)	35	1
unheated	2 slices (1.9 oz)	89	4

CANDY

FOOD	PORTION	CALORIES	FAT
3 Musketeers Bar	2.1 oz	260	8
5th Avenue	1 (2.1 oz)	290	13
After Eight Dark Chocolate Wafer Thin Mints (Rowntree)	1	35	1
Almond Joy	1.76 oz	250	14
Alpine White Bar w/ Almonds (Nestle)	1.25 oz	200	13
Baby Ruth Bar	2.2 oz	300	13
Bar None	1.5 oz	240	14
Barat Bar	1 (2 oz)	340	24
Bit-O-Honey	1.7 oz	200	4
Breath Savers Sugar Free			
Cinnamon	1 candy	2	0
Peppermint	1 candy	2	0
Spearmint	1 candy	2	0
Wintergreen	1 candy	2	0
Butter Mints (Kraft)	1	8	0
Butterfinger Bar	2.1 oz	280	12
Caramel Nip (Pearson's)	1 oz	120	3
Caramello	1 (1.6 oz)	220	11
Caramels (Kraft)	1	30	1
Caramels Chocolate (Estee)	1	30	1
Caramels Vanilla (Estee)	1	30	1

FOOD	PORTION	CALORIES	FAT
Charleston Chew! (Pearson's)			
Chocolate	½ bar	120	3
Strawberry	½ bar	120	3
Vanilla	½ bar	120	3
Chocolate Bar Almond (Estee)	2 squares	60	4
Chocolate Bar Coconut (Estee)	2 squares	60	4
Chocolate Bar Fruit & Nut (Estee)	2 squares	60	4
Chocolate Bar Peanut (Estee)	2 squares	60	4
Chocolate Coated Raisins (Estee)	10 pieces	30	1
Chocolate Covered Cherries (Cella's)	1 oz	126	4
Chocolate Fudgies (Kraft)	1	35	1
Chocolate Parfait (Pearson's)	4 pieces	120	3
Chocolate Parfait (Pearson's)	1 oz	120	3
Chocolaty Peanut Bar (Lance)	2 oz	320	18
Chunky	1.4 oz	210	12
Coffee Nip (Pearson's)	1 oz	120	3
Coffioca Mocha Parfait (Pearson's)	1 oz	120	3
Coffioca Parfait (Pearson's)	4 pieces	120	3
Crunch Chocolate Bar (Estee)	2 squares	45	3
Crunch 'N Munch (Franklin)			
Candied	1.25 oz	170	7
Caramel	1.25 oz	160	5
Maple Walnut	1.25 oz	160	6
Toffee	1.25 oz	160	6
Dark Chocolate Bar (Estee)	2 squares	60	5
Dark Chocolate Mint Bar (Estee)	2 squares	60	5
Estee-ets (Estee)	5 pieces	35	2
Fruit & Nut Bar (Cadbury)	1 oz	150	8
Fruit & Nut Mix (Estee)	4 pieces	35	2
Golden Almond	½ bar	260	17

FOOD	PORTION	CALORIES	FAT
Golden III	½ bar	250	15
Goobers	1⅜ oz	220	13
Gum Drops (Estee)	4 pieces	25	0
Gummy Bears (Estee)	3 pieces	20	0
Hard Candy (Estee)	2	25	0
Hershey Bar	1 (1.55 oz)	240	14
Hersey Bar w/ Almonds	1 (1.45 oz)	230	14
Hershey's Kisses	9 pieces	220	13
Holidays Peanut	1 oz	140	6
Holidays Plain	1 oz	140	6
Junior Mints	12 pieces	120	3
Kit Kat Wafer	1 (1.63 oz)	250	13
Krackel	1 (1.55 oz)	230	13
Laffy Taffy (Beich's)			
Apple Chews	1 oz	110	1
Banana Chews	1 oz	110	1
Grape Chews	1 oz	110	1
Passion Punch Chews	1 oz	110	1
Strawberry Chews	1 oz	110	1
Sweet & Sour Cherry Chews	1 oz	110	1
Watermelon Chews	1 oz	110	1
Licorice Nip (Pearson's)	1 oz	120	3
Life Saver Lollipops All Flavors	1	45	0
Life Saver Sugar Free	1	8	0
Lifesaver Holes Sunshine Fruits	1 candy	2	0
Lifesaver Holes Tangerine	1 candy	2	0
Lifesavers			
Christmas Lollipops	1	40	0
Easter Pops	1	40	0
Fancy Fruits	1 candy	8	0

FOOD	PORTION	CALORIES	FAT
Fruit Juicers Citrus Fruits	1 candy	8	0
Fruit Juicers Easter Egg-Sortments	1 candy	10	0
Fruit Juicers Fruit Punch	1 candy	8	0
Fruit Juicers Grape	1 candy	8	0
Fruit Juicers Lollipops	1	40	0
Fruit Juicers Mixed Berries	1 candy	8	0
Fruit Juicers Strawberry	1 candy	8	0
Gummi Savers Grape	1 candy	12	0
Gummi Savers Mixed Berry	1 candy	12	0
Sunshine Fruits	1 candy	8	0
Tropical Fruits	1 candy	8	0
Valentine Pops	1	40	0
Wild Cherry	1 candy	8	0
Lollipops (Estee)	1	25	0
Lollipops Sugar Free (Louis Sherry)	1	18	0
M&M's Peanut	1.7 oz	250	13
M&M's Plain	1.7 oz	240	10
Mars Bar	1.8 oz	240	12
Milk Chocolate Bar (Estee)	2 squares	60	4
Milky Way II	1 bar (2 oz)	193	8
Milky Way Bar	2.2 oz	290	11
Mint Parfait (Pearson's)	4 pieces	120	3
Mounds	1 (1.9 oz)	260	14
Mr. GoodBar	1 (1.75 oz)	290	19
Munch Bar	1.4 oz	220	14
NECCO Mint Lozenges	1 piece	12	tr
Nestle Crunch Bar	1.4 oz	210	10
Nestle Milk Chocolate Bar	1.45 oz	220	13

FOOD	PORTION	CALORIES	FAT
Nestle Milk Chocolate w/ Almonds Bar	1.45 oz	230	14
Nip Carmel (Pearson's)	4 pieces	120	3
Nip Coffee (Pearson's)	4 pieces	120	3
Nip Licorice (Pearson's)	4 pieces	120	3
Oh Henry!	2 oz	280	14
Party Mints (Kraft)	1	8	0
Peanut Bar (Lance)	1.75 oz	260	14
Peanut Brittle (Estee)	¼ oz	35	1
Peanut Brittle (Kraft)	1 oz	130	5
Peanut Butter Cups (Estee)	1	40	3
Peanut Butter Parfait (Pearson's)	4 pieces	120	3
Raisinets	1⅜ oz	180	6
Reese's Peanut Butter Cups	1.8 oz	280	17
Reese's Pieces	1.85 oz	260	11
Rolo Carmels in Milk Chocolate	8 pieces	270	12
Skittles	2 oz	320	5
Skor Toffee Bar	1 (1.4 oz)	220	14
Snickers Bar	2.2 oz	290	14
Sno-Caps Nonpareils	1 oz	140	5
Solitaires w/ Almonds	½ bag	260	17
Special Dark Sweet Chocolate Bar (Hershey oz)	1 (1.45 oz)	220	12
Starburst Fruit Chews	2 oz	240	5
Starburst Fruit Chews Strawberry	2.07 oz	240	5
Sugar Babies Tidbits	1 pkg	180	2
Sugar Daddy	1 pop	150	1
Symphony Almond Butterchips	1 (1.4 oz)	220	14
Symphony Milk Chocolate	1 (1.4 oz)	220	13
Turtles Pecan Caramel Candy (Demet's)	1 (.6 oz)	90	5

FOOD	PORTION	CALORIES	FAT
Twix Cookie Bar, Carmel	2 oz (2 bars)	140	7
Twix Cookie Bar, Peanut Butter	1.8 oz (2 bars)	130	7
Velamints	1 mint	9	0
Velamints Cocoamint	1 mint	8	0
Whatchamacallit	1 (1.8 oz)	260	13
Y&S Bites Cherry	1 oz	100	1
Y&S Nibs Cherry	1 oz	180	1
Y&S Twizzlers Strawberry	1 oz	100	1
York Peppermint Patty	1 (1.5 oz)	180	4
boiled sweets	¼ lb	327	0
candied cherries	1 cherry	12	tr
candied citron	1 oz	89	tr
candied lemon peel	1 oz	90	tr
candied orange peel	1 oz	90	tr
candied pineapple slice	1 slice (2 oz)	179	tr
candy corn	1 oz	105	0
caramels chocolate	1 oz	115	3
caramels plain	1 oz	115	3
chocolate	1 oz	145	9
chocolate crisp	1 oz	140	7
chocolate w/ almonds	1 oz	150	10
chocolate w/ peanuts	1 oz	155	11
dark chocolate	1 oz	150	10
fruit pastilles	1 tube (1.4 oz)	101	0
fudge, chocolate	1 oz	115	3
fudge, vanilla	1 oz	115	3
gum drops	1 oz	100	tr
hard candy	1 oz	110	0
jelly beans	1 oz	105	tr
marshmallow	1 oz	90	0

FOOD	PORTION	CALORIES	FAT
marzipan	3.5 oz	497	25
mint fondant	1 oz	105	0
nougat nut cream	3.5 oz	342	31

CANTALOUPE

Chiquita	1 cup	70	0
Dole	¼ melon	50	0
cubed	1 cup	57	tr
fresh	½ melon	94	1

CARAMBOLA

fresh	1	42	tr

CARAWAY

seed	1 tsp	7	tr

CARDAMOM

ground	1 tsp	6	tr

CARDOON

FRESH

cardoon, cooked	3.5 oz	22	tr
raw, shredded	½ cup	36	tr

CARIBOU

roasted	3 oz	142	4

CARISSA

fresh	1	12	tr

FOOD	PORTION	CALORIES	FAT

CAROB

carob mix	3 tsp	45	0
carob mix, as prep w/ whole milk	9 oz	195	8
flour	1 cup	185	1
flour	1 tbsp	14	tr

CARP

FRESH
cooked	3 oz	138	6
cooked	1 fillet (6 oz)	276	12
roe, raw	3½ oz	130	2

CARROTS

CANNED
Diced (Libby)	½ cup	20	0
Diced (Seneca)	½ cup	20	0
Diced Fancy (S&W)	½ cup	30	0
Julienne French Style Fancy (S&W)	½ cup	30	0
Sliced (Libby)	½ cup	20	0
Sliced (Seneca)	½ cup	20	0
Sliced Fancy (S&W)	½ cup	30	0
Sliced Water Pack (S&W)	½ cup	30	0
Whole Tiny Fancy (S&W)	½ cup	30	0
slices	½ cup	17	tr
slices, low sodium	½ cup	17	tr

FRESH
Dole	1 med	40	1
baby, raw	1 (½ oz)	6	tr
raw	1 (2.5 oz)	31	tr

FOOD	PORTION	CALORIES	FAT
raw, shredded	½ cup	24	tr
slices, cooked	½ cup	35	tr
FROZEN			
Crinkle Sliced (Hanover)	½ cup	35	0
Harvest Fresh Baby (Green Giant)	½ cup	18	0
Whole Baby (Birds Eye)	½ cup	40	tr
slices, cooked	½ cup	26	tr
JUICE			
canned	6 oz	73	tr

CASABA

cubed	1 cup	45	tr
fresh	⅒ melon	43	tr

CASHEWS

Cashews (Beer Nuts)	1 oz	170	13
Cashews (Lance)	1⅛ oz	190	15
Fancy (Planters)	1 oz	170	14
Honey Roasted (Planters)	1 oz	170	12
Honey Toasted (Lance)	1⅛ oz	200	14
Unsalted Halves (Planters)	1 oz	170	14
Whole Salted (Guy's)	1 oz	170	14
cashew butter w/o salt	1 tbsp	94	8
dry roasted	1 oz	163	13
dry roasted, salted	1 oz	163	13
oil roasted	1 oz	163	14
oil roasted, salted	1 oz	163	14

CASSAVA

fresh, raw	3.5 oz	120	tr

FOOD	PORTION	CALORIES	FAT

CATFISH

channel, breaded & fried	3 oz	194	11

CATSUP

Estee	1 tbsp	6	0
Heinz	1 tbsp	16	0
Heinz Hot	1 tbsp	14	0
Heinz Lite	1 tbsp	8	0
Hunt's	1 tbsp	15	tr
Hunt's No Salt Added	1 tbsp	20	tr
Smucker's	1 tsp	8	0
Weight Watchers	2 tsp	8	0
catsup	1 tbsp	16	tr
catsup	1 pkg (.2 oz)	6	tr
low sodium	1 tbsp	16	tr

CAULIFLOWER

FRESH			
Dole	⅛ med head	18	0
cooked	½ cup	15	tr
raw	½ cup	12	tr
FROZEN			
Cauliflower (Birds Eye)	⅔ cup	23	tr
Cauliflower (Hanover)	½ cup	20	0
Cauliflower in Cheddar Cheese Sauce (Budget Gourmet)	5 oz	110	5
Cauliflower w/ Cheddar Cheese Sauce (Budget Gourmet)	1 pkg	130	9
Cauliflower w/ Cheese Sauce (Birds Eye)	½ cup	113	6

FOOD	PORTION	CALORIES	FAT
Cuts (Green Giant)	½ cup	12	0
Florets (Hanover)	½ cup	20	0
In Cheese Sauce (Green Giant)	½ cup	60	2
One Serve in Cheese Sauce (Green Giant)	1 pkg	80	3
cooked	½ cup	17	tr
JARRED			
Hot & Spicy (Vlasic)	1 oz	4	0
Sweet (Vlasic)	1 oz	35	0

CAVIAR

FOOD	PORTION	CALORIES	FAT
black granular	1 oz	71	5
black granular	1 tbsp	40	3
red granular	1 oz	71	5
red granular	1 tbsp	40	3

CELERIAC

FOOD	PORTION	CALORIES	FAT
fresh, cooked	3.5 oz	25	tr
fresh, raw	½ cup	31	tr

CELERY

FOOD	PORTION	CALORIES	FAT
DRIED			
seed	1 tsp	8	tr
FRESH			
Dole	2 med stalks	20	0
diced, cooked	½ cup	13	tr
raw	1 stalk (1.3 oz)	6	tr
raw, diced	½ cup	10	tr

CELTUCE

FOOD	PORTION	CALORIES	FAT
raw	3.5 oz	22	tr

FOOD	PORTION	CALORIES	FAT

CEREAL

COOKED

FOOD	PORTION	CALORIES	FAT
5-Bran Kashi (Kashi)	2.5 oz	281	6
Barley Plus (Erewhon)	1 oz	110	1
Bear Mush (Arrowhead)	1 oz	100	0
Brown Rice Cream (Erewhon)	1 oz	110	1
Bulgar Wheat (Arrowhead)	2 oz	200	1
Cracked Wheat Cereal (Arrowhead)	2 oz	180	1
Cream of Rice (Nabisco)	1 oz	100	0
Cream of Wheat Instant (Nabisco)	1 oz	100	tr
Cream of Wheat Quick (Nabisco)	1 oz	100	tr
Cream of Wheat Regular (Nabisco)	1 oz	100	0
Enriched White Hominy Grits Quick (Aunt Jemima)	3 tbsp	101	tr
Enriched White Hominy Grits Quick (Quaker)	3 tbsp	101	tr
Enriched White Hominy Grits Regular (Aunt Jemima)	3 tbsp	101	tr
Enriched White Hominy Grits Regular (Quaker)	3 tbsp	101	tr
Enriched Yellow Hominy Quick Grits (Quaker)	3 tbsp	101	tr
Farina (H-O)	3 tbsp	120	0
Farina Instant (H-O)	1 pkg	110	0
Farina, as prep (Pillsbury)	⅔ cup	80	tr
Four Grain Cereal (Arrowhead)	2 oz	94	1
High Fiber Hot Cereal, as prep (Ralston)	⅓ cup	90	1
Hominy Quick Grits, uncooked (Albers)	¼ cup	150	0
Instant Grits White Hominy (Quaker)	1 pkt	79	tr

FOOD	PORTION	CALORIES	FAT
Instant Grits w/ Imitation Bacon Bits (Quaker)	1 pkt	101	tr
Instant Grits w/ Imitation Ham Bits (Quaker)	1 pkt	99	tr
Instant Grits w/ Real Cheddar Cheese (Quaker)	1 pkt	104	1
Kashi (Kashi)	2 oz	177	1
Mix'n Eat Cream of Wheat (Nabisco)			
Brown Sugar Cinnamon	1 pkg (1.25 oz)	130	0
Apple & Cinnamon	1 pkg (1.25 oz)	130	0
Maple Brown Sugar	1 pkg (1.25 oz)	130	0
Our Original	1 pkg (1.25 oz)	100	0
Oat Bran (Quaker)	⅓ cup	92	2
Oat Bran Natural Apples & Cinnamon (Health Valley)	¼ cup	100	tr
Oat Bran Natural Raisins & Spice (Health Valley)	¼ cup	100	tr
Oat Bran w/ Toasted Wheat Germ (Erewhon)	1 oz	115	2
Oat Groats (Arrowhead)	2 oz	220	4
Oat Steel Cut (Arrowhead)	2 oz	220	4
Oatmeal Instant			
(H-O)	½ cup	130	2
(H-O)	1 pkg	110	2
Apple Cinnamon (Erewhon)	1.25 oz	145	3
Apple Cinnamon (H-O)	1 pkg	130	2
Apple Date & Almond (Arrowhead)	1 oz	130	3
Apple Raisin (Erewhon)	1.3 oz	150	3
Apple Spice (Arrowhead)	1 oz	130	2
Apples & Cinnamon, cooked (Quaker)	1 pkg	118	2
Cinnamon & Spice, cooked (Quaker)	1 pkg	164	2

FOOD	PORTION	CALORIES	FAT
Cinnamon Raisin & Almond (Arrowhead)	1 oz	140	3
Dates & Walnuts (Erewhon)	1.2 oz	130	3
Extra Fortified Apples & Spice, cooked (Quaker)	1 pkg	133	2
Extra Fortified Raisins & Cinnamon, cooked (Quaker)	1 pkg	129	2
Extra Fortified Regular, cooked (Quaker)	1 pkg	95	2
Maple & Brown Sugar, cooked (Quaker)	1 pkg	152	2
Maple Brown Sugar (H-O)	1 pkg	160	2
Maple Spice (Erewhon)	1.2 oz	140	3
Peaches & Cream Flavors, cooked (Quaker)	1 pkg	129	2
Raisin & Spice (H-O)	1 pkg	150	2
Raisin & Spice, cooked (Quaker)	1 pkg	149	2
Raisin, Dates & Walnuts, cooked (Quaker)	1 pkg	141	4
Regular (Arrowhead)	1 oz	100	2
Regular, cooked (Quaker)	1 pkg	94	2
Strawberries & Cream Flavors, cooked (Quaker)	1 pkg	129	2
Sweet 'n Mellow (H-O)	1 pkg	150	2
With Added Oat Bran (Erewhon)	1.25 oz	125	3
Oats Gourmet (H-O)	⅓ cup	100	2
Oats 'n Fiber (H-O)	1 pkg	110	2
Oats 'n Fiber (H-O)	⅓ cup	100	2
Oats 'n Fiber Apple & Bran (H-O)	1 pkg	130	2
Oats 'n Fiber Raisin & Bran (H-O)	1 pkg	150	2
Oats, Old Fashion, cooked (Quaker)	⅔ cup	99	2
Oats, Old Fashioned, not prep (Roman Meal)	⅓ cup (1 oz)	100	4

FOOD	PORTION	CALORIES	FAT
Oats, Quick (H-O)	½ cup	130	2
Oats, Quick, cooked (Quaker)	⅔ cup	99	2
Oats, Quick, not prep (Roman Meal)	⅓ cup (1 oz)	100	2
Oats, Wheat, Dates, Raisins, Almonds Cereal, not prep (Roman Meal)	⅓ cup (1.3 oz)	140	3
Oats, Wheat, Honey, Coconut, Almonds Cereal, not prep (Roman Meal)	⅓ cup (1.3 oz)	150	6
Oats, Wheat, Rye Flax Cereal, not prep (Roman Meal)	⅓ cup (1 oz)	90	1
Original Cereal w/ Wheat, Rye, Bran, Flax, not prep (Roman Meal)	⅓ cup (1 oz)	80	tr
Rice & Shine (Arrowhead)	¼ oz	160	1
Seven Grain Cereal (Arrowhead)	1 oz	100	1
Total Oatmeal (General Mills)			
Apple Cinnamon Almond Instant	1.5 oz pkg	150	4
Apple Cinnamon Instant	1.25 oz pkg	130	2
Mixed Nut Instant	1.3 oz pkg	140	4
Quick	1 oz pkg	90	2
Regular Flavor Instant	1 oz pkg	90	2
Wheat Hearts, as prep (General Mills)	¾ cup	110	1
White Corn Grits (Arrowhead)	2 oz	200	1
Whole Wheat Hot Natural Cereal, cooked (Mother's)	⅔ cup	92	1
Whole Wheat Hot Natural Cereal, cooked (Quaker)	⅔ cup	92	1
Yellow Corn Grits (Arrowhead)	2 oz	200	1
corn grits, instant, as prep	1 pkg (.8 oz)	82	tr
corn grits, quick	1 cup	579	2
corn grits, quick	1 tbsp	36	tr
corn grits, quick, cooked	1 cup	146	1

FOOD	PORTION	CALORIES	FAT
corn grits, regular	1 cup	579	2
corn grits, regular, cooked	1 cup	146	1
farina, cooked	¾ cup	87	tr
farina, dry	1 tbsp	40	0
oatmeal, cooked	1 cup	145	2
oatmeal, dry	1 cup	311	5
oatmeal instant, cooked w/o salt	1 cup	145	2
oatmeal quick, cooked w/o salt	1 cup	145	2
oatmeal regular, cooked w/o salt	1 cup	145	2
READY-TO-EAT			
100% Bran (Nabisco)	⅓ cup	70	2
100% Natural Bran w/ Apples & Cinnamon (Health Valley)	¼ cup	100	1
7-Grain Crunch (Loma Linda)	½ cup	110	1
7-Grain No Sugar Added (Loma Linda)	1 cup	110	1
All-Bran (Kellogg's)	⅓ cup (1 oz)	70	1
All-Bran w/ Extra Fiber (Kellogg's)	½ cup (1 oz)	50	0
Almond Delight (Ralston)	¾ cup	110	2
Alpha-Bits (Post)	1 cup	112	tr
Apple Cinnamon Squares (Kellogg's)	½ cup (1 oz)	90	0
Apple Corns (Arrowhead)	1 oz	100	1
Apple Jacks (Kellogg's)	1 cup (1 oz)	110	0
Apple Raisin Crisp (Kellogg's)	⅔ cup (1 oz)	130	0
Arrowhead Crunch (Arrowhead)	1 oz	120	3
Aztec (Erewhon)	1 oz	100	0
Batman (Ralston)	1 cup	110	1
Blue Corn Flakes 100% Organic (Health Valley)	½ cup	90	tr
Blueberry Squares (Kellogg's)	½ cup (1 oz)	90	0

FOOD	PORTION	CALORIES	FAT
BooBerry (General Mills)	1 cup	110	1
Bran (Loma Linda)	⅓ cup	90	tr
Bran Buds (Kellogg's)	⅓ cup (1 oz)	70	1
Bran Cereal w/ Dates 100% Organic (Health Valley)	¼ cup	100	1
Bran Cereal w/ Raisins 100% Organic (Health Valley)	¼ cup	100	1
Bran Flakes (Arrowhead)	1 oz	100	1
Bran Flakes (Kellogg's)	⅔ cup (1 oz)	90	0
Bran News (Ralston)	¾ cup	100	0
Breakfast With Barbie (Ralston)	1 cup	110	1
Brown Sugar & Honey Body Buddies (General Mills)	1 cup	110	tr
Cap'n Crunch (Quaker)	¾ cup	113	2
Cap'n Crunch's Crunchberries (Quaker)	¾ cup	113	2
Cap'n Crunch's Peanut Butter Crunch (Quaker)	¾ cup	119	3
Cheerios (General Mills)	1¼ cup	110	2
Chex Corn (Ralston)	1 cup	110	0
Chex Double (Ralston)	⅔ cup	100	0
Chex Honey Graham (Ralston)	⅔ cup	110	1
Chex Honey Nut Oat (Ralston)	½ cup	100	1
Chex Multi-Bran (Ralston)	⅔ cup	90	0
Chex Rice (Ralston)	1⅛ cup	110	0
Chex Wheat (Ralston)	⅔ cup	100	0
Cinnamon Mini Buns (Kellogg's)	¾ cup (1 oz)	110	1
Cinnamon Toast Crunch (General Mills)	1 cup	120	3
Circus Fun (General Mills)	1 cup	110	1
Clusters (General Mills)	½ cup	100	3
Cocoa Krispies (Kellogg's)	¾ cup (1 oz)	110	0

FOOD	PORTION	CALORIES	FAT
Cocoa Pebbles (Post)	⅞ cup	112	1
Cocoa Puffs (General Mills)	1 cup	110	1
Common Sense Oat Bran (Kellogg's)	¾ cup (1 oz)	100	2
Common Sense Oat Bran w/ Raisins (Kellogg's)	¾ cup (1 oz)	130	1
Cookie-Crisp Chocolate Chip (Ralston)	1 cup	110	1
Cookie-Crisp Vanilla Wafer (Ralston)	1 cup	110	1
Corn Flakes (Arrowhead)	1 oz	110	1
Corn Flakes (Kellogg's)	1 cup (1 oz)	100	0
Corn Pops (Kellogg's)	1 cup (1 oz)	110	0
Country Corn Flakes (General Mills)	1 cup	110	tr
Cracklin' Oat Bran (Kellogg's)	½ cup (1 oz)	110	3
Crispix (Kellogg's)	1 cup (1 oz)	110	0
Crispy Brown Rice (Erewhon)	1 oz	110	1
Crispy Brown Rice, Low Sodium (Erewhon)	1 oz	110	1
Crispy Critters (Post)	1 cup	112	tr
Crispy Wheats 'n Raisins (General Mills)	¾ cup	110	1
Crunchy Not Oh!s (Quaker)	1 cup	127	4
Dinersaurs (Ralston)	1 cup	110	1
Double Dip Crunch (Kellogg's)	⅔ cup (1 oz)	120	2
Fiber 7 Flakes 100% Organic (Health Valley)	½ cup	90	tr
Fiber 7 Flakes w/ Raisins 100% Organic (Health Valley)	½ cup	90	tr
Fiberwise (Kellogg's)	⅔ cup (1 oz)	90	1
Fortified Oat Flakes (Post)	⅔ cup	105	tr
Frankenberry (General Mills)	1 cup	110	1
Froot Loops (Kellogg's)	1 cup (1 oz)	110	1
Frosted Flakes (Kellogg's)	¾ cup (1 oz)	110	0

FOOD	PORTION	CALORIES	FAT
Frosted Krispies (Kellogg's)	¾ cup (1 oz)	110	0
Frosted Mini-Wheats (Kellogg's)	4 biscuits (1 oz)	100	0
Frosted Mini-Wheats Bite Size (Kellogg's)	½ cup	100	0
Fruit & Fiber Dates, Raisins & Walnuts (Post)	½ cup	89	tr
Fruit & Fiber Harvest Medley (Post)	½ cup	88	tr
Fruit & Fiber Mountain Trail (Post)	½ cup	87	1
Fruit & Fiber Peach, Raisin, Almond (Post)	½ cup	85	tr
Fruit & Fiber Tropical Fruit (Post)	½ cup	90	1
Fruit & Fitness (Health Valley)	1 cup	220	4
Fruit Lites Wheat (Health Valley)	½ cup	45	1
Fruit Lites Corn (Health Valley)	½ cup	45	0
Fruit Lites Rice (Health Valley)	½ cup	45	1
Fruit Muesli (Ralston)			
Raisins, Walnuts & Cranberries	½ cup	150	3
Raisins, Apples & Almonds	½ cup	150	2
Raisins, Dates & Almonds	½ cup	140	2
Raisins, Peaches & Pecans	½ cup	150	3
Fruit 'n Wheat (Erewhon)	1 oz	100	1
Fruit Wheats Apple (Nabisco)	1 oz	90	0
Fruitful Bran (Kellogg's)	⅔ cup (1.4 oz)	120	0
Fruity Marshmallow Krispies (Kellogg's)	1¼ cups (1.3 oz)	140	0
Fruity Pebbles (Post)	⅞ cup	112	1
Golden Grahams (General Mills)	¾ cup	110	1
Grape-Nuts (Post)	¼ cup	104	tr
Grape-Nuts Flakes (Post)	⅞ cup	104	tr
Healthy Crunch Almond Date (Health Valley)	¼ cup	110	3

FOOD	PORTION	CALORIES	FAT
Healthy Crunch Apple Cinnamon (Health Valley)	¼ cup	110	3
Healthy O's 100% Organic (Health Valley)	¾ cup	90	1
Honey Buc Wheat Crisp (General Mills)	¾ cup	110	tr
Honey Graham Oh!s (Quaker)	1 cup	122	3
Honey Nut Cheerios (General Mills)	1 cup	110	1
Honeycomb (Post)	1⅓ cup	110	tr
Hot Wheels (Ralston)	1 cup	110	1
Ice Cream Cones Chocolate Chip (General Mills)	¾ cup	110	2
Ice Cream Cones Vanilla (General Mills)	¾ cup	110	2
Just Right Fiber Nuggets (Kellogg's)	⅔ cup (1 oz)	100	1
Just Right w/ Raisins, Dates & Nuts (Kellogg's)	¾ cup (1.3 oz)	140	1
Kaboom (General Mills)	1 cup	110	1
Kashi Brittles Sesame/Maple (Kashi)	3½ oz	473	19
Kashi Puffed (Kashi)	¾ oz	74	1
Kenmei (Kellogg's)	¾ cup (1 oz)	110	1
King Vitaman (Quaker)	1½ cup	110	1
Life (Quaker)	⅔ cup	101	2
Life Cinnamon (Quaker)	⅔ cup	101	2
Lites Puffed Corn (Health Valley)	½ cup	50	0
Lites Puffed Rice (Health Valley)	½ cup	50	0
Lites Puffed Wheat (Health Valley)	½ cup	50	0
Lucky Charms (General Mills)	1 cup	110	1
Maple Corns (Arrowhead)	1 oz	100	1
Morning Funnies (Ralston)	1 cup	110	1
Muesli (Ralston)	½ cup	160	3

FOOD	PORTION	CALORIES	FAT
Mueslix Crispy Blend (Kellogg's)	⅔ cup (1.5 oz)	150	2
Mueslix Golden Crunch (Kellogg's)	½ cup (1.2 oz)	120	2
Natural Bran Flakes (Post)	⅔ cup	87	tr
Natural Raisin Bran (Post)	½ cup	83	tr
Natural Sugar & Honey Body Buddies (General Mills)	1 cup	110	1
Nature O's (Arrowhead)	1 oz	110	1
Nintendo Cereal System (Ralston)	1 cup	110	1
Nut & Honey Crunch (Kellogg's)	⅔ cup (1 oz)	110	1
Nut & Honey Crunch O's (Kellogg's)	⅔ cup (1 oz)	110	2
Nutri-Grain Almond Raisin (Kellogg's)	⅔ cup (1.4 oz)	140	2
Nutri-Grain Raisin Bran (Kellogg's)	1 cup (1.4 oz)	130	1
Nutri-Grain Wheat (Kellogg's)	⅔ cup (1 oz)	90	0
Oat Bran Flakes (Arrowhead)	1 oz	110	2
Oat Bran Flakes 100% Organic (Health Valley)	½ cup	100	tr
Oat Bran Flakes w/ Almonds & Dates 100% Organic (Health Valley)	½ cup	100	tr
Oat Bran Flakes w/ Raisins 100% Organic (Health Valley)	½ cup	100	tr
Oat Bran O'S 100% Organic (Health Valley)	½ cup	110	tr
Oat Bran O'S Fruit & Nuts (Health Valley)	½ cup	110	3
Oat Brand Options (Ralston)	¾ cup	130	1
Oatbake Honey Bran (Kellogg's)	⅓ cup (1 oz)	110	3
Oatbake Raisin Nut (Kellogg's)	⅓ cup (1 oz)	110	3
Orangeola Almonds & Dates (Health Valley)	¼ cup	110	3
Orangeola Bananas & Hawaiian Fruit (Health Valley)	¼ cup	120	4

FOOD	PORTION	CALORIES	FAT
Pac-Man (General Mills)	1 cup	110	tr
Popeye Sweet Crunch (Quaker)	1 cup	113	2
Poppets (US Mills)	1 oz	110	1
Post Toasties (Post)	1¼ cup	108	tr
Product 19 (Kellogg's)	1 cup (1 oz)	100	0
Puffed Corn (Arrowhead)	½ oz	50	0
Puffed Millet (Arrowhead)	½ oz	50	0
Puffed Rice (Arrowhead)	½ oz	50	0
Puffed Wheat (Arrowhead)	½ oz	50	0
Quaker 100% Natural	¼ cup	127	6
Quaker 100% Natural Apples & Cinnamon	¼ cup	126	5
Quaker 100% Natural Raisins & Date	¼ cup	123	5
Quaker Crunchy Bran	⅔ cup	89	1
Quaker Oat Squares	½ cup	105	2
Quaker Puffed Rice	1 cup	54	tr
Quaker Puffed Wheat	1 cup	50	tr
Quaker Shredded Wheat	2 biscuits	132	1
Raisin Bran (Erewhon)	1 oz	100	0
Raisin Bran (Kellogg's)	¾ cup (1.4 oz)	120	1
Raisin Bran Flakes 100% Organic (Health Valley)	½ cup	100	tr
Raisin Grape-Nuts (Post)	¼ cup	101	tr
Raisin Squares (Kellogg's)	½ cup (1 oz)	90	0
Real Oat Bran Almond Crunch (Health Valley)	¼ cup	110	3
Real Oat Bran Hawaiian Fruit (Health Valley)	¼ cup	130	3
Real Oat Bran Raisin Nut (Health Valley)	¼ cup	130	3
Rice Bran O's (Health Valley)	½ cup	110	1

FOOD	PORTION	CALORIES	FAT
Rice Bran w/ Almonds & Dates (Health Valley)	½ cup	110	3
Rice Brand Options (Ralston)	⅔ cup	120	2
Rice Krispies (Kellogg's)	1 cup (1 oz)	110	0
Rice Toasties (Post)	¾ oz	81	tr
Ruskets Biscuits (Loma Linda)	2 biscuits	110	tr
Shredded Wheat (Sunshine)	1 biscuit	90	1
Shredded Wheat Bite Size (Sunshine)	⅔ cup	110	1
Shredded Wheat 'n Bran (Nabisco)	⅔ cup	90	1
Shredded Wheat Spoon Size (Nabisco)	⅔ cup	90	1
Shredded Wheat w/ Oat Bran (Nabisco)	⅔ cup	100	1
Slimer! And the Real Ghostbusters (Ralston)	1 cup	110	1
Special K (Kellogg's)	1 cup (1 oz)	100	0
Sprouts 7 Bananas & Hawaiian Fruit (Health Valley)	¼ cup	90	1
Sprouts 7 Raisin (Health Valley)	¼ cup	90	1
Strawberry Squares (Kellogg's)	½ cup (1 oz)	90	0
Sugar Sparkled Flakes (Post)	¾ cup	108	tr
Sunflakes Multi-Grain (Ralston)	1 cup	100	1
Super Golden Crisp (Post)	⅞ cup	104	tr
Super-O's (Erewhon)	1 oz	110	0
Swiss Breakfast Raisin Nut (Health Valley)	¼ cup	100	3
Swiss Breakfast Tropical Fruit (Health Valley)	¼ cup	100	3
Team (Nabisco)	1 cup	110	1
Teenage Mutant Ninja Turtles (Ralston)	1 cup	110	1
Total (General Mills)	1 cup	110	1

FOOD	PORTION	CALORIES	FAT
Total Corn Flakes (General Mills)	1 cup	110	1
Trix (General Mills)	1 cup	110	1
Uncle Sam Cereal (US Mills)	1 oz	110	1
Weetabix	2 (1.3 oz)	142	1
Wheat Flakes (Arrowhead)	1 oz	110	1
Wheat Flakes (Erewhon)	1 oz	100	0
Wheaties (General Mills)	1 cup	110	1
Whole Grain Shredded Wheat (Kellogg's)	½ cup (1 oz)	90	0
all bran	½ cup (1 oz)	76	1
bran flakes	¾ cup (1 oz)	90	1
corn flakes	1¼ cup (1 oz)	110	tr
corn flakes, low sodium	1 cup	100	tr
crispy rice	1 cup	111	tr
fortified oat flakes	1 cup	177	1
granola	¼ cup	138	8
puffed rice	1 cup	57	tr
puffed wheat	1 cup	44	tr
shredded wheat	1 biscuit	83	tr
sugar-coated corn flakes	¾ cup (1 oz)	110	1
WITH ½ CUP 1% MILK			
Cheerios (General Mills)	1 cup + milk	160	3
Crispy Wheats 'n Raisins (General Mills)	¾ cup + milk	160	3
Honey Buc Wheat Crisp (General Mills)	¾ cup + milk	160	2
Honey Nut Cheerios (General Mills)	1 cup + milk	160	3
Total (General Mills)	1 cup + milk	160	3
Total Corn Flakes (General Mills)	1 cup + milk	160	3
Trix (General Mills)	1½ cup + milk	160	2
Wheaties (General Mills)	1 cup + milk	160	3

FOOD	PORTION	CALORIES	FAT
WITH ½ CUP 2% MILK			
Alpha-Bits (Post)	1 cup + milk	172	3
BooBerry (General Mills)	1 cup + milk	170	4
Cinnamon Toast Crunch (General Mills)	1 cup + milk	180	6
Cocoa Puffs (General Mills)	1 cup + milk	170	4
Frankenberry (General Mills)	1 cup + milk	170	4
Fruity Pebbles (Post)	⅞ cup + milk	173	3
Honeycomb (Post)	1⅓ cup + milk	171	3
Oats, Old Fashioned, as prep (Roman Meal)	⅓ cup + milk	160	4
Oats, Quick, as prep (Roman Meal)	⅓ cup + milk	160	4
Oats, Wheat, Dates, Raisins, Almonds Cereal, as prep (Roman Meal)	⅓ cup + milk	170	4
Oats, Wheat, Honey, Coconut, Almonds Cereal, as prep (Roman Meal)	⅓ cup + milk	190	7
Oats, Wheat, Rye Flax Cereal, as prep (Roman Meal)	⅓ cup + milk	120	3
Original Cereal w/ Wheat, Rye, Bran, Flax, as prep (Roman Meal)	⅓ cup + milk	120	2
Pac-Man (General Mills)	1 cup + milk	170	3
Shredded Wheat (Sunshine)	1 biscuit + milk	150	4
Shredded Wheat Bite Size (Sunshine)	⅔ cup + milk	170	4
Total Oatmeal (General Mills)			
Apple Cinnamon Almond Instant	1.5 oz pkg + milk	210	7
Apple Cinnamon Instant	1.25 oz pkg + milk	190	5
Quick	1 oz pkg + milk	150	5

FOOD	PORTION	CALORIES	FAT
Regular Flavor Instant	1 oz pkg + milk	150	5
WITH ½ CUP SKIM MILK			
BooBerry (General Mills)	1 cup + milk	150	1
Brown Sugar & Honey Body Buddies (General Mills)	1 cup + milk	150	1
Cheerios (General Mills)	1 cup + milk	150	2
Circus Fun (General Mills)	1 cup + milk	150	1
Clusters (General Mills)	½ cup + milk	140	3
Cocoa Puffs (General Mills)	1 cup + milk	150	1
Count Chocula (General Mills)	1 cup + milk	150	1
Country Corn Flakes (General Mills)	1 cup + milk	150	1
Crispy Wheats 'n Raisins (General Mills)	¾ cup + milk	150	1
Frankenberry (General Mills)	1 cup + milk	150	1
Fruit & Fiber Harvest Medley (Post)	½ cup + milk	131	1
Fruit & Fiber Peach, Raisin, Almond (Post)	½ cup + milk	129	1
Golden Grahams (General Mills)	¾ cup + milk	150	1
Grape-Nuts (Post)	¼ cup + milk	148	tr
Honey Buc Wheat Crisp (General Mills)	¾ cup + milk	150	1
Honey Nut Cheerios (General Mills)	1 cup + milk	150	1
Ice Cream Cones Chocolate Chip (General Mills)	¾ cup + milk	150	2
Ice Cream Cones Vanilla (General Mills)	¾ cup + milk	150	2
Kaboom (General Mills)	1 cup + milk	150	1
Lucky Charms (General Mills)	1 cup + milk	150	1
Muesli (Ralston)	½ cup + milk	200	3
Natural Raisin Bran (Post)	½ cup + milk	127	tr

FOOD	PORTION	CALORIES	FAT
Natural Sugar & Honey Body Buddies (General Mills)	1 cup + milk	150	1
Oatmeal Raisin Crisp (General Mills)	½ cup + milk	150	2
Pac-Man (General Mills)	1 cup + milk	150	1
Raisin Grape-Nuts (Post)	1 cup + milk	144	tr
Shredded Wheat (Sunshine)	1 biscuit + milk	135	1
Shredded Wheat Bite Size (Sunshine)	⅔ cup + milk	200	1
Shredded Wheat 'n Bran (Nabisco)	1 oz + milk	150	1
Shredded Wheat Spoon Size (Nabisco)	1 oz + milk	150	1
Total (General Mills)	1 cup + milk	150	1
Total Corn Flakes (General Mills)	1 cup + milk	150	1
Total Oatmeal (General Mills)			
Apple Cinnamon Almond Instant	1.5 oz pkg + milk	190	4
Apple Cinnamon Instant	1.25 oz pkg + milk	170	2
Mixed Nut Instant	1.3 oz pkg + milk	180	4
Quick	1 oz pkg + milk	130	2
Regular Flavor Instant	1 oz pkg + milk	130	2
Trix (General Mills)	1 cup + milk	150	1
Trix (General Mills)	1½ cup + milk	150	1
Wheaties (General Mills)	1 cup + milk	150	1
WITH ½ CUP WHOLE MILK Brown Sugar & Honey Body Buddies (General Mills)	1 cup + milk	185	4
Circus Fun (General Mills)	1 cup + milk	185	5
Clusters (General Mills)	½ cup + milk	175	7
Country Corn Flakes (General Mills)	1 cup + milk	185	4

FOOD	PORTION	CALORIES	FAT
Fortified Oat Flakes (Post)	⅔ cup + milk	181	5
Golden Grahams (General Mills)	¾ cup + milk	185	5
Ice Cream Cones Chocolate Chip (General Mills)	¾ cup + milk	185	6
Ice Cream Cones Vanilla (General Mills)	¾ cup + milk	185	6
Kaboom (General Mills)	1 cup + milk	185	5
Lucky Charms (General Mills)	1 cup + milk	185	5
Oatmeal Raisin Crisp (General Mills)	½ cup + milk	185	6
Shredded Wheat (Sunshine)	1 biscuit + milk	165	5
Shredded Wheat Bite Size (Sunshine)	⅔ cup + milk	225	5
Sugar Sparkled Flakes (Post)	¾ cup + milk	184	4
Total Oatmeal Mixed Nut Instant (General Mills)	1.3 oz pkg + milk	215	8
Trix (General Mills)	1 cup + milk	185	5

CHAYOTE

FRESH			
cooked	1 cup	38	1
raw	1 (7 oz)	49	1
raw, cut up	1 cup	32	tr

CHEESE
(*See also* CHEESE DISHES, CHEESE SUBSTITUTES, COTTAGE CHEESE, CREAM CHEESE)

NATURAL			
Asiago (Frigo)	1 oz	110	9
Baby Swiss (Cracker Barrel)	1 oz	110	9
Babybel (Fromageries Bel)	1 oz	91	7
Babybel (Fromageries Bel)	8 oz	726	57
Babybel, Mini (Fromageries Bel)	¾ oz	74	6

FOOD	PORTION	CALORIES	FAT
Blue (Frigo)	1 oz	100	8
Blue (Kraft)	1 oz	100	9
Blue (Sargento)	1 oz	100	8
Bonbel (Fromageries Bel)	1 oz	100	8
Bonbel (Fromageries Bel)	8 oz	790	65
Bonbel, Mini (Fromageries Bel)	¾ oz	74	6
Bonbino (Fromageries Bel)	1 oz	103	9
Bonbino (Fromageries Bel)	8 oz	822	68
Breakfast (Marin French Cheese)	1 oz	86	7
Brick (Kraft)	1 oz	110	9
Brick (Land O'Lakes)	1 oz	110	8
Brick (Sargento)	1 oz	105	8
Brie (Marin French Cheese)	1 oz	86	7
Brie (Sargento)	1 oz	95	8
Burger Cheese (Sargento)	1 oz	106	9
Cajun (Sargento)	1 oz	110	9
Camembert (Marin French Cheese)	1 oz	86	7
Camembert (Sargento)	1 oz	114	9
Cheda-Jack Reduced Fat Low Sodium (Dorman)	1 oz	80	5
Chedarella (Land O'Lakes)	1 oz	100	8
Cheddar			
(Armour)	1 oz	110	9
(Cabot)	1 oz	110	9
(Dorman)	1 oz	110	9
(Frigo)	1 oz	110	9
(Fromageries Bel)	8 oz	883	73
(Fromageries Bel)	1 oz	110	9
(Kraft)	1 oz	110	9
(Land O'Lakes)	1 oz	110	9

FOOD	PORTION	CALORIES	FAT
Bristol Gold Light	1 oz	70	4
Light w/ Simplesse (White Clover)	1 oz	80	4
Lite (Frigo)	1 oz	80	5
Lower Salt (Armour)	1 oz	110	9
Reduced Fat Low Sodium (Dorman)	1 oz	80	5
Cheddar Mild			
Low Sodium White (Weight Watchers)	1 oz	80	5
Low Sodium Yellow (Weight Watchers)	1 oz	80	5
Reduced Fat (Kraft Light)	1 oz	80	5
Shredded (Weight Watchers)	1 oz	80	5
White (Weight Watchers)	1 oz	80	5
Yellow (Weight Watchers)	1 oz	80	5
Cheddar New York (Sargento)	1 oz	114	9
Cheddar Sharp			
Nut Log (Sargento)	1 oz	97	7
Reduced Fat (Kraft Light)	1 oz	80	5
Reduced Fat White (Cracker Barrel Light)	1 oz	80	5
White (Weight Watchers)	1 oz	80	5
Yellow (Weight Watchers)	1 oz	80	5
Cheddar Shredded (Polly-O)	1 oz	110	9
Ched-R-Lo (Alpine Lace)	1 oz	80	5
Cherve (Brier Run)	1 oz	61	5
Colbi-Lo (Alpine Lace)	1 oz	80	5
Colby			
(Dorman)	1 oz	110	9
(Kraft)	1 oz	110	9
(Land O'Lakes)	1 oz	110	9
(Sargento)	1 oz	112	9

FOOD	PORTION	CALORIES	FAT
Colby *(cont.)*			
(Weight Watchers)	1 oz	80	5
And Monterey Jack Reduced Fat Shredded (Kraft Light)	1 oz	80	5
Lower Salt (Armour)	1 oz	110	9
Light w/ Simplesse (White Clover)	1 oz	80	4
Reduced Fat (Kraft Light)	1 oz	80	5
Colby-Jack (Sargento)	1 oz	109	9
Edam			
(Dorman)	1 oz	100	8
(Fromageries Bel)	1 oz	100	8
(Fromageries Bel)	8 oz	800	66
(Holland Farm)	1 oz	97	8
(Kraft)	1 oz	90	7
(Land O'Lakes)	1 oz	110	8
(May-Bud)	1 oz	100	8
(Sargento)	1 oz	101	8
Farmer (Friendship)	4 oz	160	12
Farmer (Holland Farm)	1 oz	102	8
Farmer No Salt Added (Friendship)	4 oz	160	12
Farmers Cheese (May-Bud)	1 oz	90	7
Farmers Cheese (Sargento)	1 oz	102	8
Farmers Cheese (White Clover)	1 oz	90	7
Feta (Frigo)	1 oz	100	8
Feta (Sargento)	1 oz	75	6
Feta (White Clover)	1 oz	90	7
Finland Swiss (Sargento)	1 oz	107	8
Fior di Latte (Polly-O)	1 oz	80	6
Fontina (Sargento)	1 oz	110	9
French Onion (Bristol Gold Light)	1 oz	70	4
Fruit Moos Apricot (Dannon)	3.5 oz	150	8

FOOD	PORTION	CALORIES	FAT
Fruit Moos Banana (Dannon)	3.5 oz	150	8
Fruit Moos Raspberry (Dannon)	3.5 oz	150	8
Fruit Moos Strawberry (Dannon)	3.5 oz	150	8
Garlic & Herb (Bristol Gold Light)	1 oz	70	4
Gjetost (Sargento)	1 oz	132	8
Gorgonzola (Sargento)	1 oz	100	8
Gouda			
(Dorman)	1 oz	100	8
(Fromageries Bel)	1 oz	110	9
(Fromageries Bel)	8 oz	880	73
(Holland Farm)	1 oz	103	8
(Kraft)	1 oz	110	8
(Land O'Lakes)	1 oz	110	8
(May-Bud)	1 oz	100	8
(Sargento)	1 oz	101	8
Mini (Fromageries Bel)	¾ oz	80	6
Mini Reduced Calorie (Fromageries Bel)	¾ oz	45	3
Grated (Polly-O)	1 oz	130	10
Gruyere (Sargento)	1 oz	117	9
Havarti (Casino)	1 oz	120	11
Havarti (Sargento)	1 oz	118	11
Hoop (Friendship)	4 oz	84	tr
Horseradish (Bristol Gold Light)	1 oz	70	4
Impastata (Frigo)	1 oz	60	5
Italian Style Grated Cheese (Sargento)	1 oz	108	8
Jalapeno Vitalait (Cabot)	1 oz	70	4
Jarlsberg ((Norseland)	1 oz	100	7
Jarlsberg (Sargento)	1 oz	100	7
Limburger (Sargento)	1 oz	93	8

FOOD	PORTION	CALORIES	FAT
Limburger Little Gem Size (Mohawk Valley)	1 oz	90	8
Monterey Jack			
(Armour)	1 oz	110	9
(Cabot)	1 oz	80	5
(Dorman)	1 oz	100	8
(Holland Farm)	1 oz	102	9
(Kraft)	1 oz	110	9
(Land O'Lakes)	1 oz	110	9
(May-Bud)	1 oz	100	9
(Sargento)	1 oz	106	9
(Weight Watchers)	1 oz	80	5
Hot Pepper (Land O'Lakes)	1 oz	110	7
Light w/ Simplesse (White Clover)	1 oz	70	4
Lower Salt (Armour)	1 oz	110	9
Reduced Fat (Kraft Light)	1 oz	80	5
Reduced Fat Low Sodium (Dorman)	1 oz	80	5
With Caraway Seeds (Kraft)	1 oz	100	8
With Jalapeno Peppers (Kraft)	1 oz	110	9
With Peppers Reduced Fat (Kraft Light)	1 oz	80	5
Monti-Jack-Lo (Alpine Lace)	1 oz	80	5
Mozzarella			
(Weight Watchers)	1 oz	70	4
Lite Low Moisture, Whole Milk (Frigo)	1 oz	60	2
Lite Sandwich Slices (Polly-O)	1 oz	70	4
Low Moisture (Kraft)	1 oz	90	7
Low Moisture Part Skim (Frigo)	1 oz	80	5
Low Moisture Part Skim (Sargento)	1 oz	79	5

FOOD	PORTION	CALORIES	FAT
Low Moisture Whole Milk (Frigo)	1 oz	90	7
Low Moisture Whole Milk (Sargento)	1 oz	90	7
Part Skim (Dorman)	1 oz	90	7
Part Skim (Land O'Lakes)	1 oz	80	5
Part Skim (Polly-O)	1 oz	80	5
Part Skim Low Moisture (Alpine Lace)	1 oz	70	5
Part Skim Low Moisture (Kraft)	1 oz	80	5
Part Skim Shredded (Polly-O)	1 oz	80	6
Reduced Fat (Kraft Light)	1 oz	80	4
Reduced Fat Low Sodium (Dorman)	1 oz	80	4
Shredded (Weight Watchers)	1 oz	80	5
Smoked (Polly-O)	1 oz	85	7
Whole Milk (Polly-O)	1 oz	90	6
Whole Milk Sandwich Slices (Polly-O)	1 oz	90	6
Whole Milk Shredded (Polly-O)	1 oz	90	6
With Pizza Spices (Sargento)	1 oz	79	5
Muenster			
(Alpine Lace)	1 oz	100	9
(Dorman)	1 oz	110	9
(Holland Farm)	1 oz	102	9
(Land O'Lakes)	1 oz	100	9
Light w/ Simplesse (White Clover)	1 oz	70	4
Low Sodium (Dorman)	1 oz	110	9
Red Rind (Sargento)	1 oz	104	9
Reduced Fat Low Sodium (Dorman)	1 oz	80	5
Nacho (Sargento)	1 oz	106	9
Naturally Slender (Northfield)	1 oz	90	7

FOOD	PORTION	CALORIES	FAT
Parmazest (Frigo)	1 oz	120	7
Parmesan			
(Dorman)	1 oz	110	7
And Romano Dry Grated (Frigo)	1 oz	130	9
And Romano Grated (Frigo)	1 oz	110	7
And Romano Grated (Sargento)	1 oz	111	7
Dry Grated (Frigo)	1 oz	130	9
Grated (Frigo)	1 oz	110	7
Grated (Kraft)	1 oz	130	9
Grated (Polly-O)	1 oz	130	9
Grated (Sargento)	1 oz	129	9
Natural (Kraft)	1 oz	100	7
Whole (Frigo)	1 oz	110	7
Pizza Shredded (Frigo)	1 oz	65	3
Port Wine Cup Cheese (Weight Watchers)	1½ tbsp (1 oz)	70	3
Port Wine Nut Log (Sargento)	1 oz	97	7
Provo-Lo (Alpine Lace)	1 oz	70	5
Provolone			
(Dorman)	1 oz	90	7
(Frigo)	1 oz	100	7
(Kraft)	1 oz	100	7
(Land O'Lakes)	1 oz	100	8
(Sargento)	1 oz	100	8
Lite (Frigo)	1 oz	70	4
Reduced Fat Low Sodium (Dorman)	1 oz	80	4
Quark (Brier Run)	1 oz	34	3
Queso Blanco (Sargento)	1 oz	104	9
Queso de Papa (Sargento)	1 oz	114	9
Ricotta Lite (Polly-O)	2 oz	80	4

FOOD	PORTION	CALORIES	FAT
Ricotta			
Lite (Sargento)	1 oz	25	tr
Low Fat Low Salt (Frigo)	1 oz	30	1
Part Skim (Frigo)	1 oz	40	3
Part Skim (Polly-O)	2 oz	90	6
Part Skim (Sargento)	1 oz	32	2
Part Skim No Salt (Polly-O)	2 oz	90	6
Whole Milk (Frigo)	1 oz	60	5
Whole Milk (Polly-O)	2 oz	100	7
Whole Milk (Sargento)	1 oz	53	4
Whole Milk & Whey (Sargento)	1 oz	40	3
Whole Milk No Salt (Polly-O)	2 oz	100	7
Romano			
(Dorman)	1 oz	100	7
(Sargento)	1 oz	110	8
Dry Grated (Frigo)	1 oz	130	9
Grated (Casino)	1 oz	130	9
Grated (Frigo)	1 oz	110	8
Grated (Polly-O)	1 oz	130	10
Natural (Casino)	1 oz	100	7
Whole (Frigo)	1 oz	110	8
Schloss (Marin French Cheese)	1 oz	86	7
Sharp Cheddar Cup Cheese (Weight Watchers)	1 oz	70	3
Sheep's Milk (Hallow Road Farms)	1 oz	45	3
Smoke (Bristol Gold Light)	1 oz	70	4
Smokestick (Sargento)	1 oz	103	7
String (Frigo)	1 oz	80	5
String (Polly-O)	1 oz	90	6
String (Sargento)	1 oz	79	5

FOOD	PORTION	CALORIES	FAT
String Lite (Frigo)	1 oz	60	2
String Smoked (Sargento)	1 oz	79	5
String w/ Jalapeno Peppers (Kraft)	1 oz	80	5
Swiss			
(Casino)	1 oz	110	8
(Dorman)	1 oz	100	8
(Frigo)	1 oz	110	8
(Kraft)	1 oz	110	8
(Land O'Lakes)	1 oz	110	8
(Sargento)	1 oz	107	8
Aged (Kraft)	1 oz	110	8
Almond Nut Log (Sargento)	1 oz	94	7
No Salt Added (Dorman)	1 oz	100	8
Reduced Fat (Kraft Light)	1 oz	90	5
Reduced Fat Low Sodium (Dorman)	1 oz	90	5
Very Low (Kraft)	1 oz	110	8
Swiss-Lo (Alpine Lace)	1 oz	100	7
Taco (Sargento)	1 oz	109	9
Taco Shredded (Frigo)	1 oz	110	9
Taco Shredded (Kraft)	1 oz	110	9
Tilsiter (Sargento)	1 oz	96	7
Tybo Red Wax (Sargento)	1 oz	98	7
Vitalait (Cabot)	1 oz	70	4
Wine (Bristol Gold Light)	1 oz	70	4
bel paese	3.5 oz	391	30
blue	1 oz	100	8
blue, crumbled	1 cup	477	39
brick	1 oz	105	8
brie	1 oz	95	8

FOOD	PORTION	CALORIES	FAT
caerphilly	1.4 oz	150	13
camembert	1 oz	85	7
camembert	1 wedge (1⅓ oz)	114	9
caraway	1 oz	107	8
cheddar	1 oz	114	9
cheddar, reduced fat	1.4 oz	104	6
cheddar, shredded	1 cup	455	37
cheshire	1 oz	110	9
cheshire, reduced fat	1.4 oz	108	6
colby	1 oz	112	9
derby	1.4 oz	161	14
double gloucester	1.4 oz	162	14
edam	1 oz	101	8
edam, reduced fat	1.4 oz	92	4
emmentaler	3.5 oz	403	30
feta	1 oz	75	6
fontina	1 oz	110	9
fromage frais	1.6 oz	51	3
gjetost	1 oz	132	8
goat, hard	1 oz	128	10
goat, semi-soft	1 oz	103	8
goat, soft	1 oz	76	6
gorgonzola	3.5 oz	376	31
gouda	1 oz	101	8
gruyere	1 oz	117	9
lancashire	1.4 oz	149	12
leicester	1.4 oz	160	14
limburger	1 oz	93	8
lymeswold	1.4 oz	170	16
monterey	1 oz	106	9

FOOD	PORTION	CALORIES	FAT
mozzarella	1 oz	80	6
mozzarella	1 lb	1276	98
mozzarella, low moisture	1 oz	90	7
mozzarella, part skim	1 oz	72	5
mozzarella, part skim, low moisture	1 oz	79	5
muenster	1 oz	104	9
parmesan, grated	1 tbsp	23	2
parmesan, grated	1 oz	129	9
parmesan, hard	1 oz	111	7
port du salut	1 oz	100	8
provolone	1 oz	100	8
quark, 20% fat	3.5 oz	116	5
quark, 40% fat	3.5 oz	167	11
quark, made w/ skim milk	3.5 oz	78	tr
ricotta	½ cup	216	16
ricotta	1 cup	428	32
ricotta, part skim	½ cup	171	10
ricotta, part skim	1 cup	340	19
romadur, 40% fat	3.5 oz	289	20
romano	1 oz	110	8
roquefort	1 oz	105	9
stilton, blue	1.4 oz	164	14
stilton, white	1.4 oz	145	13
swiss	1 oz	107	8
tilsit	1 oz	96	7
wensleydale	1.4 oz	151	13
yogurt cheese	1 oz	20	0
PROCESSED Alpine Lace American	1 oz	80	7

FOOD	PORTION	CALORIES	FAT
Free N'Lean American	1 oz	35	0
Free N'Lean Cheddar	1 oz	40	0
Free N'Lean Cheese Spread	1 oz	30	0
Free N'Lean Cheese Spread w/ Jalapeno	1 oz	30	0
Free N'Lean Mozzarella	1 oz	40	0
Free N'Lean Party Spread w/ Garlic & Herbs	1 oz	30	0
American Cheese White (Hoffman's)	1 oz	110	9
Borden			
American Singles	1 oz	90	7
American Slices	1 oz	110	9
Lite Line Mozzarella	1 oz	50	2
Lite Line Sharp Cheddar	1 oz	50	2
Lite Line Swiss	1 oz	50	2
Swiss Slices	1 oz	100	8
Cheez Whiz	1 oz	80	6
Cheez Whiz Mild Mexican	1 oz	80	6
Cheez Whiz w/ Jalapeno Peppers	1 oz	80	6
Churney			
Cheese Fudge w/ Walnuts	1 oz	120	4
Diet Snack Cheddar Flavored	1 oz	70	3
Diet Snack Port Wine Flavored	1 oz	70	3
Maple Walnut Cheese Fudge	1 oz	118	4
Mint Cheese Fudge w/ Walnuts	1 oz	117	4
Cracker Barrel			
Cheese Ball Sharp Cheddar w/ Almonds	1 oz	100	7
Cheese Log Port Wine w/ Almonds	1 oz	90	6
Cheese Log Sharp Cheddar w/ Almonds	1 oz	90	6

FOOD	PORTION	CALORIES	FAT
Cracker Barrel *(cont.)*			
Cheese Log Smokey Cheddar w/ Almonds	1 oz	90	6
Extra Sharp Cheddar	1 oz	90	7
Port Wine Cheddar	1 oz	100	7
Sharp Cheddar	1 oz	100	7
With Bacon	1 oz	90	7
Dorman's Lo-Chol Cheddar	1 oz	100	7
Dorman's Lo-Chol Colby	1 oz	100	7
Dorman's Lo-Chol Mozzarella	1 oz	90	6
Dorman's Lo-Chol Muenster	1 oz	100	7
Dorman's Lo-Chol Swiss	1 oz	100	7
Easy Cheese Sharp Cheddar Spread	1 oz	80	6
Formagg			
American Swiss Slices	¾ oz	70	5
American White Slices	¾ oz	70	5
American Yellow Slices	¾ oz	70	5
Cheddar	1 oz	70	5
Grated Italian Pasta Topping	1 oz	100	7
Monterey Jack	1 oz	70	5
Monterey Jack Jalapeno Flavored	1 oz	70	5
Mozzarella	1 oz	70	5
Pizza Topper	1 oz	70	5
Provolone	1 oz	70	5
Ricotta	1 oz	130	5
Shredded Cheddar	1 oz	70	5
Shredded Mozzarella	1 oz	70	5
Shredded Parmesan	1 oz	70	4
Shredded Provolone	1 oz	70	5
Shredded Salad Topping	1 oz	70	5
Shredded Swiss	1 oz	70	5

FOOD	PORTION	CALORIES	FAT
Swiss	1 oz	70	5
Frigo Imitation Cheddar	1 oz	90	7
Frigo Imitation Mozzarella	1 oz	90	7
Fromageries Bel			
Cheddar Cheese Wedges	1 oz	72	6
Cheddar Cheese Wedges Reduced Calorie	¾ oz	35	2
Gruyere Cheese Wedges	1 oz	72	6
Gruyere Cheese Wedges Reduced Calorie	¾ oz	35	2
Harvest Moon American	1 oz	70	4
Kraft			
American Cheese Spread	1 oz	80	7
American Grated	1 oz	130	7
American Singles	1 oz	90	7
American Singles White	1 oz	90	7
Cheese Food w/ Garlic	1 oz	90	7
Cheese Food w/ Jalapeno Peppers	1 oz	90	7
Cheese Spread w/ Bacon	1 oz	80	7
Cheez 'N Bacon Singles	1 oz	90	7
Deluxe American Cheese	1 oz	110	9
Deluxe Pimento Cheese	1 oz	100	8
Deluxe Swiss Cheese	1 oz	90	7
Free Singles	1 oz	45	5
Jalapeno Cheese Spread	1 oz	80	6
Jalapeno Pepper Spread	1 oz	70	5
Jalapeno Singles	1 oz	90	7
Light Singles	1 oz	70	4
Light Singles American	1 oz	70	4
Light Singles Sharp Cheddar	1 oz	70	4
Light Singles Swiss	1 oz	70	3

FOOD	PORTION	CALORIES	FAT
Kraft *(cont.)*			
Monterey Jack Singles	1 oz	90	7
Olives & Pimento Spread	1 oz	60	5
Pimento Singles	1 oz	90	7
Pimento Spread			
Pineapple Spread	1 oz	70	5
Sharp Singles	1 oz	100	8
Swiss Singles	1 oz	90	7
Lactaid American	3.5 oz	328	25
Land O'Lakes			
American	1 oz	110	9
American & Swiss	1 oz	100	8
Cheddar & Bacon	1 oz	110	9
Extra Sharp Cheddar	1 oz	100	9
Golden Velvet Cheese Spread	1 oz	80	6
Italian Herb Cheese Food	1 oz	90	7
Jalapeno Cheese Spread	1 oz	90	7
Jalapeno Jack	1 oz	90	8
Onion Cheese Food	1 oz	90	7
Pepperoni Cheese Food	1 oz	90	7
Salami Cheese Food	1 oz	90	7
Laughing Cow Cheesebits	1	13	1
Light N' Lively Singles American	1 oz	70	4
Light N' Lively Singles American White	1 oz	70	4
Light N' Lively Singles Sharp Cheddar	1 oz	70	4
Light N' Lively Singles Swiss	1 oz	70	3
Lunch Wagon Sandwich Slices Made w/ Vegetable Oil	1 oz	90	7
Michael's Country Gourmet Spread French Onion	1 oz	48	5

FOOD	PORTION	CALORIES	FAT
Garden Vegetable	1 oz	48	5
Garlic & Herbs	1 oz	48	5
Mohawk Valley Limburger Cheese Spread	1 oz	70	6
Nippy Cheese Food	1 oz	90	7
Old English Sharp American	1 oz	110	9
Old English Sharp Cheese Spread	1 oz	90	7
Roka Blue Spread	1 oz	70	6
Sargento			
American Hot Pepper	1 oz	106	9
American Sharp Spread	1 oz	106	9
American w/ Pimento	1 oz	106	9
Imitation Cheddar	1 oz	85	6
Imitation Mozzarella	1 oz	80	6
Process Brick	1 oz	95	9
Process Swiss	1 oz	95	7
Smart Beat American	1 slice (⅔ oz)	35	2
Smart Beat Low Sodium	1 slice (⅔ oz)	35	2
Smart Beat Sharp	1 slice (⅔ oz)	35	2
Spreadery			
Medium Cheddar	1 oz	70	4
Mild Mexican w/ Jalapeno Peppers	1 oz	70	4
Nacho	1 oz	70	4
Port Wine	1 oz	70	4
Sharp Cheddar	1 oz	70	4
Vermont White Cheddar	1 oz	70	4
Squeez-A-Snak Garlic	1 oz	80	7
Squeez-A-Snak Hickory Smoke	1 oz	80	7
Squeez-A-Snak Sharp	1 oz	80	7
Squeez-A-Snak w/ Bacon	1 oz	90	7

FOOD	PORTION	CALORIES	FAT
Squeez-A-Snak w/Jalapeno Pepper	1 oz	80	6
Super Sharp (Hoffman's)	1 oz	110	8
Swisson Rye Cheese Food (Hoffman's)	1 oz	90	7
Velveeta			
Cheese Spread	1 oz	80	6
Light Singles	1 oz	70	4
Mexican Hot	1 oz	80	6
Mexican Wild	1 oz	80	6
Pimento	1 oz	80	6
Shredded	1 oz	100	7
Shredded Hot Mexican w/ Jalapeno Peppers	1 oz	100	7
Shredded Mild Mexican w/ Jalapeno Peppers	1 oz	100	7
Slices	1 oz	90	6
Weight Watchers			
American Slices Low Sodium White	2 slices (⅔ oz)	35	1
American Slices Low Sodium Yellow	2 slices (⅔ oz)	35	1
American Slices White	2 slices (⅔ oz)	35	1
American Slices Yellow	2 slices (⅔ oz)	35	1
Sharp Cheddar Slices	2 slices (⅔ oz)	35	1
Swiss Slices	2 slices (⅔ oz)	35	1
Wispride Port Wine	1 oz	100	7
Wispride Sharp Cheddar	1 oz	100	7
american	1 oz	106	9
american, cheese food	1 oz	93	7
american, cheese food	1 pkg (8 oz)	745	56
american, cheese food, cold pack	1 oz	94	7
american, cheese food, cold pack	1 pkg (8 oz)	752	56

FOOD	PORTION	CALORIES	FAT
american, cheese spread	1 oz	82	6
american, cheese spread	1 jar (5 oz)	412	30
pimento	1 oz	106	9
swiss	1 oz	95	7
swiss, cheese food	1 oz	92	7
swiss, cheese food	1 pkg (8 oz)	734	55

CHEESE DISHES

FROZEN

Mozzarella Cheese Nuggets (Banquet)	2.5 oz	230	12

HOME RECIPE

welsh rarebit, as prep w/ 1 white toast	1 slice	228	16

TAKE-OUT

cheese omelette, as prep w/ 2 eggs	1 (6.8 oz)	519	44
fondue	½ cup	303	18
macaroni & cheese	6.3 oz	320	19

CHEESE SUBSTITUTES

Cheeztwin	1 oz	90	6
Delicia American & Caraway	1 oz	80	6
Delicia American Cheese	1 oz	80	6
Delicia American w/ Hot Peppers	1 oz	80	6
Delicia Colby Longhorn	1 oz	80	6
Delicia Hickory Smoked American	1 oz	80	6
Golden Image American	1 oz	90	6
Golden Image Colby	1 oz	110	9
Golden Image Mild Cheddar	1 oz	110	9
Lite Line Low Cholesterol Cheese Food Substitute	1 oz	90	7

FOOD	PORTION	CALORIES	FAT
mozzarella	1 oz	70	3

CHERIMOYA

fresh	1	515	2

CHERRIES

CANNED			
sour in heavy syrup	½ cup	232	tr
sour in light syrup	½ cup	189	tr
sour water packed	1 cup	87	tr
sweet in heavy syrup	½ cup	107	tr
sweet in light syrup	½ cup	85	tr
sweet juice pack	½ cup	68	tr
sweet water pack	½ cup	57	tr
DRIED			
Bing (Chukar)	2 oz	160	1
Rainer (Chukar)	2 oz	160	1
Tart (Chukar)	2 oz	170	0
Tart 'N Sweet (Chukar)	2 oz	180	0
FRESH			
Dole	1 cup	90	1
sour	1 cup	51	tr
sweet	10	49	1
FROZEN			
sour unsweetened	1 cup	72	1
sweet sweetened	1 cup	232	tr
JUICE			
Dole Pure & Light	6 oz	90	tr
Juice Works Cherry	6 oz	100	0
Sipps Wild Cherry	8.45 oz	130	0
Smucker's Black Cherry	8 oz	130	0

FOOD	PORTION	CALORIES	FAT

CHERVIL

seed	1 tsp	1	tr

CHESTNUTS

chinese, cooked	1 oz	44	tr
chinese, dried	1 oz	103	tr
chinese, raw	1 oz	64	tr
chinese, roasted	1 oz	68	tr
cooked	1 oz	37	tr
dried, peeled	1 oz	105	1
japanese, cooked	1 oz	16	tr
japanese, dried	1 oz	102	tr
japanese, raw	1 oz	44	tr
japanese, roasted	1 oz	57	tr
raw, peeled	1 oz	56	tr
roasted	1 cup	350	3
roasted	1 oz	70	1

CHEWING GUM

Beech-Nut Cinnamon	1 piece	10	0
Beech-Nut Fruit	1 piece	10	0
Beech-Nut Peppermint	1 piece	10	0
Beech-Nut Spearmint	1 piece	10	0
Big Red	1 stick	10	tr
Bubble Yum Fruit Juice Variety	1 piece	20	0
Bubble Yum Luscious Lime	1 piece	25	0
Care*Free Sugarless All Flavors	1 piece	8	0
Care*Free Sugarless Bubble Gum All Flavors	1 piece	10	0
Extra Sugar Free Cinnamon	1 piece	8	tr

FOOD	PORTION	CALORIES	FAT
Extra Sugar Free Spearmint & Peppermint	1 stick	8	tr
Extra Sugar Free Winter Fresh	1 piece	8	tr
Freedent Spearmint, Peppermint, & Cinnamon	1 stick	10	tr
Fruit Stripe	1 piece	8	0
Fruit Stripe Bubble Gum	1 piece	8	0
Fruit Stripe Variety Pack	1 piece	8	0
Hubba Bubba Bubble Gum Cola	1 piece	23	tr
Hubba Bubba Bubble Gum Sugarfree Original	1 piece	14	tr
Hubba Bubba Bubble Gum Sugarfree Grape	1 piece	13	tr
Hubba Bubba Original	1 piece	23	tr
Hubba Bubba Strawberry, Grape, Raspberry	1 piece	23	tr
Wrigley's Doublemint	1 piece	10	tr
Wrigley's Juicy Fruit	1 stick	10	tr
Wrigley's Spearmint	1 stick	10	tr

CHIA SEEDS

dried	1 oz	134	7

CHICKEN

(*see also* CHICKEN DISHES, CHICKEN SUBSTITUTES, DINNER, HOT DOG)

CANNED

Chunk Style Mixin' Chicken (Swanson)	2.5 oz	130	8
White (Swanson)	2.5 oz	100	4
White & Dark (Swanson)	2.5 oz	100	4
chicken spread	1 tbsp	25	2
chicken spread	1 oz	55	3

FOOD	PORTION	CALORIES	FAT
chicken spread, barbeque flavored	1 oz	55	3
w/ broth	1 can (5 oz)	234	11
w/ broth	½ can (2.5 oz)	117	6
FRESH			
Breast Oven Stuffer Roaster w/ skin, cooked (Perdue)	1 oz	42	2
Breast Quarters Fresh Young w/ skin, cooked (Perdue)	1 oz	48	3
Breast Skinless & Boneless Oven Stuffer Roaster, cooked (Perdue)	1 oz	31	tr
Breast Skinless & Boneless, cooked (Perdue)	1 oz	30	tr
Breast Split Fresh Young w/ skin, cooked (Perdue)	1 oz	45	3
Breast Tender Skinless & Boneless w/ skin, cooked (Perdue)	1 oz	29	tr
Breast Thin-Sliced Skinless & Boneless Oven Stuffer, cooked (Perdue)	1 oz	31	tr
Breast Whole Fresh Young w/ skin, cooked (Perdue)	1 oz	45	3
Cornish Hen Dark Meat w/ skin, cooked (Perdue)	1 oz	43	3
Cornish Hen White Meat w/ skin, cooked (Perdue)	1 oz	42	3
Drumsticks Fresh Young w/ skin, cooked (Perdue)	1 oz	42	2
Drumsticks Oven Stuffer, Roaster w/ skin, cooked (Perdue)	1 oz	41	2
Ground Fresh Young, cooked (Perdue)	1 oz	49	3
Leg Quarters Fresh Young w/ skin, cooked (Perdue)	1 oz	49	4
Legs Fresh Young w/ skin, cooked (Perdue)	1 oz	51	4

FOOD	PORTION	CALORIES	FAT
Soup & Stew Baking Hen Dark Meat w/ skin, cooked (Perdue)	1 oz	41	3
Soup & Stew Baking Hen White Meat w/ skin, cooked (Perdue)	1 oz	41	2
Thighs Fresh Young w/ skin, cooked (Perdue)	1 oz	57	4
Thighs Skinless & Boneless, cooked (Perdue)	1 oz	30	2
Thighs Skinless & Boneless Oven Stuffer Roaster, cooked (Perdue)	1 oz	34	2
Whole Fresh Young Dark Meat w/ skin, cooked (Perdue)	1 oz	47	3
Whole Fresh Young White Meat w/ skin, cooked (Perdue)	1 oz	43	2
Whole Oven Stuffer Roaster Dark Meat w/ skin, cooked (Perdue)	1 oz	49	3
Whole Oven Stuffer Roaster White Meat w/ skin, cooked (Perdue)	1 oz	44	2
Wing Drumettes Fresh Young w/ skin, cooked (Perdue)	1 oz	50	3
Wingettes Oven Stuffer Roaster w/ skin, cooked (Perdue)	1 oz	52	3
Wings Fresh Young w/ skin, cooked (Perdue)	1 oz	54	4
broiler/fryer			
back w/ skin, batter dipped, fried	½ back (2.5 oz)	238	16
back w/ skin, floured, fried	1.5 oz	146	9
back w/ skin, roasted	1 oz	96	7
back w/ skin, stewed	½ back (2.1 oz)	158	11
back w/o skin, fried	½ back (2 oz)	167	9
breast w/ skin, batter dipped, fried	½ breast (4.9 oz)	364	18
breast w/ skin, batter dipped, fried	2.9 oz	218	11

FOOD	PORTION	CALORIES	FAT
breast w/ skin, roasted	2 oz	115	5
breast w/ skin, roasted	½ breast (3.4 oz)	193	8
breast w/ skin, stewed	½ breast (3.9 oz)	202	8
breast w/o skin, fried	½ breast (3 oz)	161	4
breast w/o skin, roasted	½ breast (3 oz)	142	3
breast w/o skin, stewed	2 oz	86	2
dark meat w/ skin, batter dipped, fried	5.9 oz	497	31
dark meat w/ skin, floured, fried	3.9 oz	313	19
dark meat w/ skin, roasted	3.5 oz	256	16
dark meat w/ skin, stewed	3.9 oz	256	16
dark meat w/o skin, fried	1 cup (5 oz)	334	16
dark meat w/o skin, roasted	1 cup (5 oz)	286	14
dark meat w/o skin, stewed	3 oz	165	8
dark meat w/o skin, stewed	1 cup (5 oz)	269	13
drumstick w/ skin, batter dipped, fried	1 (2.6 oz)	193	11
drumstick w/ skin, floured, fried	1 (1.7 oz)	120	7
drumstick w/ skin, roasted	1 (1.8 oz)	112	6
drumstick w/ skin, stewed	1 (2 oz)	116	6
drumstick w/o skin, fried	1 (1.5 oz)	82	3
drumstick w/o skin, roasted	1 (1.5 oz)	76	2
drumstick w/o skin, stewed	1 (1.6 oz)	78	3
leg w/ skin, batter dipped, fried	1 (5.5 oz)	431	26
leg w/ skin, floured, fried	1 (3.9 oz)	285	16
leg w/ skin, roasted	1 (4 oz)	265	15
leg w/ skin, stewed	1 (4.4 oz)	275	16
leg w/o skin, fried	1 (3.3 oz)	195	9
leg w/o skin, roasted	1 (3.3 oz)	182	8

FOOD	PORTION	CALORIES	FAT
broiler/fryer *(cont.)*			
leg w/o skin, stewed	1 (3.5 oz)	187	8
light meat w/ skin, batter dipped, fried	4 oz	312	17
light meat w/ skin, floured, fried	2.7 oz	192	9
light meat w/ skin, roasted	2.8 oz	175	9
light meat w/ skin, stewed	3.2 oz	181	9
light meat w/o skin, fried	1 cup (5 oz)	268	8
light meat w/o skin, roasted	1 cup (5 oz)	242	6
light meat w/o skin, stewed	1 cup (5 oz)	223	6
neck w/ skin, stewed	1 (1.3 oz)	94	7
neck w/o skin, stewed	1 (.6 oz)	32	1
skin, batter dipped, fried	4 oz	449	33
skin, floured, fried	from ½ chicken (2 oz)	281	24
skin, floured, fried	1 oz	166	14
skin, roasted	from ½ chicken (2 oz)	254	23
skin, stewed	2.5 oz	261	24
thigh w/ skin, batter dipped, fried	1 (3 oz)	238	14
thigh w/ skin, floured, fried	1 (2.2 oz)	162	9
thigh w/ skin, roasted	1 (2.2 oz)	153	10
thigh w/ skin, stewed	1 (2.4 oz)	158	10
thigh w/o skin, fried	1 (1.8 oz)	113	5
thigh w/o skin, roasted	1 (1.8 oz)	109	6
thigh w/o skin, stewed	1 (1.9 oz)	107	5
wing w/ skin, batter dipped, fried	1 (1.7 oz)	159	11
wing w/ skin, floured, fried	1 (1.1 oz)	103	7
wing w/ skin, roasted	1 (1.2 oz)	99	7
wing w/ skin, stewed	1 (1.4 oz)	100	7
w/ skin, floured, fried	½ chicken (11 oz)	844	47

FOOD	PORTION	CALORIES	FAT
w/ skin, fried	½ chicken (16.4 oz)	1347	81
w/ skin, roasted	½ chicken (10.5 oz)	715	41
w/ skin, stewed	½ chicken (11.7 oz)	730	42
w/ skin, neck & giblets, batter dipped, fried	1 chicken (2.3 lbs)	2987	180
w/ skin, neck & giblets, roasted	1 chicken (1.5 lbs)	1598	90
w/ skin, neck & giblets, stewed	1 chicken (1.6 lbs)	1625	93
w/o skin, fried	1 cup	307	13
w/o skin, roasted	1 cup (5 oz)	266	10
w/o skin, stewed	1 oz	54	3
w/o skin, stewed	1 cup (5 oz)	248	9
capon w/ skin, neck & giblets, roasted	1 chicken (3.1 lbs)	3211	165
roaster dark meat w/o skin, roasted	1 cup (5 oz)	250	12
roaster light meat w/o skin, roasted	1 cup (5 oz)	214	6
roaster w/ skin, roasted	½ chicken (1.1 lbs)	1071	64
roaster w/ skin, neck & giblets, roasted	1 chicken (2.4 lbs)	2363	140
roaster w/o skin, roasted	1 cup (5 oz)	469	28
stewing dark meat w/o skin, stewed	1 cup (5 oz)	361	21
stewing w/ skin, stewed	½ chicken (9.2 oz)	744	49
stewing w/ skin, stewed	6.2 oz	507	34
stewing w/ skin, neck & giblets, stewed	1 chicken (1.3 lbs)	1636	107

FROZEN PREPARED

Banquet
Boneless Breast Tenders	2.25 oz	150	6

FOOD	PORTION	CALORIES	FAT
Banquet *(cont.)*			
Boneless Chicken Nuggets	2.5 oz	200	13
Boneless Chicken Nuggets w/ Cheddar	2.5 oz	240	17
Boneless Chicken Patties	2.5 oz	190	12
Boneless Chicken Sticks	2.5 oz	210	14
Boneless Drum-Snackers	2.5 oz	210	14
Boneless Fried Breast Tenders	2.25 oz	160	7
Boneless Southern Fried Chicken Nuggets	2.5 oz	210	14
Boneless Southern Fried Chicken Patties	2.5 oz	200	12
Fried Chicken Breast Portions	5.75 oz	220	11
Fried Chicken Thighs & Drumsticks	6.25 oz	250	14
Hot'n Spicy Chicken Nuggets	2.5 oz	240	18
Hot'n Spicy Fried Chicken	6.4 oz	330	19
Hot'n Spicy Snack'n Chicken	3.75 oz	140	9
Original Fried Chicken	5.6 oz	290	17
Southern Fried Chicken	5.6 oz	290	17
Country Skillet			
Chicken Chunks	3 oz	260	16
Chicken Nuggets	3 oz	250	15
Chicken Patties	3 oz	230	15
Southern Fried Chicken Chunks	3 oz	270	18
Southern Fried Chicken Patties	3 oz	240	15
Healthy Balance			
Baked Boneless Breast Nuggets	2.25 oz	120	4
Baked Boneless Breast Patties	2.25 oz	120	4
Baked Boneless Breast Tenders	2.25 oz	120	4
Swanson			
Chicken Duet Gourmet Nuggets Pizza Style	3 oz	210	12

FOOD	PORTION	CALORIES	FAT
Chicken Nibbles	3.25 oz	300	19
Chicken Nuggets	3 oz	230	14
Fried Chicken Breast Portion	4.5 oz	360	20
Pre-fried Chicken Parts	3.25 oz	270	16
Thighs & Drumsticks	3.25 oz	290	18
Weaver			
Batter Dipped Breast	3.5 oz	250	16
Batter Dipped Thighs/Drums	3.5 oz	245	16
Batter Dipped Wings	3.5 oz	270	19
Breast Fillets	3.5 oz	195	10
Breast Fillets Strips	3.5 oz	200	9
Chicken Croquettes	3.5 oz	245	15
Chicken Nuggets	4 pieces	240	14
Crispy Dutch Frye Breasts	3.5 oz	285	18
Crispy Dutch Frye Thighs/Drums	3.5 oz	295	20
Crispy Dutch Frye Wings	3.5 oz	360	25
Crispy Light Fried Chicken	2.9 oz	160	9
Mini-Drums Crispy	3 oz	205	11
Mini-Drums Herbs 'n Spice	3 oz	205	11
Rondelets Cheese	3 oz	215	13
Rondelets Homestyle	3 oz	185	10
Rondelets Italian	3 oz	200	11
Rondelets Original	3 oz	185	10
Thigh Fillets Strips	3.5 oz	240	14
Weight Watchers Chicken Nuggets	5.9 oz	220	7
READY-TO-USE			
Carl Buddig	1 oz	60	4
Dutch Family Roll	1 oz	61	15
Longacre Roll	1 oz	65	17

FOOD	PORTION	CALORIES	FAT
Louis Rich			
Deluxe Oven Roasted Breast	1 slice (28 g)	30	tr
Oven Roasted Breast	1 slice (28 g)	39	2
Smoked Breast	1 slice (28 g)	31	tr
Mr. Turkey Breast	1 slice (1 oz)	32	1
Oscar Mayer Oven Roasted Breast	1 slice (28 g)	29	tr
Oscar Mayer Smoked Breast	1 slice (28 g)	26	tr
Perdue Done It!			
BBQ Breast Half	1 oz	46	2
BBQ Drumsticks	1 oz	53	2
BBQ Half Dark Meat	1 oz	57	4
BBQ Half White Meat	1 oz	40	1
BBQ Thighs	1 oz	59	3
BBQ Wings	1 oz	62	4
Breast Roasted	1 oz	45	2
Cornish Hen Roasted Dark Meat	1 oz	45	3
Cornish Hen Roasted White Meat	1 oz	39	1
Cutlets	3.5 oz	250	14
Drumsticks Roasted	1 oz	40	1
Nuggets Cheese	1 (.67 oz)	54	4
Nuggets Fun Shaped	1 (.73 oz)	54	3
Nuggets Original	1 (.67 oz)	48	3
Tenders	1 oz	62	3
Thighs Roasted	1 oz	46	2
Whole or Half Roasted Dark Meat	1 oz	51	3
Whole or Half Roasted White Meat	1 oz	37	1
Wings Garlic & Herb	1 oz	61	4
Wings Hot & Spicy	1 oz	60	4
Wampler Longacre			
Breast Deli Sliced Browned Roasted	1 oz	49	11

FOOD	PORTION	CALORIES	FAT
Breast Meat	1 oz	38	2
Breast Stuffed w/ Breading	8 oz	472	94
Breast Stuffed w/ Cordon Blue	6.5 oz	429	39
Diced Breast	1 oz	38	2
Roll Diced Breast	1 oz	49	11
Roll Sliced	1 oz	63	16
Weaver			
Bologna	3.5 oz	240	20
Breast Hickory Smoked	3.5 oz	125	4
Breast Oven Roasted	3.5 oz	120	4
White Meat Roll	3.5 oz	130	6
Weight Watchers			
Roasted & Smoked Breast	2 slices (¾ oz)	25	1
Roasted & Smoked Deli Thin Ham	5 slices (⅓ oz)	10	tr
Roasted Ham	2 slices (¾ oz)	25	1
chicken roll light meat	1 pkg (6 oz)	271	13
chicken roll light meat	2 oz	90	4
poultry salad sandwich spread	1 tbsp	109	2
poultry salad sandwich spread	1 oz	238	4
TAKE-OUT			
boneless, breaded & fried w/ barbecue sauce	6 pieces (4.6 oz)	330	18
boneless, breaded & fried w/ honey	6 pieces (4 oz)	339	18
boneless, breaded & fried w/ mustard sauce	6 pieces (4.6 oz)	323	17
boneless, breaded & fried w/ sweet & sour sauce	6 pieces (4.6 oz)	346	18
breast & wing, breaded & fried	2 pieces (5.7 oz)	494	30
drumstick, breaded & fried	2 pieces (5.2 oz)	430	27
thigh, breaded & fried	2 pieces (5.2 oz)	430	27

FOOD	PORTION	CALORIES	FAT

CHICKEN DISHES
(see also CHICKEN SUBSTITUTES, DINNER)

CANNED

FOOD	PORTION	CALORIES	FAT
Chicken & Dumplings (Swanson)	7.5 oz	220	11
Chicken Ala King (Swanson)	5.25 oz	190	12
Chicken Stew (Chef Boyardee)	7 oz	140	5
Chicken Stew (Swanson)	7⅝ oz	160	7

FROZEN

FOOD	PORTION	CALORIES	FAT
Banquet Family Entrees Dumplings & Chicken	7 oz	280	14
Banquet Entree Chicken & Noodles	8.5 oz	240	10
Budget Gourmet Orange Glazed Chicken	1 pkg	250	34
Dining Light Chicken Ala King	9 oz	240	7
Dining Light Chicken w/ Noodles	9 oz	240	7
Healthy Choice Chicken A L'Orange	9 oz	240	2
Healthy Choice Glazed Chicken	8.5 oz	220	3
Healthy Choice Mandarin Chicken	11 oz	260	2
Kibun Chicken Pasta Salad w/ dressing	½ pkg	220	9
Kibun Chicken Pasta Salad w/o dressing	½ pkg	150	2
Le Menu Entree LightStyle Chicken A La King	8.25 oz	240	5
Le Menu Entree LightStyle Chicken Dijon	8 oz	240	7
Le Menu Entree LightStyle Empress Chicken	8.25 oz	210	5
Le Menu Entree LightStyle Herb Roast Chicken	7.75 oz	260	6
MicroMagic Chicken Sandwich	1 pkg (4.5 oz)	390	16
Ovenstuffs Chicken Turnover	1 (4.75 oz)	350	16

FOOD	PORTION	CALORIES	FAT
HOME RECIPE			
chicken & noodles	1 cup	365	18
chicken a la king	1 cup	470	34
READY-TO-USE			
Salad (Wampler Longacre)	1 oz	65	16
The Spreadables Chicken Salad	¼ can	100	6
TAKE-OUT			
chicken & dumplings	¾ cup	256	12
chicken cacciatore	¾ cup	394	24
chicken paprikash	1½ cup	296	10
chicken pie w/ top crust	1 slice (5.6 oz)	472	31
fillet sandwich plain	1	515	29
fillet sandwich w/ cheese, mayonnaise, tomato, lettuce	1	632	39

CHICKEN SUBSTITUTES

FOOD	PORTION	CALORIES	FAT
Chick Sticks, frzn (Worthington)	3.5 oz	232	14
Chick-Ketts, frzn (Worthington)	3.5 oz	199	9
Chik-Nuggets (Loma Linda)	5 nuggets (3 oz)	228	11
Chik-Patties (Loma Linda)	1 patty (3 oz)	226	12
Meatless Chicken (Loma Linda)	2 slices (2 oz)	93	3
Meatless Chicken Supreme, mix not prep (Loma Linda)	¼ cup	50	tr
Meatless Fried Chicken (Loma Linda)	1 piece (2 oz)	180	14
Meatless Fried Chicken w/ Gravy (Loma Linda)	2 pieces (3 oz)	140	10
Spicy-Chik Minidrums (Loma Linda)	5 pieces (3 oz)	230	13

CHICKPEAS

FOOD	PORTION	CALORIES	FAT
CANNED			
Chick Peas (Hanover)	½ cup	100	1

FOOD	PORTION	CALORIES	FAT
Chick Peas Spanish Style (Goya)	7.5 oz	150	2
Garbanzo (Green Giant)	½ cup	90	2
Garbanzo Beans Water Pack (S&W)	½ cup	105	1
Garbanzo Lite 50% Less Salt (S&W)	½ cup	110	0
Garbanzo Premium Large (S&W)	½ cup	110	1
chickpeas	1 cup	285	3
DRIED			
Garbonzo (Arrowhead)	2 oz	200	3
Garbanzo (Hurst Brand)	1 cup	288	4
cooked	1 cup	269	4
raw	1 cup	729	12

CHICORY

FRESH			
greens, raw, chopped	½ cup	21	tr
roots, raw, cut up	½ cup	33	tr
witloof, raw	½ cup	7	tr

CHILI

CANNED			
Chef Boyardee			
Beef Chili w/ Beans	7.5 oz	330	17
Chili Con Carne w/ Beans	7 oz	340	20
Chili Hot Dog Sauce w/ Beef	1 oz	30	1
Chili Mac	7 oz	230	10
Hot Chili Con Carne w/ Beans	7 oz	350	21
Dennison's			
Chili Beans in Chili Gravy	7.5 oz	180	1
Chili Con Carne w/ Beans	7.5 oz	310	15
Chili Con Carne w/o Beans	7.5 oz	300	19

FOOD	PORTION	CALORIES	FAT
Cook-off Chili w/ Beans	7.5 oz	340	19
Chunky Chili w/ Beans	7.5 oz	310	14
Hot Chili Con Carne w/ Beans	7.5 oz	310	16
Gebhardt Hot w/ Beans	1 cup	470	27
Gebhardt Plain	1 cup	530	43
Gebhardt w/ Beans	1 cup	495	28
Health Valley			
Mild Vegetarian w/ Beans	5 oz	160	3
Mild Vegetarian w/ Beans No Salt Added	5 oz	160	3
Mild Vegetarian w/ Lentils	5 oz	140	4
Mild Vegetarian w/ Lentils No Salt Added	5 oz	140	4
Spicy Vegetarian w/ Beans	5 oz	160	4
Healthy Choice Spicy w/ Beans & Ground Turkey	½ can (7.5 oz)	210	5
Healthy Choice Turkey w/ Beans	½ can (7.5 oz)	200	5
Hunt's Chili Beans	4 oz	100	tr
Just Rite Hot w/ Beans	4 oz	195	10
Just Rite w/ Beans	4 oz	200	11
Just Rite w/o Beans	4 oz	180	11
Luck's Hot Chili Beans	7.5 oz	200	2
Manwich Chili Fixin's, as prep	8 oz	290	14
S&W Chili Beans	½ cup	130	1
S&W Chili Makin's Original	½ cup	100	1
Van Camp's Chili Weenee	1 cup	309	16
Van Camp's Chili w/ Beans	1 cup	352	23
Van Camp's Chili w/o Beans	1 cup	412	36
Wolf Brand Chili-Mac	7.5 oz	317	20
Wolf Brand Extra Spicy w/ Beans	7.5 oz	324	21
Wolf Brand Extra Spicy w/o Beans	7.5 oz	363	25

FOOD	PORTION	CALORIES	FAT
Wolf Brand Plain	7.5 oz	330	22
Wolf Brand w/ Beans	7.5 oz	345	22
Wolf Brand w/o Beans	1 cup	387	27
chili w/ beans	1 cup	286	14
DRIED			
Gebhardt Chili Powder	1 tsp	15	tr
Gebhardt Chili Quik Seasoning	1 tsp	10	tr
Oscar Mayer Chili Con Carne Concentrate	1 oz	78	6
powder	1 tsp	8	tr
FROZEN			
Swanson Homestyle Chili Con Carne	8.25 oz	270	10
TAKE-OUT			
con carne w/ beans	8.9 oz	254	8

CHINESE CABBAGE
(see CABBAGE)

CHINESE FOOD
(see ORIENTAL FOOD)

CHINESE PRESERVING MELON

cooked	½ cup	11	tr

CHIPS
(see also POPCORN, PRETZELS, SNACKS)

CORN			
Arrowhead			
Blue Corn Curls	1 oz	120	2
Blue Corn Curls Unsalted	1 oz	120	2
Yellow Corn Chips	¾ oz	90	1
Yellow Corn Chips w/ Cheese	¾ oz	90	2

FOOD	PORTION	CALORIES	FAT
Health Valley	1 oz	160	11
Health Valley No Salt Added	1 oz	160	11
Health Valley w/ Cheddar Cheese	1 oz	160	10
Lance	1 pkg (1.75 oz)	260	17
Lance BBQ	1 pkg (1.75 oz)	280	16
Weight Watchers Corn Snacker	½ oz	60	2
Weight Watchers Corn Snackers Nacho Cheese	½ oz	60	2
Wise			
Corn Crunchies	1 oz	160	10
Crispy Corn Chips	1 oz	160	10
Crispy Corn Chips Nacho Cheese	1 oz	160	10
POTATO			
Cottage Fries No Salt Added	1 oz	160	11
Eagle	1 oz	150	10
Health Valley			
Country Ripple	1 oz	160	10
Country Ripple No Salt Added	1 oz	160	10
Dip Chips	1 oz	160	10
Dip Chips No Salt Added	1 oz	160	10
Natural	1 oz	160	10
Natural No Salt Added	1 oz	160	10
Kelly's			
Bar-B-Q	1 oz	150	9
Crunchy	1 oz	150	9
Rippled	1 oz	150	9
Sour Cream n' Onion	1 oz	150	9
Unsalted	1 oz	150	10
Lance			
BBQ	1 pkg (1⅛ oz)	190	12
Cajun Style	1 pkg (1 oz)	160	10

FOOD	PORTION	CALORIES	FAT
Lance *(cont.)*			
Ripple	1 pkg (1⅛ oz)	190	15
Ripple	1 oz	160	13
Sour Cream & Onion	1 pkg (1⅛ oz)	190	12
Lay's	1 oz	150	10
Lay's Jalapeno & Cheddar	1 oz	150	9
New York Deli	1 oz	160	11
Old Dutch Foods			
Augratin	1 oz	150	8
BBQ	1 oz	140	8
Dill Flavored	1 oz	150	8
Onion & Garlic	1 oz	150	9
Ripple	1 oz	150	9
Sour Cream & Onion	1 oz	150	10
Pringle's			
Butter 'n Herbs	1 oz	170	13
Cheez-ums	1 oz	170	13
Idaho Rippled	1 oz	170	12
Idaho Rippled French Onion	1 oz	170	12
Idaho Rippled Taco 'n Cheddar	1 oz	170	12
Light	1 oz	150	8
Light B-B-Q	1 oz	150	8
Rippled	1 oz	170	12
Sour Cream & Onion	1 oz	170	12
Ripple Sour Cream & Onion	1 oz	170	11
Ruffles	1 oz	150	10
Ruffles Bar-B-Q	1 oz	150	9
Ruffles Sour Cream & Onion	1 oz	150	9
Weight Watchers			
Great Snackers Barbecue	½ oz	70	3

FOOD	PORTION	CALORIES	FAT
Great Snackers Cheddar Cheese	½ oz	70	3
Great Snackers Sour Cream & Onion	½ oz	70	3
Wise Natural	1 oz	160	11
Wise Ripple Barbecue	1 oz	150	10
potato	10 chips	105	7
potato	1 oz	148	10
sticks	1 oz pkg	148	10
sticks	½ cup	94	6
TORTILLA			
Doritos	1 oz	140	6
Doritos Cool Ranch	1 oz	140	7
Doritos Nacho Cheese	1 oz	140	7
La FAMOUS	1 oz	140	7
La FAMOUS No Salt Added	1 oz	140	7
Lance Jalapeno Cheese	1 pkg (1⅛ oz)	160	8
Lance Nacho	1 pkg (1⅛ oz)	160	8
Wise Bravos	1 oz	150	8

CHITTERLINGS

pork, simmered	3 oz	258	24

CHIVES

fresh, chopped	1 tbsp	1	tr
fresh, chopped	1 tsp	0	tr
freeze-dried	1 tbsp	1	tr

CHOCOLATE
(see also CANDY, CAROB, COCOA, ICE CREAM TOPPINGS, MILK DRINKS)

BAKING			
German Sweet (Bakers)	1 oz	144	10

FOOD	PORTION	CALORIES	FAT
Premium Baking Bar Semi-Sweet (Hershey)	1 oz	140	8
Premium Baking Bar Unsweetened (Hershey)	1 oz	190	16
Semi-Sweet (Bakers)	1 oz	136	9
Unsweetened (Bakers)	1 oz	142	15
baking	1 oz	145	15
CHIPS			
Chocolate Flavored Chips (Bakers)	¼ cup	196	9
German Sweet Chocolate Chips (Bakers)	¼ cup	203	12
Milk Chocolate Chips (Hershey)	1 oz	150	12
Milk Chocolate Chunks (Hershey)	1 oz	160	9
Mint Chocolate Chips (Hershey)	¼ cup	230	12
Real Semi-Sweet Chocolate Chips (Bakers)	¼ cup	201	12
Semi-Sweet Chocolate Chips, Miniature (Hershey)	¼ cup	220	12
Semi-Sweet Chocolate Chips, Regular (Hershey)	¼ cup	220	12
Semi-Sweet Chunks (Hershey)	1 oz	140	8
Vanilla Milk Chips (Hershey)	¼ cup	240	14
MIX			
Hershey Chocolate Milk Mix	3 tbsp	90	4
powder	2–3 heaping tsp	75	1
powder, as prep w/ whole milk	9 oz	226	9
SYRUP			
Estee	1 tbsp	20	tr
Hershey's	2 tbsp	80	1
chocolate	1 cup	653	3
chocolate	2 tbsp	82	tr
chocolate, as prep w/ whole milk	9 oz	232	9

FOOD	PORTION	CALORIES	FAT

CHOCOLATE MILK
(*see* CHOCOLATE, COCOA, MILK DRINKS)

CHUTNEY

apple	1.2 oz	68	0
apple cranberry	1 tbsp	16	0
tomato	1.2 oz	54	0

CILANTRO

fresh	¼ cup	1	tr

CINNAMON

ground	1 tsp	6	tr

CISCO

fresh, raw	3 oz	84	2
smoked	3 oz	151	10
smoked	1 oz	50	3

CLAMS

CANNED

Chopped Clams Liquid & Solids (Doxsee)	6.5 oz	90	tr
Clam Juice (Doxsee)	3 oz	4	0
Fancy Chopped Clams (S&W)	2 oz	28	0
Fancy Minced Clams (S&W)	2 oz	28	0
Minced & Chopped Clams (Gorton's)	½ can	70	1
Minced Clams Liquid & Solids (Snow's)	6.5 oz	90	tr
Quahogs (American Original Foods)	4 oz	66	tr
Whole Baby (Empress)	4 oz	60	1

FOOD	PORTION	CALORIES	FAT
Whole Baby Chowder Clams (S&W)	2 oz	33	0
liquid only	3 oz	2	tr
liquid only	1 cup	6	tr
meat only	3 oz	126	2
meat only	1 cup	236	3
FRESH			
cooked	3 oz	126	2
cooked	20 sm	133	2
raw	20 sm	133	2
raw	9 lg	133	2
raw	3 oz	63	1
FROZEN			
Breaded Clams (Van De Kamp's)	2.25 oz	210	11
Fried (Mrs. Paul's)	2.5 oz	200	9
Microwave Chrunchy Clam Strips (Gorton's)	3.5 oz	330	22
Microwave Fried Clams (Mrs. Paul's)	2.5 oz	260	15
HOME RECIPE			
breaded & fried	20 sm	379	21
breaded & fried	3 oz	171	9
TAKE-OUT			
breaded & fried	¾ cup	451	26

CLOVES

ground	1 tsp	7	tr

COCOA
(*see also* CHOCOLATE)

Carnation Hot Cocoa 70 Calorie	3 tsp (21 g)	70	tr

FOOD	PORTION	CALORIES	FAT
Carnation Hot Cocoa Milk Chocolate	1 pkg or 4 heaping tsp (1 oz)	110	1
Carnation Hot Cocoa Natural Mint	1 pkg or 4 heaping tsp	110	1
Carnation Hot Cocoa Rich Chocolate	1 pkg or 4 heaping tsp	110	1
Carnation Hot Cocoa Rich Chocolate w/ Marshmallows	1 pkg or 4 heaping tsp	110	1
Carnation Hot Cocoa Sugar Free Mint	1 pkg or 4 heaping tsp	50	tr
Carnation Hot Cocoa Sugar Free Rich Chocolate	1 pkg or 4 heaping tsp	50	tr
Hershey's Cocoa	⅓ cup	120	4
Hershey's European Cocoa	1 oz	90	3
Hills Bros. Hot Cocoa Sugar Free, as prep w/ water	6 oz	60	2
Hills Bros. Hot Cocoa, as prep w/ water	6 oz	110	2
Nestle Hot Cocoa Mix	1 oz	110	1
Nestle Hot Cocoa Mix, as prep w/ 2% milk	6 oz	210	5
Nestle Hot Cocoa Mix, as prep w/ skim milk	6 oz	180	1
Nestle Hot Cocoa Mix, as prep w/ whole milk	6 oz	230	8
Nestle Hot Cocoa Mix w/ Marshmallows	1 oz	120	1
Nestle Hot Cocoa Mix w/ Marshmallows, as prep w/ 2% milk	6 oz	220	5
Nestle Hot Cocoa Mix w/ Marshmallows, as prep w/ skim milk	6 oz	190	1
Nestle Hot Cocoa Mix w/ Marshmallows, as prep w/ whole milk	6 oz	240	8

FOOD	PORTION	CALORIES	FAT
Swiss Miss Cocoa Diet, as prep	4 oz	20	tr
Swiss Miss Cocoa Lite, as prep	6 oz	70	tr
Swiss Miss Cocoa Sugar Free, as prep	6 oz	60	tr
Swiss Miss Cocoa Sugar Free w/ Sugar Free Marshmallows, as prep	6 oz	50	tr
Swiss Miss Hot Cocoa Bavarian Chocolate, as prep	6 oz	110	3
Swiss Miss Hot Cocoa Double Rich, as prep	4 oz	110	1
Swiss Miss Hot Cocoa Milk Chocolate, as prep	6 oz	110	1
Swiss Miss Hot Cocoa w/ Mini Marshmallows, as prep	4 oz	110	1
Weight Watchers	1 pkg	60	0
hot cocoa	1 cup	218	9
mix, as prep w/ water	7 oz	103	1
mix w/ Nutrasweet, as prep w/ water	7 oz	48	tr
powder	1 oz	102	1

COCONUT

FOOD	PORTION	CALORIES	FAT
Angel Flake Bag (Bakers)	⅓ cup	116	8
Angel Flake Can (Bakers)	⅓ cup	114	9
Cream of Coconut (Coco Lopez)	2 tbsp	120	5
Premium Shred (Bakers)	⅓ cup	136	10
coconut water	1 cup	46	tr
coconut water	1 tbsp	3	tr
cream, canned	1 cup	568	52
cream, canned	1 tbsp	36	3
dried, sweetened, flaked	7 oz pkg	944	64
dried, sweetened, flaked	1 cup	351	24
dried, sweetened, flaked, canned	1 cup	341	24

FOOD	PORTION	CALORIES	FAT
dried, sweetened, shredded	1 cup	466	33
dried, sweetened, shredded	7 oz pkg	997	71
dried, toasted	1 oz	168	13
dried, unsweetened	1 oz	187	18
fresh	1 piece (1.5 oz)	159	15
fresh, shredded	1 cup	283	27
milk, canned	1 cup	445	48
milk, canned	1 tbsp	30	3
milk, frozen	1 cup	486	50
milk, frozen	1 tbsp	30	3

COD

CANNED

atlantic	3 oz	89	1
atlantic	1 can (11 oz)	327	3

DRIED

atlantic	3 oz	246	2

FRESH

atlantic, cooked	1 fillet (6.3 oz)	189	2
atlantic, cooked	3 oz	89	1
pacific, baked	3 oz	95	1
roe, raw	3.5 oz	130	2

FROZEN

Fishmarket Fresh (Gorton's)	5 oz	110	1
Light Fillets (Mrs. Paul's)	1 fillet	240	11
Lightly Breaded Cod (Van De Kamp's)	1 piece	290	19
Microwave Lightly Breaded Cod (Van De Kamp's)	5 oz	290	19
Today's Catch Cod (Van De Kamp's)	5 oz	110	0

FOOD	PORTION	CALORIES	FAT

COFFEE
(see also COFFEE BEVERAGES, COFFEE SUBSTITUTES)

INSTANT

Kava	1 tsp	2	0
cappuccino mix, as prep w/ water	7 oz	62	2
decaffeinated	1 rounded tsp	4	0
decaffeinated, as prep w/ water	6 oz	4	0
fresh mix, as prep w/ water	7 oz	57	3
mocha mix, as prep w/ water	7 oz	51	2
regular	1 rounded tsp	4	0
regular, as prep w/ water	6 oz	4	0
regular w/ chicory	1 rounded tsp	6	0
regular w/ chicory, as prep w/ water	6 oz	6	0

REGULAR

brewed	6 oz	4	0

COFFEE BEVERAGES
(see also COFFEE SUBSTITUTES)

Chock O'ccino Cinnamon	8 oz	120	2
Chock O'ccino Coffee	8 oz	120	2
Chock O'ccino Mocha	8 oz	120	2
International Coffee (General Foods)			
Cafe Amaretto	6 oz	51	3
Cafe Francais	6 oz	55	3
Cafe Irish Creme	6 oz	55	3
Cafe Vienna	6 oz	59	2
Irish Mocha Mint	6 oz	51	2
Orange Cappuccino	6 oz	59	10
Sugar Free Cafe Francais	6 oz	35	2
Sugar Free Cafe Irish Creme	6 oz	31	3

FOOD	PORTION	CALORIES	FAT
Sugar Free Cafe Vienna	6 oz	29	3
Sugar Free Irish Mocha Mint	6 oz	28	2
Sugar Free Orange Cappuccino	6 oz	29	2
Sugar Free Suisse Mocha	6 oz	29	2
Suisse Mocha	6 oz	53	3

COFFEE SUBSTITUTES

Postum Instant, as prep	6 oz	11	tr
Postum Instant Coffee Flavored, as prep	6 oz	11	tr
powder	1 tsp	9	tr
powder, as prep w/ milk	6 oz	121	6
powder, as prep w/ water	6 oz	9	tr

COFFEE WHITENERS
(*see also* MILK SUBSTITUTES)

LIQUID

Coffee Rich	1 tbsp	20	2
Coffee-Mate	1 oz	31	2
Grand Union	1 tbsp	24	2
nondairy, frzn	1 tbsp	20	2

POWDER

Coffee-Mate	1 pkg (3 g)	16	tr
Coffee-Mate	1 tsp	10	tr
Cremora	1 tsp	12	1
N-Rich Creamer	1 tsp	10	tr
Weight Watchers Dairy Creamer Instant Non-fat Dry Milk	1 pkg	10	0
nondairy	1 tsp	11	tr

FOOD	PORTION	CALORIES	FAT

COLLARDS

FOOD	PORTION	CALORIES	FAT
fresh, cooked	½ cup	17	tr
fresh, raw, chopped	½ cup	6	tr
frozen, chopped, cooked	½ cup	31	tr

COOKIES

(*see also* BROWNIE, CAKE, DOUGHNUT, PIE)

FOOD	PORTION	CALORIES	FAT
HOME RECIPE			
chocolate chip	4 (1.5 oz)	185	11
peanut butter	4 (1.7 oz)	245	14
shortbread	2 (1 oz)	145	8
MIX			
Chocolate Chip (Duncan Hines)	2	130	5
Chocolate Chip (Estee)	1	50	3
Golden Sugar (Duncan Hines)	2	130	6
Oatmeal Raisin (Duncan Hines)	2	130	6
Peanut Butter (Duncan Hines)	2	140	7
READY-TO-EAT			
7-Grain Oatmeal (Frookie)	1	45	2
Almond Crescents (Sunshine)	2	70	3
Almond Toast (Stella D'Oro)	1	56	1
Almost Home Oatmeal Raisin (Nabisco)	1	70	3
Almost Home Real Chocolate Chip (Nabisco)	1	60	3
Aloha (LU)	1	75	5
Amaranth (Health Valley)	1	70	3
Amaretti (Stella D'Oro)	1	28	5
Angel Bars (Stella D'Oro)	1	74	5
Angel Puffs (Stella D'Oro)	1	13	tr

FOOD	PORTION	CALORIES	FAT
Angel Wings (Stella D'Oro)	1	74	5
Angelica Goodies (Stella D'Oro)	1	104	4
Anginetti (Stella D'Oro)	1	30	1
Animal Crackers (FFV)	9	110	3
Animal Crackers (Sunshine)	7	70	2
Animal Crackers Barnum's (Nabisco)	5	60	2
Animal Frackers (Frookie)	6	60	2
Anisette Sponge (Stella D'Oro)	1	52	tr
Anisette Toast (Stella D'Oro)	1	46	tr
Anisette Toast Jumbo (Stella D'Oro)	1	109	1
Apple Cinnamon Oat Bran (Frookie)	1 lg	120	4
Apple Cinnamon Oat Bran (Frookie)	1	45	2
Apple Cinnamon (Lance)	1 pkg (1 oz)	120	5
Apple Fruitins (Frookie)	1	60	1
Apple Oatmeal Bar (Lance)	1 pkg (1.65 oz)	190	7
Apple Pastry Dietetic (Stella D'Oro)	1	90	4
Apple Raisin Bar (Weight Watchers)	1	100	3
Arrowroot Biscuit National (Nabisco)	1	20	1
Baked Apple Bar (Sunbelt)	1 pkg (1.31 oz)	130	2
Bakers Bonus Oatmeal (Nabisco)	1	80	3
Barre Chocolat (LU)	1	65	3
Bavarian Fingers (Sunshine)	1	70	3
Beacon Hill Chocolate Chocolate Walnut (Pepperidge Farm)	1	120	7
Biscos Sugar Wafers (Nabisco)	4	70	3
Biscos Waffle Cremes (Nabisco)	1	40	2
Blueberry (Lance)	1 pkg (1 oz)	120	4
Bonnie (Lance)	1 pkg (¾ oz)	100	4
Bordeaux (Pepperidge Farm)	2	70	3
Breakfast Treats (Stella D'Oro)	1	102	4

FOOD	PORTION	CALORIES	FAT
Brown Edge Wafers (Nabisco)	2½	70	2
Brownie Chocolate Nut (Pepperidge Farm)	2	110	7
Brownie Nut Large Cookie (Pepperidge Farm)	1	140	8
Brussels (Pepperidge Farm)	2	110	5
Brussels Mint (Pepperidge Farm)	2	130	7
Bugs Bunny Graham (Nabisco)	5	60	2
Butter Chessman (Pepperidge Farm)	2	90	4
Butter Flavored (Sunshine)	2	60	2
Buttercup (Keebler)	3	70	3
Cappucino (Pepperidge Farm)	1	50	3
Capri (Pepperidge Farm)	1	80	5
Caramel Patties (FFV)	2	150	7
Champagne (Pepperidge Farm)	2	110	6
Chantilly (Pepperidge Farm)	1	80	2
Chesapeake Chocolate Chunk Pecan (Pepperidge Farm)	1	120	7
Cheyenne Peanut Butter Milk Chocolate Chunk (Pepperidge Farm)	1	110	6
Chinese Dessert (Stella D'Oro)	1	172	9
Chip-A-Roos (Sunshine)	1	60	3
Chips Ahoy! (Nabisco)			
Chewy	1	60	3
Chocolate Chocolate Chunk	1	90	5
Chocolate Chocolate Walnut	1	100	6
Chocolate Chunk Pecan	1	100	6
Chunky Chocolate Chip	1	90	5
Mini	6	70	3
Oatmeal Chocolate Chip	1	90	5
Pure Chocolate Chip	1	50	2

FOOD	PORTION	CALORIES	FAT
Sprinkled	1	60	3
Striped	1	90	5
Chips Chocolat (LU)	1	85	5
Chocolate (Weight Watchers)	3	80	3
Chocolate Chip (Archway)	1	60	3
Chocolate Chip (Drake's)	2 (1 oz)	140	6
Chocolate Chip (Duncan Hines)	2	110	5
Chocolate Chip (Frookie)	1	45	2
Chocolate Chip (Frookie)	1 lg	120	4
Chocolate Chip (Lance)	1 pkg (1 oz)	135	7
Chocolate Chip (Nutra/Balance)	1 (2 oz)	260	14
Chocolate Chip (Pepperidge Farm)	2	100	5
Chocolate Chip (Weight Watchers)	2	90	2
Chocolate Chip Fudge (Lance)	1 pkg (1 oz)	130	5
Chocolate Chip Large (Pepperidge Farm)	1	130	6
Chocolate Chip Mint (Frookie)	1	45	2
Chocolate Chip Snaps (Nabisco)	3	70	2
Chocolate Chocolate Chip (Drake's)	2 (1 oz)	130	5
Chocolate Chunk Pecan (Pepperidge Farm)	1	70	4
Chocolate Cookiesaurus (Sunshine)	7	120	5
Chocolate Fudge Sandwich (Keebler)	1	80	4
Chocolate Laced Pirouettes (Pepperidge Farm)	2	70	4
Chocolate Sandwich (Weight Watchers)	2	90	3
Chocolate Snaps (Nabisco)	4	70	2
Chocolu (LU)	1	55	3
Choc-O-Lunch (Lance)	1 oz	130	5
Choc-O-Mint (Lance)	1.25 oz	180	10

FOOD	PORTION	CALORIES	FAT
Coated Graham (Lance)	1.31 oz	180	9
Coconut (Drake's)	2 (1 oz)	130	5
Coconut Dietetic (Stella D'Oro)	1	50	2
Coconut Macaroons (Drake's)	1 (1 oz)	135	7
Coconut Macaroons (Stella D'Oro)	1	63	4
Commodore (Keebler)	1	60	2
Como Delight (Stella D'Oro)	1	141	7
Cookie Break (Nabisco)	1	50	2
Cookie Caramel Bars (Little Debbie)	1 pkg (1.17 oz)	170	8
Cookie Mates (Keebler)	2	50	2
Cookie 'N Fudge Party Grahams (Nabisco)	1	45	2
Cookies 'N Fudge Striped Shortbread (Nabisco)	1	60	3
Cookies 'N Fudge Striped Wafers (Nabisco)	1	70	4
Craquelin (LU)	1	55	3
Creme Filled Chocolate (Little Debbie)	1 pkg (1.8 oz)	250	12
Creme Filled Wafers Assorted (Estee)	1	30	2
Creme Filled Wafers Chocolate (Estee)	1	20	1
Creme Filled Wafers Vanilla (Estee)	1	20	1
Crokine (LU)	2	19	0
Dakota Milk Chocolate Oatmeal (Pepperidge Farm)	1	110	6
Date Pecan (Pepperidge Farm)	2	110	5
Devil's Food Cakes (Nabisco)	1	70	1
Dinosaur Grrrahams (Mother's)	1	70	2
Dixi Vanilla (Sunshine)	2	130	5
Egg Biscuits (Stella D'Oro)	1	43	1

FOOD	PORTION	CALORIES	FAT
Egg Biscuits Dietetic (Stella D'Oro)	1	40	1
Egg Jumbo (Stella D'Oro)	1	46	tr
Euphrates (LU)	2	40	2
Famous Chocolate Wafers (Nabisco)	2	70	2
Fancy Fruit Chunks (Health Valley)			
Apricot Almond	2	90	4
Date Pecan	2	90	4
Raisin Oat Bran	2	70	2
Tropical Fruit	2	90	3
Fancy Peanut Chunks (Health Valley)	2	90	3
Fat Free (Health Valley)			
Apple Spice	3	75	tr
Apricot Delight	3	75	tr
Date Delight	3	75	tr
Hawaiian Fruit	3	75	tr
Jumbos Apple Raisin	1	70	tr
Jumbos Raisin	1	70	tr
Jumbos Raspberry	1	70	tr
Raisin Oatmeal	3	75	tr
Fiber Jumbos Blueberry Nut (Health Valley)	1	100	3
Fiber Jumbos Chunky Pecan (Health Valley)	1	100	3
Fiber Jumbos Raisin Nut (Health Valley)	1	100	3
Fig Bar (Lance)	1.5 oz	150	2
Fig Bar (Mother's)	1 oz	100	2
Fig Bars (Sunshine)	1	50	1
Fig Fruitins (Frookie)	1	60	1
Fig Newtons (Nabisco)	1	60	1
Fig Pastry Dietetic (Stella D'Oro)	1	95	4

FOOD	PORTION	CALORIES	FAT
Fortune (La Choy)	1	15	tr
French Vanilla Creme (Keebler)	1	80	4
Fruit & Fitness (Health Valley)	5	200	6
Fruit Filled Apricot-Raspberry (Pepperidge Farm)	2	100	4
Fruit Filled Strawberry (Pepperidge Farm)	2	100	5
Fruit Filled Bar Apple (Weight Watchers)	1	80	tr
Fruit Filled Bar Raspberry (Weight Watchers)	1	80	tr
Fruit Jumbos Almond Date (Health Valley)	1	70	3
Fruit Jumbos Oat Bran (Health Valley)	1	70	2
Fruit Jumbos Raisin Nut (Health Valley)	1	70	3
Fruit Jumbos Tropical Fruit (Health Valley)	1	70	3
Fruit Slices (Stella D'Oro)	1	59	2
Fudge (Estee)	1	30	1
Fudge Bar (Tastykake)	1	240	8
Fudge Chips Chocolate (LU)	1	75	4
Fudge Dipped Grahams (Sunshine)	2	80	4
Fudge Family Bears Chocolate w/ Vanilla Filling (Sunshine)	1	70	3
Fudge Family Bears Peanut Butter (Sunshine)	1	70	3
Fudge Family Bears Vanilla w/ Fudge Filling (Sunshine)	1	60	3
Fudge Striped Shortbread (Sunshine)	3	160	8
Gaufrettes (LU)	2	85	4
Geneva (Pepperidge Farm)	2	130	6

FOOD	PORTION	CALORIES	FAT
Ginger Boys Calcium Enriched (FFV)	6	120	3
Ginger Snaps (Bakery Wagon)	4–5 (1 oz)	140	6
Ginger Snaps (Sunshine)	3	60	2
Ginger Snaps Old Fashioned (Nabisco)	2	60	1
Ginger Spice (Frookie)	1	45	2
Gingerman (Pepperidge Farm)	2	70	3
Gingersnaps (Archway)	1	35	1
Golden Bars (Stella D'Oro)	1	111	5
Golden Fruit (Sunshine)	1	70	1
Graham (Nabisco)	2	60	1
Graham Amaranth (Health Valley)	7	110	3
Graham Chocolate (Nabisco)	1	50	3
Graham Honey (Health Valley)	7	100	4
Graham Honey (Honey Maid)	2	60	1
Graham Honey Fiber Enriched (Keebler)	2	90	2
Graham Kitchen Rich (Keebler)	2	60	2
Graham Oat Bran (Health Valley)	7	120	3
Grahamy Bears (Sunshine)	4	60	2
Hazelnut (Pepperidge Farm)	2	110	6
Hermit (Drake's)	1 (2 oz)	230	7
Heyday Caramel & Peanut (Nabisco)	1	110	6
Heyday Fudge (Nabisco)	1	110	6
Holiday Trinkets (Stella D'Oro)	1	37	2
Homeplate (Keebler)	1	60	2
Honey Jumbos Crisp Cinnamon (Health Valley)	1	70	4
Honey Jumbos Crisp Peanut Butter (Health Valley)	1	70	2

FOOD	PORTION	CALORIES	FAT
Honey Jumbos Fancy Oat Bran (Health Valley)	2	130	4
Hostess Assortment (Stella D'Oro)	1	41	2
Hydrox	1	50	2
Hydrox Doubles Peanut Butter	1	60	2
Iced Gingerbread (Sunshine)	3	70	3
Ideal Bars (Nabisco)	1	90	5
Irish Oatmeal (Pepperidge Farm)	2	90	5
Jelly Tarts (FFV)	2	110	4
Jingles (Sunshine)	3	70	3
Keebies (Keebler)	1	80	3
Kichel Dietetic (Stella D'Oro)	1	8	tr
Krisp Kreem Wafers (Keebler)	2	50	3
Lady Stella Assortment (Stella D'Oro)	1	42	2
Lemon Coolers (Sunshine)	2	60	2
Lemon Nut Crunch (Pepperidge Farm)	2	110	7
Le Petit-Beurre (LU)	1	40	1
Lido (Pepperidge Farm)	1	90	5
Linzer (Pepperidge Farm)	1	120	4
Little Schoolboy (LU)	1	65	3
Lorna Doone	2	70	4
Love Cookies Dietetic (Stella D'Oro)	1	110	6
Mallomars	1	60	3
Mallopuffs (Sunshine)	1	70	2
Malt (Lance)	1.25 oz	190	10
Mandarin Chocolate Chip (Frookie)	1	45	2
Margherite Chocolate (Stella D'Oro)	1	73	3
Margherite Vanilla (Stella D'Oro)	1	72	3
Marie LU (LU)	1	50	2

FOOD	PORTION	CALORIES	FAT
Marshmallow Puffs (Nabisco)	1	90	4
Marshmallow Twirls (Nabisco)	1	130	5
Milano (Pepperidge Farm)	2	120	6
Milk Chocolate Chip (Duncan Hines)	2	110	5
Milk Chocolate Macadamia (Pepperidge Farm)	2	140	8
Milk Lunch (LU)	1	35	1
Mini Chocolate Chip (Sunshine)	2	70	4
Mint Milano (Pepperidge Farm)	2	150	7
Mint Sandwich (FFV)	2	160	7
Molasses (Archway)	1	100	2
Molasses Crisps (Pepperidge Farm)	2	70	3
Molasses Iced (Bakery Wagon)	1	100	4
My Goodness Banana Nut (Nabisco)	1	90	3
My Goodness Chocolate Chip & Raisin (Nabisco)	1	90	3
My Goodness Oatmeal Raisin (Nabisco)	1	90	3
Mystic Mint	1	90	5
Nantucket Chocolate Chunk (Pepperidge Farm)	1	120	6
Nassau (Pepperidge Farm)	1	80	5
Newtons Apple (Nabisco)	1	70	2
Newtons Raspberry (Nabisco)	1	70	2
Newtons Strawberry (Nabisco)	1	70	2
Nilla Wafers (Nabisco)	3	60	2
Nut-O-Lunch (Lance)	1 oz	140	5
Nutter Butter Peanut Butter (Nabisco)	1	70	3
Nutter Butter Peanut Creme (Nabisco)	2	80	4
Oat Bran Animal (Health Valley)	7	110	4

FOOD	PORTION	CALORIES	FAT
Oat Bran Fruit & Nut (Health Valley)	2	110	4
Oat Bran Muffin (Frookie)	1	45	2
Oat Bran Muffin (Frookie)	1 lg	120	4
Oat Bran w/ Nuts & Raisins (Sunshine)	1	60	3
Oatmeal (Archway)	1	110	3
Oatmeal (Drake's)	2 (1 oz)	120	5
Oatmeal (Lance)	1 pkg (1 oz)	130	5
Oatmeal (Little Debbie)	1 pkg (2.75 oz)	340	12
Oatmeal (Mother's)	1	60	3
Oatmeal Apple Filled (Archway)	1	90	1
Oatmeal Calcium Enriched (FFV)	5	130	5
Oatmeal Country Style (Sunshine)	1	70	3
Oatmeal Creme (Drake's)	1 (2 oz)	240	9
Oatmeal Date Filled (Archway)	1	100	2
Oatmeal Date Filled (Bakery Wagon)	1	90	3
Oatmeal Large (Pepperidge Farm)	1	120	6
Oatmeal Raisin (Duncan Hines)	2	110	5
Oatmeal Raisin (Frookie)	1	45	2
Oatmeal Raisin (Frookie)	1 lg	120	4
Oatmeal Raisin (Nutra/Balance)	1 (2 oz)	240	9
Oatmeal Raisin (Pepperidge Farm)	2	110	5
Oatmeal Raisin (Weight Watchers)	2	90	tr
Oatmeal Raisin Bar (Tastykake)	1	224	8
Oatmeal Soft (Bakery Wagon)	1	100	5
Oatmeal Spice (Weight Watchers)	3	80	2
Old Fashion Chocolate Chip (Keebler)	1	80	4
Old Fashion Double Fudge (Keebler)	1	80	4
Old Fashion Oatmeal (Keebler)	1	80	4
Old Fashion Peanut Butter (Keebler)	1	80	4

FOOD	PORTION	CALORIES	FAT
Old Fashion Sugar (Keebler)	1	80	3
Old Fashioned Chocolate Chip (Pepperidge Farm)	2	100	5
Orange Milano (Pepperidge Farm)	2	150	7
Oreo	1	50	2
Oreo Big Stuf	1	200	9
Oreo Double Stuf	1	70	4
Oreo Fudge Covered	1	110	6
Oreo Mini	5	70	3
Oreo White Fudge Covered	1	110	6
Original Pirouettes (Pepperidge Farm)	2	70	4
Orleans (Pepperidge Farm)	3	90	6
Orleans Sandwich (Pepperidge Farm)	2	120	8
Palmito (LU)	1	50	3
Pantry Molasses (Nabisco)	1	80	3
Paris (Pepperidge Farm)	2	100	5
Peacan Shortbread (Nabisco)	1	80	5
Peach-Apricot Pastry (Stella D'Oro)	1	96	4
Peach-Apricot Pastry Dietetic (Stella D'Oro)	1	90	4
Peanut Butter & Jelly Sandwiches (Little Debbie)	1 pkg (1.13 oz)	150	7
Peanut Butter Bars (Little Debbie)	1 pkg (1.83 oz)	290	18
Peanut Butter Creme Filled Wafer (Lance)	1 pkg (1.75 oz)	240	10
Peanut Butter Naturals (Sunbelt)	1 pkg (1.2 oz)	170	10
Peanut Butter Sandwich (FFV)	2	170	8
Peanut Butter Wafers (Drake's)	1 (2.25 oz)	324	16
Peanut Clusters (Little Debbie)	1 pkg (1.44 oz)	210	11
Pecan Crunch (Archway)	1	35	1

FOOD	PORTION	CALORIES	FAT
Pecan Shortbread (Pepperidge Farm)	1	70	5
Pfeffernusse (Stella D'Oro)	1	34	tr
Pims (LU)	1	50	1
Pinwheels (Nabisco)	1	130	5
Pitter Patter (Keebler)	1	90	4
Prune Pastry Dietetic (Stella D'Oro)	1	90	4
Pure Chocolate Middles (Nabisco)	1	80	5
Raisin Bran (Pepperidge Farm)	2	110	5
Raisin Oatmeal (Archway)	1	35	1
Regal Grahams (FFV)	2	140	7
Roman Egg Biscuits Anise (Stella D'Oro)	1	138	5
Roman Egg Biscuits Rum & Brandy (Stella D'Oro)	1	138	5
Roman Egg Biscuits Vanilla (Stella D'Oro)	1	138	5
Royal Dainty (FFV)	2	120	6
Royal Nuggets Dietetic (Stella D'Oro)	1	1	tr
Sandwich Cookies Chocolate (Estee)	1	50	2
Sandwich Cookies Original (Estee)	1	45	2
Sandwich Cookies Peanut Butter (Estee)	1	50	3
Sante Fe Oatmeal Raisin (Pepperidge Farm)	1	100	4
Sausalito Milk Chocolate Macadamia (Pepperidge Farm)	1	120	7
Schoks-Chocolate (LU)	1	70	4
School House (Sunshine)	15	120	4
Sea Flappers (Sunshine)	7	140	6
Select Assortment (Archway)	1	60	2
Sesame (Stella D'Oro)	1	48	2
Sesame Dietetic (Stella D'Oro)	1	43	2

FOOD	PORTION	CALORIES	FAT
Seville (Pepperidge Farm)	2	100	5
Shortbread (Pepperidge Farm)	2	150	8
Shortbread (Weight Watchers)	3	80	2
Snack Wafer Chocolate (Estee)	1	80	4
Snack Wafer Chocolate Coated (Estee)	1	130	7
Snack Wafer Strawberry (Estee)	1	80	4
Snack Wafer Vanilla (Estee)	1	80	4
Social Tea (Nabisco)	3	70	2
Soft'n Chewy Chocolate Chip (Tastykake)	1	188	8
Soft'n Chewy Chocolate Chocolate Chip (Tastykake)	1	199	7
Soft'n Chewy Oatmeal Raisin (Tastykake)	1	207	8
Southport (Pepperidge Farm)	2	170	10
Sprinkles Rainbow Topping (Sunshine)	1	70	2
Strawberry (Lance)	1 pkg (1 oz)	120	4
Suddenly S'Mores (Nabisco)	1	100	4
Sugar (Pepperidge Farm)	2	100	5
Sugar Wafers Assorted (Sunshine)	2	90	4
Sugar Wafers Chocolate (Sunshine)	2	90	4
Sugar Wafers Chocolate (Tastyklake)	1 pkg	367	19
Sugar Wafers Peanut Butter (Sunshine)	2	80	4
Sugar Wafers Vanilla (Sunshine)	2	90	4
Sugar Wafers Vanilla (Tastykake)	1 pkg	366	20
Sugared Egg Biscuits (Stella D'Oro)	1	73	1
Swiss Fudge (Stella D'Oro)	1	68	3
T. C. Rounds (FFV)	2	160	8
Taffy Creme Sandwich (Mother's)	1–2 (1 oz)	140	8

FOOD	PORTION	CALORIES	FAT
Tahiti (Pepperidge Farm)	1	90	6
Tango (FFV)	2	160	5
Teddy Grahams (Nabisco)			
Bearwich Chocolate & Vanilla Creme	4	70	3
Bearwich Cinnamon & Vanilla Creme	4	70	3
Bearwich Vanilla & Chocolate Creme	4	70	3
Chocolate Graham	11	60	2
Cinnamon Graham	11	60	2
Honey Graham	11	60	2
Vanilla Graham	11	60	2
The Great Tofu (Health Valley)	2	90	3
The Great Wheat Free (Health Valley)	2	80	3
Trolley Cakes Devilsfood (FFV)	2	120	2
Tru Blu Chocolate (Sunshine)	2	160	7
Tru Blu Lemon (Sunshine)	1	70	3
Tru Blu Vanilla (Sunshine)	1	8	3
Van-O-Lunch (Lance)	1 oz	140	4
Vanilla Fig Bars (FFV)	1	60	1
Vanilla Shortbread (Tastykake)	1	57	3
Vanilla Wafers (FFV)	8	120	5
Vanilla Wafers (Keebler)	4	80	4
Vanilla Wafers (Sunshine)	3	70	3
Vienna Finger (Sunshine)	12	70	3
Whole Wheat Fig Bars (FFV)	1	60	1
Zurich (Pepperidge Farm)	1	60	2
animal crackers	1 box (2.4 oz)	299	9
chocolate chip	4 (1.5 oz)	180	9
chocolate chip	1 box (1.9 oz)	233	12

FOOD	PORTION	CALORIES	FAT
chocolate sandwich	4 (1.4 oz)	195	8
digestive biscuits, plain	2	141	7
fig bars	4 (2 oz)	210	4
graham	2 squares	60	1
oatmeal raisin	4 (1.8 oz)	245	10
shortbread	4 (1 oz)	155	8
vanilla sandwich	4 (1.4 oz)	195	8
vanilla wafers	10 (1.25 oz)	185	7
REFRIGERATED			
Chocolate Chip (Pillsbury)	1	70	3
Oatmeal Raisin (Pillsbury)	1	60	2
Peanut Butter (Pillsbury)	1	70	3
Sugar (Pillsbury)	1	70	3
chocolate chip	4 (1.7 oz)	225	11
sugar	4 (1.7 oz)	235	12

CORIANDER

FOOD	PORTION	CALORIES	FAT
leaf, dried	1 tsp	2	tr
leaf, fresh	¼ cup	1	tr
seed	1 tsp	5	tr

CORN
(*see also* BRAN, CEREAL, CORNMEAL, FLOUR)

FOOD	PORTION	CALORIES	FAT
CANNED			
50% Less Salt No Sugar Added (Green Giant)	½ cup	50	1
Corn (Green Giant)	½ cup	70	0
Cream Style (Green Giant)	½ cup	100	tr
Cream Style (Libby)	½ cup	80	0
Cream Style (Owatonna)	½ cup	100	1

FOOD	PORTION	CALORIES	FAT
Cream Style, Diet (S&W)	½ cup	100	1
Cream Style Premium Homestyle (S&W)	½ cup	105	1
Deli Corn (Green Giant)	½ cup	80	tr
Golden Kernel 50% Less Salt (Green Giant)	½ cup	70	tr
Golden Vacuum Packed (Green Giant)	½ cup	80	0
Mexi Corn (Green Giant)	½ cup	80	tr
No Salt No Sugar (Green Giant)	½ cup	80	tr
Sweet 'N Natural (S&W)	½ cup	90	1
Sweet Select (Green Giant)	½ cup	60	1
White Vacuum Packed (Green Giant)	½ cup	80	0
Whole Kernel (Libby)	½ cup	80	1
Whole Kernel (Seneca)	½ cup	80	1
Whole Kernel in Brine (Owatonna)	½ cup	90	1
Whole Kernel Natural Pack (Libby)	½ cup	80	1
Whole Kernel Natural Pack (Seneca)	½ cup	80	1
Whole Kernel Tender Young (S&W)	½ cup	90	1
Whole Kernel Vacuum Pack (Owatonna)	½ cup	100	1
Whole Kernel Water Pack (S&W)	½ cup	80	1
cream style	½ cup	93	1
w/ red & green peppers	½ cup	86	1
white	½ cup	66	1
yellow	½ cup	66	1
DRIED			
Blue (Arrowhead)	2 oz	210	3
Yellow (Arrowhead)	2 oz	210	2
FRESH			
on the cob, cooked, w/ butter	1 ear	155	3

FOOD	PORTION	CALORIES	FAT
white, cooked	½ cup	89	1
yellow, cooked	1 ear (2.7 oz)	83	1
yellow, cooked	½ cup	89	1
FROZEN			
Corn Cob (Bird's Eye)	1 ear (4.4 oz)	120	tr
Cob Corn (Ore Ida)	1 ear (5.3 oz)	190	tr
Corn Cob Little Ears (Birds Eye)	2 ears (4.6 oz)	126	1
Cob Corn Mini-Gold (Ore Ida)	1 (2.65 oz)	90	tr
Corn on the Cob Natural Ears (Birds Eye)	1 ear (5.7 oz)	156	1
Cream Style (Green Giant)	½ cup	110	1
Fritters (Mrs. Paul's)	2	240	9
Harvest Fresh Niblets (Green Giant)	½ cup	80	1
Harvest Fresh White Shoepeg (Green Giant)	½ cup	90	1
In Butter Sauce (Green Giant)	½ cup	100	2
Nibblers Corn on the Cob (Green Giant)	2 ears	120	1
Niblet Ears (Green Giant)	1 ear	120	1
Niblets (Green Giant)	½ cup	90	tr
One Serve Corn on the Cob (Green Giant)	1 pkg	120	1
One Serve Niblets in Butter Sauce (Green Giant)	1 pkg	120	2
Super Sweet Nibblers Corn on the Cob (Green Giant)	2 ears	90	2
Super Sweet Niblet (Green Giant Select)	½ cup	60	1
Super Sweet Niblet Ears (Green Giant)	1 ear	90	2
White (Green Giant Select)	½ cup	90	1
White in Butter Sauce (Green Giant)	½ cup	100	2

FOOD	PORTION	CALORIES	FAT
White Shoepeg (Hanover)	½ cup	80	0
White Sweet (Hanover)	½ cup	80	0
Whole Kernel Cut (Birds Eye)	½ cup	82	tr
Whole Kernel Tendersweet (Birds Eye)	½ cup	82	tr
Yellow Sweet (Hanover)	½ cup	80	0
cooked	½ cup	67	tr
on the cob, cooked	1 ear (2.2 oz)	59	tr
SHELF STABLE Golden Whole Kernel (Pantry Express)	½ cup	60	tr
TAKE-OUT fritters	1 (1 oz)	62	2
scalloped	½ cup	258	7

CORN CHIPS
(see CHIPS)

CORNISH HENS
(see CHICKEN)

CORNMEAL

FOOD	PORTION	CALORIES	FAT
Albers White	1 oz	100	0
Albers Yellow	1 oz	100	0
Blue (Arrowhead)	2 oz	210	3
Enriched White (Aunt Jemima)	3 tbsp	102	1
Enriched White (Quaker)	3 tbsp	102	1
Enriched Yellow (Aunt Jemima)	3 tbsp	102	1
Enriched Yellow (Quaker)	3 tbsp	102	1
Hi-lysine (Arrowhead)	2 oz	210	2
Yellow (Arrowhead)	2 oz	210	2

FOOD	PORTION	CALORIES	FAT
corn crits, cooked	1 cup	146	tr
corn grits, uncooked	1 cup	579	2
degermed	1 cup	506	2
self-rising, degermed	1 cup	489	2
whole grain	1 cup	442	4
MIX			
Bolted White (Aunt Jemima)	3 tbsp	99	1
Buttermilk Self-Rising White (Aunt Jemima)	3 tbsp	101	1
Corn Bread (Arrowhead)	1 oz	100	1
Corny Dog Batter (Golden Dipt)	1 oz	100	0
Hush Puppy Deluxe (Golden Dipt)	1.25 oz	120	0
Hush Puppy w/ Onion (Golden Dipt)	1.25 oz	120	0
Jalapeno Hush Puppy (Golden Dipt)	1.25 oz	120	0
Self-Rising White (Aunt Jemina)	3 tbsp	98	1
Self-Rising White Enriched Bolted (Aunt Jemina)	3 tbsp	99	1
Self-Rising Yellow (Aunt Jemima)	3 tbsp	100	1

CORNSALAD

raw	1 cup	12	tr

CORNSTARCH

Argo	1 cup	460	tr
Argo	1 tbsp	30	0
Kingsford's	1 cup	460	tr
Kingsford's	1 tbsp	30	tr
cornstarch	⅓ cup	164	tr

COTTAGE CHEESE

Borden	½ cup	120	5

FOOD	PORTION	CALORIES	FAT
Borden 5% Dry Curd	½ cup	80	1
Borden Unsalted	½ cup	120	5
Breakstone 2%	4 oz	100	2
Breakstone 4% Small Curd	4 oz	110	5
Breakstone 4% w/ Pineapple	4 oz	140	5
Breakstone Dry Curd No Salt Added	4 oz	90	0
Cabot	4 oz	120	5
Cabot Light	4 oz	90	1
Formagg	1 oz	80	2
Friendship California Style	½ cup	120	5
Friendship Lactose Reduced Lowfat	½ cup	90	1
Friendship Large Curd Pot Style Lowfat	½ cup	100	2
Friendship Lowfat	½ cup	90	1
Friendship Lowfat No Salt Added	½ cup	90	1
Friendship 'N Fruit	6 oz	100	1
Friendship w/ Pineapple	½ cup	140	4
Knudsen 2%	4 oz	100	2
Knudsen 2% w/ Fruit Cocktail	4 oz	130	2
Knudsen 2% w/ Mandarin Orange	4 oz	110	2
Knudsen 2% w/ Peach	4 oz	170	2
Knudsen 2% w/ Pear	4 oz	110	2
Knudsen 2% w/ Pineapple	4 oz	170	2
Knudsen 2% w/ Spiced Apple	4 oz	180	2
Knudsen 2% w/ Strawberry	4 oz	170	2
Knudsen 4% Large Curd	4 oz	120	5
Knudsen 4% Small Curd	4 oz	120	5
Knudsen Nonfat	4 oz	90	0
Lactaid 1%	4 oz	72	1
Land O'Lakes	4 oz	120	5

FOOD	PORTION	CALORIES	FAT
Land O'Lakes 2%	4 oz	100	2
Light N'Lively 1%	4 oz	80	2
Light N'Lively 1% Garden Salad	4 oz	80	2
Light N'Lively 1% Peach & Pineapple	4 oz	100	1
Lite-Line Lowfat 1½%	½ cup	90	2
Sargento Pot Cheese	1 oz	26	tr
Sealtest 2%	4 oz	100	2
Weight Watchers 1%	½ cup	90	1
Weight Watchers 2%	½ cup	100	2
creamed	4 oz	117	5
creamed	1 cup	217	9
creamed w/ fruit	4 oz	140	4
dry curd	4 oz	96	tr
dry curd	1 cup	123	1
lowfat 1%	4 oz	82	1
lowfat 1%	1 cup	164	2
lowfat 2%	4 oz	101	2
lowfat 2%	1 cup	203	4

COTTONSEED

FOOD	PORTION	CALORIES	FAT
kernels, roasted	1 tbsp	51	4

COUSCOUS

FOOD	PORTION	CALORIES	FAT
Couscous Lemon Thyme Salad Mix, as prep (Nile Spice)	½ cup	103	5
Golden Couscous Lentil Curry Soup Mix, as prep (Nile Spice)	10 oz	220	tr
Golden Couscous Tomato Minestrone Soup Mix, as prep (Nile Spice)	10 oz	200	0
Golden Couscous Vegetable Chicken Soup Mix, as prep (Nile Spice)	10 oz	220	5

FOOD	PORTION	CALORIES	FAT
Golden Couscous Vegetable Parmesan Soup Mix, as prep (Nile Spice)	10 oz	200	3
Whole Wheat Lentil & Onion Couscous Pilaf, as prep (Nile Spice)	½ cup	153	4
cooked	½ cup	101	tr
dry	½ cup	346	tr

COWPEAS

FOOD	PORTION	CALORIES	FAT
CANNED			
common	1 cup	184	1
DRIED			
catjang, cooked	1 cup	200	1
catjang, raw	1 cup	572	3
FRESH			
leafy tips, chopped, cooked	1 cup	12	tr
leafy tips, raw, chopped	1 cup	10	tr
FROZEN			
cooked	½ cup	112	tr

CRAB

FOOD	PORTION	CALORIES	FAT
CANNED			
Dungeness Crab (S&W)	3.25 oz	81	2
blue	3 oz	84	1
blue	1 cup	133	2
FRESH			
alaska king, cooked	1 leg (4.7 oz)	129	2
alaska king, cooked	3 oz	82	1
blue, cooked	1 cup	138	2
blue, cooked	3 oz	87	2
dungeness, raw	1 crab (5.7 oz)	140	2
queen, steamed	3 oz	98	1

FOOD	PORTION	CALORIES	FAT
FROZEN			
Crab Crisp (King & Prince)	4 oz	310	19
Crab Del Rey (King & Prince)	4 oz	205	12
Deviled Crab (Mrs. Paul's)	1 cake	180	9
Deviled Crab Miniatures (Mrs. Paul's)	3.5 oz	240	12
READY-TO-USE			
crab cakes	1 cake (2.1 oz)	93	5
TAKE-OUT			
baked	1 (3.8 oz)	160	2
cake	1 (2 oz)	160	10
soft-shell, fried	1 (4.4 oz)	334	18

CRACKER CRUMBS

FOOD	PORTION	CALORIES	FAT
Corn Flake Crumbs (Kellogg's)	¼ cup (1 oz)	100	0
Cracker Meal (Golden Dipt)	1 oz	100	0
Cracker Meal (Keebler)	1 cup	100	3
Cracker Meal (Lance)	1 oz	100	1
Cracker Meal (Nabisco)	2 tbsp	50	0
Graham (Nabisco)	2 tbsp	60	1
Graham (Sunshine)	1 cup	550	14
Graham Crumbs (Keebler)	1 cup	520	14
Zesty Meal (Keebler)	1 cup	85	10

CRACKERS
(*see also* CRACKER CRUMBS)

FOOD	PORTION	CALORIES	FAT
6 Calorie Wafer (Estee)	1	6	tr
Adrienne's Gourmet Flatbread			
Caraway & Rye	2	20	tr
Classic Island	2	20	tr
Slightly Onion	2	20	tr
Ten Grain	2	20	tr

FOOD	PORTION	CALORIES	FAT
American Classic (Nabisco)			
Cracked Wheat	4	70	4
Dairy Butter	4	70	3
Golden Sesame	4	70	3
Minced Onion	4	70	3
Toasted Poppy	4	70	3
Armenian Thin Bread (Venus)	2	100	1
Bacon Flavored Thins (Nabisco)	7	70	4
Better Cheddars (Nabisco)	10	70	4
Better Cheddars Low Salt (Nabisco)	10	70	4
Bonnie (Lance)	1.2 oz	160	6
Butter Crackers (Goya)	1	40	1
Butter Thins (Pepperidge Farm)	4	70	3
Captain Wafers (Lance)	2	30	1
Captain Wafers Very Low Sodium (Lance)	2	30	1
Captain Wafers w/ Cream Cheese & Chives (Lance)	1.3 oz	170	9
Cheddar Thins (FFV)	7	70	2
Cheddar Wedges (Nabisco)	3	70	3
Cheese Crackers w/ Peanut Butter (Little Debbie)	1 pkg (1.4 oz)	210	11
Cheese-on-Wheat (Lance)	1.3 oz	180	9
Cheez-It	12	70	4
Cheez-It Low Salt	12	70	4
Cheez 'n Crackers (Handi-Snacks)	1 pkg	120	8
Cheez 'n Crackers Bacon (Handi-Snacks)	1 pkg	130	9
Chicken in a Biskit (Nabisco)	7	80	5
Club (Keebler)	2	30	2
Cracked Wheat (Pepperidge Farm)	3	100	4

FOOD	PORTION	CALORIES	FAT
Crisp Bread Dark Finn Crisp (Ryvita)	2	38	tr
Crisp Bread Dark Rye (Ryvita)	1	26	tr
Crisp Bread Dark w/ Caraway Seeds Finn Crisp (Ryvita)	2	38	tr
Crisp Bread Toasted Sesame Rye (Ryvita)	1	31	tr
Crispbread Garlic (Weight Watchers)	2	30	0
Crispy Graham (Pepperidge Farm)	4	70	2
Crown Pilot (Nabisco)	1	70	2
Double Cheddar (FFV)	7	70	2
English Water (North Castle)	1	10	0
English Water Biscuits (Pepperidge Farm)	4	70	1
Escort (Nabisco)	3	70	4
Flutters Garden Herb (Pepperidge Farm)	¾ oz	100	4
Flutters Golden Sesame (Pepperidge Farm)	¾ oz	110	5
Flutters Original Butter (Pepperidge Farm)	¾ oz	100	4
Flutters Toasted Wheat (Pepperidge Farm)	¾ oz	110	5
Garden Vegetable (Pepperidge Farm)	5	60	2
Goldfish (Pepperidge Farm)			
Cheddar Cheese	1 pkg (1.5 oz)	190	6
Cheddar Cheese	1 oz	120	4
Cheese Thins	4	50	2
Original	1 oz	130	5
Parmesan Cheese	1 oz	120	4
Pizza Flavored	1 oz	130	5
Pretzel	1 oz	110	3
Gold-N-Chee Spicy (Lance)	15	70	3

FOOD	PORTION	CALORIES	FAT
Goya Crackers	1	30	0
Ham & Cheese Crispy Wafers (FFV)	7	70	2
Harvest Crisps 5 Grain (Nabisco)	6	60	2
Harvest Crisps Oat (Nabisco)	6	60	2
Harvest Crisps Rice (Nabisco)	6	60	2
Hearty Wheat (Pepperidge Farm)	4	100	5
Herb Stoned Wheat (Health Valley)	13	55	2
Herb Stoned Wheat No Salt (Health Valley)	13	55	2
High Fiber Crisp Bread (Ryvita)	1	23	tr
Hi Ho	4	80	5
Ideal Crispbread Extra Thin	3	48	0
Ideal Crispbread Fiber Thins	2	41	1
Ideal Crispbread Oatbran Thins	2	50	0
Krispy Saltine (Sunshine)	5	60	1
Krispy Unsalted Tops (Sunshine)	5	60	1
Lanchee (Lance)	1.25 oz	180	10
Light Rye Crisp Bread (Ryvita)	1	26	tr
Light Rye Hi-Fiber Crispbread (Finn Crisp)	1	35	1
Meal Mates Sesame Bread Wafers (Nabisco)	3	70	3
Melba Toast Garlic (Keebler)	2	25	tr
Melba Toast Long (Keebler)	2	30	tr
Melba Toast Oblong (Lance)	2	30	0
Melba Toast Onion (Keebler)	2	25	tr
Melba Toast Plain (Keebler)	2	25	tr
Melba Toast Round Garlic (Lance)	2	20	1
Melba Toast Round Onion (Lance)	2	20	1
Melba Toast Round Plain (Lance)	2	20	1
Melba Toast Sesame (Keebler)	2	25	tr

FOOD	PORTION	CALORIES	FAT
Melba Toast Sesame (Lance)	2	25	1
Multi Grain (Pepperidge Farm)	4	70	2
Nekot (Lance)	1.5 oz	210	10
Nip-Chee (Lance)	1.3 oz	180	9
Nips Cheese (Nabisco)	13	70	3
Norwegian Crispbread Rye-Bran Style (Kavli)	2	30	tr
Norwegian Crispbread Thick Slice (Kavli)	1	35	tr
Norwegian Crispbread Thin Style (Kavli)	2	40	tr
Oat Bran Krisp (Ralston)	2	60	3
Oat Thins (Nabisco)	8	70	3
Ocean Crisp (FFV)	1	60	1
Oyster Crackers (Lance)	½ oz	70	2
Oyster Crackers Large (Keebler)	26	80	2
Oyster Crackers Small (Keebler)	50	80	2
Oysterettes (Nabisco)	18	60	1
Peanut Butter 'n Cheez Crackers (Handi-Snacks)	1 pkg	190	14
Peanut Butter Wheat (Lance)	1.3 oz	190	10
Pita Crisps (Tuscany)	1 oz	90	1
Pita Crisps Sesame (Tuscany)	1 oz	96	2
Premium Saltine (Nabisco)	5	60	2
Premium Plus Saltines Whole Wheat (Nabisco)	5	60	2
Premium Saltine Fat Free (Nabisco)	5	50	0
Premium Saltine Low Salt (Nabisco)	5	60	2
Premium Saltine Unsalted Tops (Nabisco)	5	60	2
Premium Soup & Oyster (Nabisco)	20	60	1
Rice Bran (Health Valley)	7	130	4

FOOD	PORTION	CALORIES	FAT
Ritz (Nabisco)	4	70	4
Ritz Whole Wheat (Nabisco)	5	70	3
Ritz Bits (Nabisco)	22	70	4
Ritz Bits Cheese (Nabisco)	22	70	4
Ritz Bits Cheese Sandwiches (Nabisco)	6	80	5
Ritz Bits Low Salt (Nabisco)	22	70	4
Ritz Bits Peanut Butter Sandwiches (Nabisco)	6	80	4
Ritz Low Salt (Nabisco)	4	70	4
Royal Lunch (Nabisco)	1	60	2
Rye-Chee (Lance)	1.5 oz	190	9
Rye Twins (Lance)	2	30	1
Rykrisp Natural	2	40	0
Rykrisp Seasoned	2	45	1
Rykrisp Seasoned Twindividuals	2	45	1
Rykrisp Sesame	2	50	2
Saltines (Lance)	2	25	1
Saltines Slug Pack (Lance)	4	50	1
Sesame (Pepperidge Farm)	4	80	4
Sesame Crisp (FFV)	2	120	3
Sesame Stoned Wheat (Health Valley)	13	55	2
Sesame Stoned Wheat No Salt Added (Health Valley)	13	55	2
Sesame Twins (Lance)	2	40	1
Seven Grain Vegetable Stoned Wheat (Health Valley)	13	55	2
Seven Grain Vegetable Stoned Wheat No Salt Added (Health Valley)	13	55	2
Snack Crackers Toasted Rye (Keebler)	2	30	2

FOOD	PORTION	CALORIES	FAT
Snack Crackers Toasted Sesame (Keebler)	2	30	2
Snack Crackers Toasted Wheat (Keebler)	2	30	2
Snack Mix Classic (Pepperidge Farm)	1 oz	140	8
Snack Mix Lightly Smoked (Pepperidge Farm)	1 oz	150	9
Snack Sticks Cheese (Pepperidge Farm)	8	130	5
Snack Sticks Pretzel (Pepperidge Farm)	8	120	3
Snack Sticks Pumpernickel (Pepperidge Farm)	8	140	6
Snack Sticks Sesame (Pepperidge Farm)	8	140	5
Snackbread High Fiber (Ryvita)	1	14	tr
Snackbread Original Wheat (Ryvita)	1	20	tr
Sociables (Nabisco)	6	70	3
Spicy Lightly Smoked (Pepperidge Farm)	1 oz	140	8
Stoned Wheat (FFV)	4	60	1
Stoned Wheat (Health Valley)	13	55	2
Stoned Wheat No Salt Added (Health Valley)	13	55	2
Swiss Cheese (Nabisco)	7	70	3
Tam Tams (Manischewitz)	10	147	8
Tam Tams No Salt (Manischewitz)	10	138	7
Tams Garlic (Manischewitz)	10	153	8
Tams Onion (Manischewitz)	10	150	8
Tams Wheat (Manischewitz)	10	150	8
Thin Wheat Snacks (Lance)	7	80	4
Tid Bits Cheese (Nabisco)	15	70	4

FOOD	PORTION	CALORIES	FAT
Toast Peanut Butter Sandwich (Planters)	6 (1.4 oz)	200	10
Toast-Chee (Lance)	1.38 oz	190	10
Toasted Bacon Snack Crackers (Keebler)	2	30	2
Toasted Onion Snack Crackers (Keebler)	2	30	2
Toasted Pumpernickel Snack Crackers (Keebler)	2	30	2
Toasted Rice (Pepperidge Farm)	4	60	2
Toasted Wheat w/ Onion (Pepperidge Farm)	4	80	3
Toasty (Lance)	1.25 oz	180	10
Toasty Crackers w/ Peanut Butter (Little Debbie)	1 pkg (.93 oz)	140	7
Town House (Keebler)	2	35	2
Triscuit (Nabisco)	3	60	2
Triscuit Bits (Nabisco)	15	60	2
Triscuit Deli-Style Rye (Nabisco)	3	60	2
Triscuit Low Salt (Nabisco)	3	60	2
Triscuit Wheat 'n Bran (Nabisco)	3	60	2
Tuc (Keebler)	3	70	4
Tuscany Toast	1 oz	95	2
Tuscany Toast Pepato	1 oz	93	2
Tuscany Toast Pesto	1 oz	96	2
Tuscany Toast Tomato	1 oz	95	2
Twigs Sesame & Cheese Sticks (Nabisco)	5	70	4
Uneeda Biscuit Unsalted Tops (Nabisco)	2	60	2
Unsalted (Estee)	4	60	2
Vegetable Thins (Nabisco)	7	70	4
Waldorf Sodium Free (Keebler)	2	30	1

FOOD	PORTION	CALORIES	FAT
Wasa Crispbread Breakfast	1	50	1
Wasa Crispbread Extra Crisp	1	25	0
Wasa Crispbread Falu Rye	1	30	0
Wasa Crispbread Fiber Plus	1	35	1
Wasa Crispbread Golden Rye	1	30	0
Wasa Crispbread Hearty Rye	1	50	0
Wasa Crispbread Light Rye	1	25	0
Wasa Crispbread Royal	½	26	0
Wasa Crispbread Savory Sesame	1	30	1
Wasa Crispbread Sesame Rye	1	30	1
Wasa Crispbread Sesame Wheat	1	60	2
Wasa Crispbread Toasted Wheat	1	50	1
Waverly (Nabisco)	4	70	3
Waverly Low Salt (Nabisco)	4	70	3
Wheat Crispy Wafers (FFV)	6	70	3
Wheat Twins (Lance)	2	30	1
Wheat Thins (Nabisco)	8	70	3
Wheat Thins Low Salt (Nabisco)	8	70	3
Wheat Thins Nutty (Nabisco)	7	70	4
Wheatswafer (Lance)	2	30	1
Wheatsworth Stone Ground (Nabisco)	4	70	3
Wholegrain Wheat (Keebler)	2	30	1
Zesta Saltine (Keebler)	2	25	1
Zesta Saltine Unsalted Top (Keebler)	2	25	1
Zings! (Nabisco)	15	70	3
Zwieback (Nabisco)	2	60	1
cheese	10 (⅓ oz)	50	3
crispbread	3	61	2
crispbread	3.5 oz	317	10

FOOD	PORTION	CALORIES	FAT
crispbread, rye	3	77	1
melba toast, plain	1	20	tr
peanut butter sandwich	1 (⅓ oz)	40	2
saltines	4	50	1
water biscuits	3	92	3
zwieback	3.5 oz	374	4

CRANBERRIES

FOOD	PORTION	CALORIES	FAT
CANNED			
Cranberry Sauce Jellied (Ocean Spray)	2 oz	90	0
Cranberry Sauce Jellied Old Fashioned (S&W)	½ cup	90	0
Cranberry Sauce Whole Berry Old Fashioned (S&W)	½ cup	90	0
CranFruit Cranberry Raspberry Sauce (Ocean Spray)	2 oz	100	0
CranFruit Cranberry Strawberry Sauce (Ocean Spray)	2 oz	100	0
CranFruit Cranberry Orange Sauce (Ocean Spray)	2 oz	100	0
Whole Berry Sauce (Ocean Spray)	2 oz	90	0
cranberry sauce sweetened	½ cup	209	tr
FRESH			
Ocean Spray	½ cup	25	0
chopped	1 cup	54	tr
JUICE			
Ocean Spray Cranberry Juice Cocktail	6 oz	100	0
Ocean Spray Cranberry Juice Cocktail Low Calorie	6 oz	40	0
Seneca Cranberry Juice Cocktail	6 oz	110	0

FOOD	PORTION	CALORIES	FAT
Seneca Cranberry Juice Cocktail frzn, as prep	6 oz	110	0
Smucker's Cranberry Juice Sparkler	10 oz	140	tr
cranberry juice cocktail	1 cup	147	tr
cranberry juice cocktail low calorie	6 oz	33	0
cranberry juice cocktail, frzn	12 oz can	821	0
cranberry juice cocktail, frzn, as prep	6 oz	102	0

CRANBERRY BEANS

CANNED			
cranberry beans	1 cup	216	1
DRIED			
cooked	1 cup	240	1
raw	1 cup	652	2

CRAYFISH

cooked	3 oz	97	1

CREAM

(see also SOUR CREAM, SOUR CREAM SUBSTITUTES, WHIPPED TOPPINGS)

LIQUID			
Half & Half (Land O'Lakes)	1 tbsp	20	2
Whipping Cream (Land O'Lakes)	1 tbsp	45	5
Whipping Cream Gourmet Heavy (Land O'Lakes)	1 tbsp	60	6
half & half	1 tbsp	20	2
half & half	1 cup	315	28
heavy whipping	1 tbsp	52	6
light coffee	1 tbsp	29	3
light coffee	1 cup	496	46

FOOD	PORTION	CALORIES	FAT
light whipping	1 tbsp	44	5
WHIPPED			
heavy whipping	1 cup	411	44
light whipping	1 cup	345	37

CREAM CHEESE

FOOD	PORTION	CALORIES	FAT
NEUFCHATEL			
Philadelphia Brand Light	1 oz	80	7
Spreadery			
Neufchatel w/ Classic Ranch Flavor	1 oz	70	7
Neufchatel w/ French Onion	1 oz	70	6
Neufchatel w/ Garden Vegetables	1 oz	70	6
Neufchatel w/ Garlic & Herb	1 oz	70	6
Neufchatel w/ Strawberries	1 oz	70	5
neufchatel	1 oz	74	7
neufchatel	1 pkg (3 oz)	221	20
REDUCED FAT			
Alpine Lace Free N'Lean	1 oz	30	0
Alpine Lace Free N'Lean w/ Chives	1 oz	30	0
Fleur De Lait			
Alouette C'est Light Herbs & Garlic	1 oz	70	6
Alouette C'est Light Spinach	1 oz	65	6
Alouette C'est Light Strawberry	1 oz	75	5
Alouette C'est Light Vegetables Julienne	1 oz	60	5
Chavrie	1 oz	50	4
Ultra Light Chives & Onions	1 oz	60	5
Ultra Light Fresh Vegetables	1 oz	60	5
Ultra Light Garlic & Spices	1 oz	60	5
Ultra Light Mixed Berry	1 oz	80	4

FOOD	PORTION	CALORIES	FAT
Ultra Light Nacho	1 oz	70	5
Ultra Light Strawberry	1 oz	70	6
Ultra Plain Light	1 oz	60	5
Formagg	1 oz	80	7
Philadelphia Brand Light	1 oz	60	5
Tofutti Better Than Cream Cheese	1 oz	80	8
Weight Watchers	2 tbsp	35	2
REGULAR			
Fleur De Lait	1 oz	100	9
Philadelphia Brand	1 oz	100	10
Philadelphia Brand w/ Pimentos	1 oz	90	9
Philadelphia Brand w/ Chives	1 oz	90	9
cream cheese	1 oz	99	10
cream cheese	1 pkg (3 oz)	297	30
SOFT			
Friendship	1 oz	103	<10
Philadelphia Brand	1 oz	100	10
Philadelphia Brand w/ Strawberries	1 oz	90	8
Philadelphia Brand w/ Chives & Onions	1 oz	100	9
Philadelphia Brand w/ Herb & Garlic	1 oz	100	9
Philadelphia Brand w/ Olives & Pimento	1 oz	90	8
Philadelphia Brand w/ Pineapple	1 oz	90	8
Philadelphia Brand w/ Smoked Salmon	1 oz	90	8
WHIPPED			
Philadelphia Brand	1 oz	100	10
Philadelphia Brand w/ Chives	1 oz	90	8
Philadelphia Brand w/ Onions	1 oz	90	8

FOOD	PORTION	CALORIES	FAT
Philadelphia Brand w/ Smoked Salmon	1 oz	90	8

CREPES

basic crepe, unfilled	1	75	2

CRESS
(*see also* WATERCRESS)

FRESH

garden, cooked	½ cup	16	tr
garden, raw	½ cup	8	tr

CROAKER

atlantic, breaded & fried	3 oz	188	11

CROISSANT

All Butter (Sara Lee)	1	170	9
All Butter Petite Size (Sara Lee)	1	120	6
Colonial Wheat Croissants (Rainbo)	1	300	19
Croissant Sandwich Quartet (Pepperidge Farm)	1	170	7
Petite All Butter (Pepperidge Farm)	1	120	6
croissant	1 (2 oz)	235	12
TAKE-OUT			
w/ egg & cheese	1	369	25
w/ egg, cheese & bacon	1	413	28
w/ egg, cheese & ham	1	475	34
w/ egg, cheese & sausage	1	524	38

CROUTONS

Cheddar & Romano Cheese (Pepperidge Farm)	½ oz	60	2

FOOD	PORTION	CALORIES	FAT
Cheese & Garlic (Pepperidge Farm)	½ oz	70	3
Croutettes (Kellogg's)	1 cup (1 oz)	100	0
Onion & Garlic (Pepperidge Farm)	½ oz	70	3
Seasoned (Pepperidge Farm)	½ oz	70	3
Sour Cream & Chive (Pepperidge Farm)	½ oz	70	3

CUCUMBER

FOOD	PORTION	CALORIES	FAT
FRESH			
raw	1 (11 oz)	39	tr
raw, sliced	½ cup	7	tr
TAKE-OUT			
cucumber salad	3.5 oz	50	tr

CUMIN

FOOD	PORTION	CALORIES	FAT
seed	1 tsp	8	tr

CURRANTS

FOOD	PORTION	CALORIES	FAT
DRIED			
zante	½ cup	204	tr
FRESH			
black	½ cup	36	tr
JUICE			
black currant nectar	3.5 oz	55	0
red currant nectar	3.5 oz	54	tr

CUSK

FOOD	PORTION	CALORIES	FAT
fresh fillet, baked	3 oz	106	1

CUSTARD

FOOD	PORTION	CALORIES	FAT
Custard (Royal)	mix for 1 serving	60	0

FOOD	PORTION	CALORIES	FAT
Flan Caramel Custard (Royal)	mix for 1 serving	60	0
baked	1 cup	305	17
custard, as prep from mix	½ cup	161	5
zabaglione (home recipe)	½ cup	159	7

CUTTLEFISH

steamed	3 oz	134	1

DANDELION GREENS

fresh, cooked	½ cup	17	tr
fresh, raw, chopped	½ cup	13	tr

DANISH PASTRY

FROZEN

Apple (Pepperidge Farm)	1	220	8
Apple (Sara Lee)	1	120	6
Apple Danish Twist (Sara Lee)	1 slice (1.9 oz)	190	10
Apple Free & Light (Sara Lee)	1 slice (2 oz)	130	0
Cheese (Pepperidge Farm)	1	240	14
Cheese (Sara Lee)	1	130	8
Cheese Danish Twist (Sara Lee)	1 slice (1.9 oz)	200	12
Cinnamon Raisin (Pepperidge Farm)	1	250	11
Cinnamon Raisin (Sara Lee)	1	150	8
Raspberry (Pepperidge Farm)	1	220	9
Raspberry Danish Twist (Sara Lee)	1 slice (1.9 oz)	200	9

READY-TO-EAT

cheese	1 (3 oz)	353	25
cinnamon	1 (3 oz)	349	17
fruit	1 (2.3 oz)	235	13

FOOD	PORTION	CALORIES	FAT
fruit	1 (3.3 oz)	335	16
plain	1 (2 oz)	220	12
plain ring	1 (12 oz)	1305	71
REFRIGERATED			
Caramel Danish w/ Nuts (Pillsbury)	1	160	8
Cinnamon Raisin Danish w/ Icing (Pillsbury)	1	150	7
Orange Danish w/ Icing (Pillsbury)	1	150	7

DATES

DRIED			
Bordo Diced	2 oz	203	1
California Deglet Noor	10	240	0
Dole Chopped	½ cup	280	0
Dole Pitted	½ cup	280	0
Dromedary Chopped	¼ cup	130	0
Dromedary Pitted	5	100	0
chopped	1 cup	489	1
whole	10	228	tr

DEER
(see VENISON)

DIETING AIDS
(see NUTRITIONAL SUPPLEMENTS)

DILL

seed	1 tsp	6	tr
sprigs, fresh	5	0	tr
sprigs, fresh	1 cup	4	tr
weed, dry	1 tsp	3	tr

FOOD	PORTION	CALORIES	FAT

DINNER
(*see also* MEXICAN FOOD, PASTA DINNERS, POT PIE, ORIENTAL FOOD)

FROZEN
(*see also* BEEF DISHES, CHICKEN DISHES, TURKEY DISHES, PASTA DINNERS)

FOOD	PORTION	CALORIES	FAT
Armour Ham Steak	11 oz	350	13
Armour Classics			
Chicken & Noodles	11 oz	230	73
Chicken Fettucini	11 oz	260	9
Chicken Mesquite	9.5 oz	370	16
Chicken Parmigiana	11.5 oz	370	19
Chicken w/ Wine & Mushroom Sauce	10.75 oz	280	11
Glazed Chicken	10.75 oz	300	16
Meat Loaf	11.25 oz	360	17
Salisbury Parmigiana	11.5 oz	410	21
Salisbury Steak	11.25 oz	350	17
Swedish Meatballs	11.25 oz	330	18
Turkey w/ Dressing & Gravy	11.5 oz	320	12
Veal Parmigiana	11.25 oz	400	22
Armour Lite			
Beef Pepper Steak	11.25 oz	220	4
Beef Strognaoff	11.25 oz	250	6
Chicken Ala King	11.25 oz	290	7
Chicken Burgundy	10 oz	210	2
Chicken Marsala	10.5 oz	250	7
Chicken Oriental	10 oz	180	1
Salisbury Steak	11.5 oz	300	11
Shrimp Creole	11.25 oz	260	2
Sweet & Sour Chicken	11 oz	240	2

FOOD	PORTION	CALORIES	FAT
Banquet			
Beans & Frankfurters Dinner	10 oz	350	14
Beef & Bean Burrito	9.5 oz	390	12
Beef Platter	9 oz	230	63
Boneless Chicken Drumsnacker Platter	7 oz	290	12
Boneless Chicken Nugget Platter	6 oz	340	16
Boneless Chicken Pattie Platter	6.75 oz	310	15
Chicken & Dumplings	10 oz	270	10
Fish Platter	8 oz	270	7
Fried Chicken Dinner	9 oz	520	29
Ham Platter	8.25 oz	200	5
Italian Style Dinner	9 oz	180	2
Meat Loaf Dinner	9.5 oz	340	19
Mexican Style Combination Dinner	11 oz	360	12
Mexican Style Dinner	11 oz	410	17
Noodles & Chicken	10 oz	170	4
Salisbury Steak Dinner	9 oz	280	13
Southern Fried Chicken Platter	8.75 oz	400	16
Spaghetti & Meat Sauce	8.75 oz	160	4
Veal Parmagian	9.25 oz	330	16
Western Style Dinner	9 oz	300	16
White Meat Fried Chicken Platter	8.75 oz	390	13
White Meat Hot'n Spicy Fried Chicken Platter	9 oz	440	15
Banquet Cookin' Bag			
Chicken Ala King	4 oz	110	5
Creamed Chipped Beef	4 oz	100	4
Gravy & Salisbury Steak	5 oz	190	14
Gravy & Sliced Beef	4 oz	100	5
Gravy & Sliced Turkey	5 oz	100	6
Turkey Chili	4 oz	80	2

FOOD	PORTION	CALORIES	FAT
Banquet Extra Helping			
Beef Dinner	15.5 oz	430	13
Chicken Nuggets w/ Barbeque Sauce	10 oz	540	19
Chicken Nuggets w/ Sweet & Sour Sauce	10 oz	540	19
Fried Chicken All White Meat	14.25 oz	760	38
Fried Chicken Dinner	14.25 oz	790	43
Meat Loaf	16.25 oz	640	34
Mexican Style Dinner	19 oz	680	25
Salisbury Steak Dinner	16.25 oz	590	28
Southern Fried Chicken Dinner	13.25 oz	790	39
Turkey Dinner	17 oz	460	12
Budget Gourmet			
Beef Cantonese	1 pkg	260	9
Beef Mexicana	1 pkg	520	18
Breast of Chicken in Wine Sauce	1 pkg	250	5
Chicken & Egg Noodle w/ Broccoli	1 pkg	440	25
Chicken Au Gratin	1 pkg	250	11
Chicken Cacciatore	1 pkg	470	27
Chicken Enchilada Suiza	1 pkg	290	12
Chicken Marsala	1 pkg	270	8
Chicken Mexicana	1 pkg	560	20
Chicken w/ Fettucini	1 pkg	400	24
French Recipe Chicken	1 pkg	240	9
Glazed Turkey	1 pkg	270	5
Ham & Asparagus Au Gratin	1 pkg	290	12
Mandarin Chicken	1 pkg	300	7
Oriental Beef	1 pkg	290	9
Pepper Steak w/ Rice	1 pkg	330	10
Roast Chicken w/ Herb Gravy	1 pkg	270	9

FOOD	PORTION	CALORIES	FAT
Roast Sirloin Supreme	1 pkg	320	15
Scallops & Shrimp Marinara	1 pkg	330	9
Seafood Newburg	1 pkg	350	13
Sirloin Beef in Herb Sauce	1 pkg	270	10
Sirloin Cheddar Melt	1 pkg	390	20
Sirloin Enchilada Ranchero	1 pkg	280	10
Sirloin Salisbury Steak	1 pkg	260	13
Sirloin Salisbury Steak Dinner	1 pkg	450	17
Sirloin Tips in Burgundy Sauce	1 pkg	340	14
Sirloin Tips w/ Country Vegetables	1 pkg	300	19
Sliced Turkey Breast w/ Herb Gravy	1 pkg	290	8
Slim Selects Beef Stroganoff	8.75 oz	280	10
Slim Selects Glazed Turkey	9 oz	270	5
Swedish Meatballs w/ Noodles	1 pkg	580	37
Sweet & Sour Chicken	1 pkg	340	5
Swiss Steak w/ Zesty Tomato Sauce	1 pkg	410	22
Turkey A La King w/ Rice	1 pkg	390	16
Veal Parmigiana	1 pkg	490	25
Yankee Pot Roast	1 pkg	360	18
Budget Gourmet Light & Healthy Chicken Breast Parmigiana	1 pkg	260	8
Herbed Chicken Breast w/ Fettucini	1 pkg	240	7
Italian Style Meatloaf	1 pkg	270	10
Pot Roast	1 pkg	210	8
Sirloin Beef in Wine Sauce	1 pkg	230	6
Sirloin Salisbury Steak	1 pkg	260	9
Special Recipe Sirloin of Beef	1 pkg	250	10
Stuffed Turkey Breast	1 pkg	230	6
Teriyaki Chicken Breast	1 pkg	310	9

FOOD	PORTION	CALORIES	FAT
Healthy Choice			
Barbecue Beef Ribs	11 oz	330	6
Beef Pepper Steak	11 oz	290	6
Breast of Turkey	10.5 oz	290	5
Cacciatore Chicken	12.5 oz	310	3
Chicken & Pasta Divan	11.5 oz	310	4
Chicken & Vegetables	11.5 oz	210	1
Chicken Dijon	11 oz	260	3
Chicken Oriental	11.25 oz	230	1
Chicken Parmigiana	11.5 oz	270	3
Herb Roasted Chicken	12.3 oz	290	4
Lemon Pepper Fish	10.7 oz	300	5
Mesquite Chicken	10.5 oz	340	1
Roasted Turkey & Mushroom Gravy	8.5 oz	200	3
Salisbury Steak	11.5 oz	300	7
Salisbury Steak w/ Mushroom Gravy	11 oz	280	6
Salsa Chicken	11.25 oz	240	2
Seafood Newburg	8 oz	200	3
Shrimp Creole	11.25 oz	230	2
Shrimp Marinara	10.25 oz	260	1
Sirloin Beef w/ Barbecue Sauce	11 oz	300	6
Sirloin Tips	11.75 oz	280	8
Sliced Turkey w/ Gravy & Dressing	10 oz	270	4
Sole Au Gratin	11 oz	270	5
Sole w/ Lemon Butter	8.25 oz	230	4
Sweet & Sour Chicken	11.5 oz	280	2
Teriyaki Pasta w/ Chicken	12.6 oz	350	3
Turkey Tetrazzini	12.6 oz	340	6
Yankee Pot Roast	11 oz	250	4

FOOD	PORTION	CALORIES	FAT
Kid Cuisine			
Chicken Nuggets	6.8 oz	360	17
Chicken Sandwiches	8.2 oz	470	17
Fish Sticks	7 oz	360	14
Fried Chicken	7.5 oz	430	22
Hot Dogs w/ Buns	6.7 oz	450	19
Mexican Style	5.7 oz	290	8
Mega Meal Chicken Nuggets	8.4 oz	470	20
Mega Meal Fried Chicken	10.8 oz	720	41
Mega Meal Hot Dog w/ Bun	8.25 oz	500	25
Le Menu			
Beef Burgundy	7.5 oz	330	23
Beef Sirloin Tips	11.5 oz	400	18
Beef Stroganoff	10 oz	430	24
Chicken A La King	10.25 oz	330	13
Chicken Cordon Bleu	11 oz	460	20
Chicken in Wine Sauce	10 oz	280	7
Chicken Parmigiana	11.75 oz	410	20
Chopped Sirloin Beef	12.25 oz	430	24
Ham Steak	10 oz	300	11
Pepper Steak	11.5 oz	370	13
Salisbury Steak	10.5 oz	370	20
Sliced Breast of Turkey w/ Mushroom Gravy	10.5 oz	300	7
Sweet & Sour Chicken	11.25 oz	400	18
Veal Parmigiana	11.25 oz	390	17
Yankee Pot Roast	10 oz	330	13
Le Menu LightStyle			
Glazed Chicken Breast	10 oz	230	3
Herb Roasted Chicken	10 oz	240	7
Salisbury Steak	10 oz	280	9

FOOD	PORTION	CALORIES	FAT
Le Menu LightStyle *(cont.)*			
Sliced Turkey	10 oz	210	5
Sweet & Sour Chicken	10 oz	250	7
Turkey Divan	10 oz	260	7
Veal Marsala	10 oz	230	3
Lean Cuisine			
Beefsteak Ranchero	9.25 oz	260	8
Breaded Breast of Chicken Parmesan	10.88 oz	270	9
Breast of Chicken Marsala w/ Vegetables	8.13 oz	190	5
Chicken A L'Orange w/ Almond Rice	8 oz	280	4
Chicken & Vegetables w/ Vermicelli	11.75 oz	250	6
Chicken in Barbeque Sauce	8.75 oz	260	6
Chicken Oriental w/ Vegetables & Vermicelli	9 oz	280	7
Chicken Italiano	9 oz	290	8
Chicken Tenderloins in Herb Cream Sauce	9.5 oz	240	5
Chicken Tenderloins in Peanut Sauce	9 oz	290	7
Fiesta Chicken	8.5 oz	240	5
Filet of Fish Divan	10.38 oz	210	5
Filet of Fish Florentine	9.62 oz	220	7
Glazed Chicken w/ Vegetable Rice	8.5 oz	260	8
Homestyle Turkey w/ Vegetables & Pasta	9.38 oz	230	5
Oriental Beef w/ Vegetables & Rice	8.63 oz	290	9
Salisbury Steak w/ Gravy & Scalloped Potatoes	9.5 oz	240	7
Sliced Turkey Breast in Mushroom Sauce	8 oz	220	6

FOOD	PORTION	CALORIES	FAT
Sliced Turkey Breast w/ Dressing	7.88 oz	200	5
Stuffed Cabbage w/ Meat in Tomato Sauce	10.75 oz	210	6
Swedish Meatballs in Gravy w/ Pasta	9.13 oz	290	8
Turkey Dijon	9.5 oz	230	5
Morton			
Beans & Franks w/ Sauce	8.5 oz	300	11
Fish w/ Mashed Potatoes & Carrots	9.25 oz	350	12
Glazed Ham	8 oz	230	3
Gravy & Charbroiled Beef Patty	9 oz	270	12
Gravy & Salisbury Steak	9 oz	270	16
Tomato Sauce & Meatloaf	9 oz	280	16
Veal Parmagian	8.75 oz	230	7
Swanson			
Beans & Franks	10.5 oz	440	19
Beef	11.25 oz	310	6
Beef in Barbecue Sauce	11 oz	460	17
Chicken Nuggets	8.75 oz	470	23
Chopped Sirloin Beef	10.75 oz	340	16
Fish & Fries Homestyle	6.5 oz	340	16
Fish 'n' Chips	10 oz	500	21
Fried Chicken BBQ Flavored	10 oz	540	22
Fried Chicken Dark Meat	9.75 oz	560	28
Fried Chicken Homestyle	7 oz	390	21
Fried Chicken White Meat	10.25 oz	550	25
Loin of Pork	10.75 oz	280	12
Macaroni & Beef	12 oz	370	15
Macaroni & Cheese	12.25 oz	370	15
Meatloaf	10.75 oz	360	15
Noodles & Chicken	10.5 oz	280	8

FOOD	PORTION	CALORIES	FAT
Swanson *(cont.)*			
Salisbury Steak	10.75 oz	400	17
Salisbury Steak Homestyle	10 oz	320	16
Scalloped Potatoes & Ham Homestyle	9 oz	300	13
Seafood Creole w/ Rice Homestyle	9 oz	240	6
Sirloin Tips in Burgundy Sauce Homestyle	7 oz	160	5
Spaghetti & Meatballs	12.5 oz	390	17
Swedish Meatballs	8.5 oz	360	20
Swiss Steak	10 oz	350	11
Turkey	8.75 oz	270	11
Turkey	11.5 oz	350	11
Turkey w/ Dressing & Potatoes Homestyle	9 oz	290	11
Veal Parmigiana	12.25 oz	430	20
Veal Parmigiana Homestyle	10 oz	330	13
Western Style	11.5 oz	430	19
Swanson Hungry-Man			
Boneless Chicken	17.75 oz	700	28
Chopped Beef Steak	16.75 oz	640	37
Fried Chicken Dark Meat	14.25 oz	860	45
Fried Chicken White Meat	14.25 oz	870	46
Salisbury Steak	16.5 oz	680	41
Sliced Beef	15.25 oz	450	12
Turkey	17 oz	550	18
Veal Parmigiana	18.25 oz	590	26
Ultra Slim-Fast			
Beef Pepper Steak	12 oz	270	4
Chicken & Vegetable	12 oz	290	3
Chicken Fettucini	12 oz	380	12

FOOD	PORTION	CALORIES	FAT
Country Style Vegetable & Beef Tips	12 oz	230	5
Mesquite Chicken	12 oz	360	1
Roasted Chicken in Mushroom Sauce	12 oz	280	6
Shrimp Creole	12 oz	240	4
Shrimp Marinara	12 oz	290	3
Sweet & Sour Chicken	12 oz	330	2
Turkey Medallions in Herb Sauce	12 oz	280	6
Van De Camp's Fillet of Fish Dinner	12 oz	300	10
Weight Watchers			
Barbecue Glazed Chicken	7 oz	200	6
Beef Sirloin Tips	7.5 oz	210	6
Beef Stroganoff	8.5 oz	280	9
Chicken Ala King	9 oz	230	4
Chicken Cordon Bleu	7.7 oz	170	5
Chicken Kiev	7 oz	190	5
Homestyle Chicken & Noodles	9 oz	240	7
Imperial Chicken	8.5 oz	210	4
London Broil	7.5 oz	110	3
Oven Baked Fish	7 oz	150	4
Southern Baked Chicken	6.3 oz	170	7
Stuffed Turkey Breast	8.5 oz	270	8
Veal Patty Parmigiana	8.2 oz	150	4

DIP

FOOD	PORTION	CALORIES	FAT
Avocado Guacamole (Kraft)	2 tbsp	50	4
Bacon & Horseradish (Breakstone)	2 tbsp	70	6
Bacon & Horseradish (Kraft)	2 tbsp	60	5
Bacon & Horseradish (Kraft Premium)	2 tbsp	50	5

FOOD	PORTION	CALORIES	FAT
Bacon & Horseradish (Sealtest)	2 tbsp	70	6
Bacon & Onion (Breakstone)	2 tbsp	70	6
Bacon & Onion (Kraft Premium)	1 tbsp	60	5
Blue Cheese (Kraft Premium)	2 tbsp	50	4
Chesapeake Clam Gourmet (Breakstone)	2 tbsp	50	4
Clam (Breakstone)	2 tbsp	50	4
Clam (Kraft)	2 tbsp	60	4
Clam (Kraft Premium)	2 tbsp	45	4
Clam (Sealtest)	2 tbsp	50	4
Creamy Cucumber (Kraft Premium)	2 tbsp	50	4
Creamy Onion (Kraft Premium)	2 tbsp	45	4
Cucumber & Onion (Breakstone)	2 tbsp	50	4
Cucumber & Onion (Sealtest)	2 tbsp	50	4
Fiesta Bean (Chi Chi's)	1 oz	32	1
Fiesta Cheese (Chi Chi's)	1 oz	37	2
French Onion (Breakstone)	2 tbsp	50	5
French Onion (Kraft)	2 tbsp	60	4
French Onion (Kraft Premium)	2 tbsp	45	4
French Onion (Sealtest)	2 tbsp	50	4
Green Onion (Kraft)	2 tbsp	60	4
Jalapeno Cheddar Gourmet (Breakstone)	2 tbsp	70	6
Jalapeno Cheese (Kraft Premium)	1 tbsp	50	4
Jalapeno Flavored Bean (Wise)	2 tbsp	25	0
Jalapeno Pepper (Kraft)	2 tbsp	50	4
Mushroom & Herb Gourmet (Breakstone)	2 tbsp	50	4
Nacho Cheese (Kraft Premium)	2 tbsp	55	4
Picante Sauce (Wise)	2 tbsp	12	0
Taco (Wise)	2 tbsp	12	0

FOOD	PORTION	CALORIES	FAT
Toasted Onion Gourmet (Breakstone)	2 tbsp	50	5

DOCK

fresh, cooked	3.5 oz	20	1
fresh, raw, chopped	½ cup	15	tr

DOGFISH

raw	3.5 oz	193	15

DOLPHINFISH

fresh, baked	3 oz	93	1
fresh fillet, baked	5.6 oz	174	1

DOUGHNUTS
(see also DUNKIN' DONUTS, WINCHELL'S)

Chocolate Dipped (Tastykake)	1	181	10
Cinnamon (Tastykake)	1	201	9
Cinnamon Apple (Earth Grains)	1	310	17
Coated Mini (Tastykake)	1	81	5
Devil's Food (Earth Grains)	1	330	21
Donut Sticks (Little Debbie)	1 pkg (1.67 oz)	200	9
Glazed Old Fashioned (Earth Grains)	1	310	18
Honey Wheat Mini (Tastykake)	1	65	3
Old Fashion Donuts (Drake's)	1 (1.7 oz)	182	8
Plain (Dutch Mill)	1 (1.75 oz)	220	10
Plain (Tastykake)	1	172	9
Powdered Old Fashioned (Earth Grains)	1	290	19
Powdered Sugar (Tastykake)	1	195	9
Powdered Sugar Donut Delites (Drake's)	7 (2.5 oz)	300	15
Powdered Sugar Mini (Tastykake)	1	58	3

FOOD	PORTION	CALORIES	FAT
Premium Fudge Iced (Tastykake)	1	350	21
Premium Honey Wheat (Tastykake)	1	342	18
Premium Orange Glazed (Tastykake)	1	357	20
cake type	1 (1.8 oz)	210	12
glazed	1 (2 oz)	235	13
jelly	1	235	10

DRESSING
(*see also* STUFFING/DRESSING)

DRINK MIXERS
(*see also* SODA, MINERAL/BOTTLED WATER)

FOOD	PORTION	CALORIES	FAT
Bitter Lemon (Schweppes)	6 oz	78	0
Bloody Mary Mix (Libby's)	6 oz	40	0
Bloody Mary Mix (Tabasco)	6 oz	56	tr
Collins Mixer (Schweppes)	6 oz	70	0
Lemon Sour (Schweppes)	6 oz	75	0
Tonic Water (Schweppes)	6 oz	64	0
Tonic Water Diet (Schweppes)	6 oz	tr	0
whiskey sour mix	2 oz	55	0

DRUM

FRESH

FOOD	PORTION	CALORIES	FAT
freshwater, baked	3 oz	130	5
freshwater fillet, baked	5.4 oz	236	10

DUCK

FOOD	PORTION	CALORIES	FAT
w/ skin, roasted	½ duck (13.4 oz)	1287	108
w/ skin, roasted	6 oz	583	49
w/o skin, roasted	3.5 oz	201	11
w/o skin, roasted	½ duck (7.8 oz)	445	25

FOOD	PORTION	CALORIES	FAT
wild w/ skin, raw	½ duck (9.5 oz)	571	41
wild breast w/o skin, raw	½ breast (2.9 oz)	102	4

DUMPLING

FROZEN
Apple Dumpling (Pepperidge Farm) | 1 (3 oz) | 260 | 13

DURIAN

| fresh | 3.5 oz | 141 | 2 |

EEL

| fresh, cooked | 3 oz | 200 | 13 |
| fresh, cooked | 1 fillet (5.6 oz) | 375 | 24 |

EGG
(*see also* EGG DISHES, EGG SUBSTITUTES)

CHICKEN
fried w/ margarine	1	91	7
frozen	1	75	5
frozen	1 cup	363	24
hard cooked	1	77	5
hard cooked, chopped	1 cup	210	14
poached	1	74	5
raw	1	75	5
scrambled plain	2	200	15
scrambled w/ whole milk & margarine	1	101	7
scrambled w/ whole milk & margarine	1 cup	365	27
white only	1	17	0
white only	1 cup	121	0
yolk, raw	1	59	5

FOOD	PORTION	CALORIES	FAT
OTHER POULTRY			
duck, raw	1	130	10
goose, raw	1	267	19
quail, raw	1	14	1
turkey, raw	1	135	9

EGG DISHES

FOOD	PORTION	CALORIES	FAT
FROZEN			
Cheese Omelet (Chefwich)	5 oz	380	17
Egg Patties w/ Cheese (Kid Cuisine)	4.8 oz	200	10
Egg, Sausage & Cheese (Great Starts)	5.5 oz	460	28
Garden Vegetable Omelet Sandwich (Weight Watchers)	1 (3.6 oz)	210	6
Ham & Cheese Handy Omelet (Weight Watchers)	4 oz	180	5
Ham & Cheese Omelet (Chefwich)	5 oz	340	14
Omelets w/ Cheese & Ham (Great Starts)	7 oz	390	29
Reduced Cholesterol Eggs w/ Mini Oatbran Muffins (Great Starts)	4.75 oz	250	12
Sausage & Cheese Omelet (Chefwich)	5 oz	400	19
Scrambled Eggs (Kid Cuisine)	4.1 oz	270	17
Scrambled Eggs & Bacon w/ Home Fries (Great Starts)	5.6 oz	340	26
Scrambled Eggs & Sausage w/ Hash Browns (Great Starts)	6.5 oz	430	34
Scrambled Eggs & Sausage w/ Hash Browns (Quaker)	1 pkg (5.7 oz)	290	20
Scrambled Eggs & Sausage w/ Pancakes (Quaker)	1 pkg (5.2 oz)	270	14
Scrambled Eggs, Cheddar Cheese & Fried Potatoes (Quaker)	1 pkg (5.9 oz)	250	13

FOOD	PORTION	CALORIES	FAT
Scrambled Eggs w/ Cheese & Cinnamon Pancakes (Great Starts)	3.4 oz	290	23
Scrambled Eggs w/ Home Fries (Great Starts)	4.6 oz	260	19
Turkey Sausage Omelet on English Muffin (Healthy Choice)	1 (4.75 oz)	210	4
Western Style Omelet (Chefwich)	5 oz	350	13
Western Style Omelet on English Muffin (Healthy Choice)	1 (4.75 oz)	200	3
HOME RECIPE			
deviled	2 halves	145	13
TAKE-OUT			
egg sandwich w/ cheese & ham	1	348	16
salad	½ cup	307	28
sandwich w/ cheese	1	340	19
scotch egg	1 (4.2 oz)	301	21

EGG SUBSTITUTES

FOOD	PORTION	CALORIES	FAT
Egg Beaters	¼ cup	25	0
Egg Beaters Cheese Omelette	½ cup	110	5
Egg Beaters Vegetable Omelette	½ cup	50	0
Egg Watchers	2 oz	50	2
Healthy Choice Cholesterol Free Egg	¼ cup	30	tr
Scramblers	3.5 oz	105	5
frozen	¼ cup	96	7
frozen	1 cup	384	27
liquid	1.5 oz	40	2
liquid	1 cup	211	8
powder	0.7 oz	88	3
powder	0.35 oz	44	1

FOOD	PORTION	CALORIES	FAT
EGGNOG			
Borden	½ cup	190	9
Borden Light	½ cup	130	2
Land O'Lakes	8 oz	300	15
eggnog	1 qt	1368	76
eggnog	1 cup	342	19
eggnog flavor mix, as prep w/ milk	9 oz	260	8
EGGPLANT			
FRESH			
cubed, cooked	½ cup	13	tr
raw, cut up	½ cup	11	tr
FROZEN			
Parmigiana (Mrs. Paul's)	5 oz	240	16
TAKE-OUT			
Baba Ghannouj	¼ cup	55	4
ELDERBERRIES			
fresh elderberries	1 cup	105	1
juice	3.5 oz	38	0
ELK			
roasted	3 oz	124	2
ENDIVE			
fresh	3.5 oz	9	tr
raw, chopped	½ cup	4	tr

FOOD	PORTION	CALORIES	FAT

ENGLISH MUFFIN

FROZEN

Egg, Beefsteak & Cheese (Great Starts)	5.9 oz	360	20
English Muffin Sandwich (Healthy Choice)	1 (4.5 oz)	200	3
Sandwich w/ Egg, Ham & Cheese (Weight Watchers)	1 (4 oz)	230	8

HOME RECIPE

cinnamon raisin	1	186	3
english muffin	1	158	2
honey bran	1	153	3
whole wheat	1	167	tr

READY-TO-EAT

Matthew's 9 Grain & Nut	1	140	4
Matthew's Cinnamon Raisin	1	160	2
Matthew's Golden White	1	140	4
Matthew's Whole Wheat	1	150	2
Pepperidge Farm Cinnamon Apple	1	140	1
Pepperidge Farm Cinnamon Chip	1	160	3
Pepperidge Farm Cinnamon Raisin	1	150	2
Pepperidge Farm Plain	1	140	1
Pepperidge Farm Sourdough	1	135	1
Roman Meal	1	146	2
Shop 'n Save	1	130	1
Thomas' Honey Wheat	1	129	1
Thomas' Raisin	1	153	2
Thomas' Regular	1	130	1
Thomas' Sourdough	1	130	1
plain, toasted	1	140	1

FOOD	PORTION	CALORIES	FAT
TAKE-OUT			
w/ butter	1	189	6
w/ cheese & sausage	1	394	24
w/ egg, cheese & bacon	1	487	31
w/ egg, cheese & canadian bacon	1	383	20

EPPAW

raw	½ cup	75	1

FALAFEL

falafel	1 (1.2 oz)	57	3
falafel	3 (1.8 oz)	170	9

FAST FOODS
(*see individual names*)

FAT
(*see also* BUTTER, BUTTER BLENDS, BUTTER SUBSTITUTES, MARGARINE, OIL)

Crisco	1 tbsp	110	12
Crisco Butter Flavor	1 tbsp	110	12
Wesson Shortening	1 tbsp	100	12
beef, cooked	1 oz	193	20
beef tallow	1 tbsp	115	13
chicken	1 cup	1846	205
chicken	1 tbsp	115	13
cocoa butter	1 tbsp	120	14
duck	1 tbsp	115	13
goose	1 tbsp	115	13
lamb, new zealand, raw	1 oz	182	19
lard	1 tbsp	115	13
lard	1 cup	1849	205

FOOD	PORTION	CALORIES	FAT
nutmeg butter	1 tbsp	120	14
pork, cooked	1 oz	200	21
pork, cured, roasted	1 oz	167	18
pork, cured, uncooked	1 oz	164	17
pork backfat	1 oz	230	25
salt pork	1 oz	212	23
shortening	1 tbsp	113	13
shortening	1 cup	1812	205
turkey	1 tbsp	115	13
ucuhuba butter	1 tbsp	120	14

FEIJOA

fresh	1 (1.75 oz)	25	tr
puree	1 cup	119	2

FENNEL

fresh, bulb	1 (8.2 oz)	72	tr
fresh, sliced	1 cup	27	tr
seed	1 tsp	7	tr

FENUGREEK

seed	1 tsp	12	tr

FIBER
(*see also* PECTIN)

Natural Delta Fiber	½ cup (1 oz)	20	tr

FIGS

CANNED Kadota Figs Whole Fancy (S&W)	½ cup	100	0
in heavy syrup	3	75	tr

FOOD	PORTION	CALORIES	FAT
in light syrup	3	58	tr
water pack	3	42	tr
DRIED			
cooked	½ cup	140	1
whole	10	477	2
FRESH			
fig	1 med	50	tr

FILBERTS

FOOD	PORTION	CALORIES	FAT
dried, blanched	1 oz	191	19
dried, unblanched	1 oz	179	18
dry roasted, unblanched	1 oz	188	19
oil roasted, unblanched	1 oz	187	18

FISH

(*see also individual names,* FISH SUBSTITUTES, RESTAURANTS AND CHAINS IN PART II)

FOOD	PORTION	CALORIES	FAT
FROZEN			
40 Crunchy Fish Sticks (Mrs. Paul's)	4 (2.75 oz)	200	10
Batter Dipped Fish & Chips (Van De Kamp's)	7 oz	440	25
Batter Dipped Fish Fillets (Mrs. Paul's)	2 fillets	330	17
Batter Dipped Fish Fillets (Van De Kamp's)	1	180	10
Batter Dipped Fish Kabobs (Van De Kamp's)	4 oz	240	15
Batter Dipped Fish Sticks (Van De Kamp's)	4	220	14
Battered Fish Portions (Mrs. Paul's)	2 portions	300	19
Battered Fish Sticks (Mrs. Paul's)	4 sticks	210	12
Breaded Fish Fillets (Van De Kamp's)	1	180	14

FOOD	PORTION	CALORIES	FAT
Breaded Fish Nuggets (Van De Kamp's)	2 oz	130	8
Breaded Fish Sticks (Van De Kamp's)	4	270	19
Combination Seafood Platter (Mrs. Paul's)	9 oz	600	33
Country Seasoned Fish Fillets (Van De Kamp's)	1	195	13
Crispy Batter Dipped Fillets (Gorton's)	2	290	19
Crispy Batter Sticks (Gorton's)	4	260	18
Crispy Crunchy Breaded Fish Portions (Mrs. Paul's)	2 portions	230	15
Crispy Crunchy Breaded Fish Sticks (Mrs. Paul's)	4 sticks	140	6
Crispy Crunchy Fish Fillets (Mrs. Paul's)	2 fillets	220	9
Crispy Crunchy Fish Sticks (Mrs. Paul's)	4 sticks	190	8
Crunchy Batter Fish Fillets (Mrs. Paul's)	2 fillets	280	14
Crunchy Fillets (Gorton's)	2	230	13
Crunchy Sticks (Gorton's)	4	210	13
Fish Cakes (Mrs. Paul's)	2	190	7
Light Fillets in Butter Sauce (Mrs. Paul's)	1 fillet	140	6
Light Recipe Lightly Breaded Fish Fillets (Gorton's)	1 fillet	180	8
Light Recipe Tempura Fillets (Gorton's)	1 fillet	200	14
Light Seafood Entrees Fish Dijon (Mrs. Paul's)	8.75 oz	200	5
Light Seafood Entrees Fish Florentine (Mrs. Paul's)	8 oz	220	8

FOOD	PORTION	CALORIES	FAT
Light Seafood Entrees Fish Mornay (Mrs. Paul's)	9 oz	230	10
Microwave Buttered Fish Fillet (Mrs. Paul's)	1 fillet	80	4
Microwave Crispy Batter Large Cut Fillets (Gorton's)	1	320	21
Microwave Entree Fillets in Herb Butter (Gorton's)	1 pkg	190	8
Microwave Fillets (Gorton's)	2	340	26
Microwave Fish Fillets (Mrs. Paul's)	1 fillet	280	19
Microwave Fish Fillet Sandwich (Mrs. Paul's)	1	280	15
Microwave Fish Sticks (Mrs. Paul's)	5	290	20
Microwave Larger Cut Fillets (Gorton's)	1	320	22
Microwave Larger Cut Ranch Fillet (Gorton's)	1	330	21
Microwave Sticks (Gorton's)	6	340	22
Potato Crisp Fillets (Gorton's)	2	300	20
Potato Crisp Sticks (Gorton's)	4	260	16
Today's Catch Fish Fillets (Van De Kamp's)	5 oz	100	4
Value Pack Portions (Gorton's)	1 portion	180	11
Value Pack Sticks (Gorton's)	4	190	9
breaded fillet, as prep	1 (2 oz)	155	7
stick, as prep	1 stick (1 oz)	76	3
HOME RECIPE			
fish loaf, cooked	3.5 oz	124	4
MIX			
Beer Batter Fry (Golden Dipt)	1 oz	100	0
Cajun Style Fish Fry (Golden Dipt)	⅔ oz	60	0

FOOD	PORTION	CALORIES	FAT
Fish & Chips Batter Mix (Golden Dipt)	1.25 oz	120	0
Fish Fry (Golden Dipt)	⅔ oz	60	0
Seafood Frying Mix (Golden Dipt)	⅔ oz	60	0
Tempura Batter Mix (Golden Dipt)	1 oz	100	0
TAKE-OUT			
kedgeree	5.6 oz	242	11
sandwich w/ tartar sauce	1	431	55
sandwich w/ tartar sauce, cheese	1	524	29
taramasalata	3.5 oz	446	46

FISH OILS
(see OILS)

FISH PASTE

fish paste	2 tsp	15	1

FISH SUBSTITUTES

Fillets, frzn (Worthington)	3.5 oz	209	11
Ocean Fillet (Loma Linda)	1 (2 oz)	160	10
Ocean Fillet (Loma Linda)	1 (1.7 oz)	130	8
Ocean Platter, mix not prep (Loma Linda)	¼ cup	50	1
Vege-Scallops (Loma Linda)	6 pieces (2.75 oz)	70	1

FLATFISH

FRESH			
cooked	3 oz	99	1
cooked	1 fillet (4.5 oz)	148	2
TAKE-OUT			
battered & fried	3.2 oz	211	11

FOOD	PORTION	CALORIES	FAT

FLAX

| Arrowhead Flax Seeds | 1 oz | 140 | 10 |

FLOUNDER

FROZEN

Crunchy Batter Fillets (Mrs. Paul's)	2 fillets	220	9
Fishmarket Fresh (Gorton's)	5 oz	110	1
Flounder Primavera (King & Prince)	4.5 oz	135	7
Flounder Primavera (King & Prince)	6 oz	180	9
Flounder Del Rey (King & Prince)	4.5 oz	163	8
Flounder Del Rey (King & Prince)	9 oz	327	16
Light Fillets (Mrs. Paul's)	1 fillet	240	10
Microwave Entree Stuffed (Gorton's)	1 pkg	350	18
Microwave Lightly Breaded (Van De Kamp's)	5 oz	290	18
Today's Catch (Van De Kamp's)	5 oz	100	1

FLOUR

All Purpose (Ballard)	1 cup	400	1
All Purpose (Ceresota)	1 cup	390	1
All Purpose (Gold Medal)	1 cup	400	1
All Purpose (Heckers)	1 cup	390	1
All Purpose (Pillsbury Best)	1 cup	400	1
All Purpose (Red Band)	1 cup	390	1
All Purpose (White Deer)	1 cup	400	1
All Purpose Unbleached (Pillsbury Best)	1 cup	400	1
Amaranth (Arrowhead)	2 oz	200	3
Barley (Arrowhead)	2 oz	200	1
Bohemian Style Rye & Wheat (Pillsbury Best)	1 cup	400	1

FOOD	PORTION	CALORIES	FAT
Bread (Pillsbury Best)	1 cup	400	2
Brown Rice Flour (Arrowhead)	2 oz	200	1
Buckwheat (Arrowhead)	2 oz	190	1
Drifted Snow (General Mills)	1 cup	400	1
Garbanzo Flour (Arrowhead)	2 oz	200	3
High Protein Better for Bread (Gold Medal)	1 cup	400	1
La Pina (Gold Medal)	1 cup	390	1
Medium Rye (Pillsbury Best)	1 cup	400	2
Millet (Arrowhead)	2 oz	185	2
Oat (Arrowhead)	2 oz	200	1
Pastry (Arrowhead)	2 oz	180	1
Rye (Arrowhead)	2 oz	190	1
Self-Rising (Aunt Jemima)	¼ cup	109	tr
Self-Rising (Ballard)	1 cup	380	1
Self-Rising (Gold Medal)	1 cup	380	1
Self-Rising (Pillsbury Best)	1 cup	380	1
Self-Rising (Red Band)	1 cup	380	1
Shake & Blend (Pillsbury Best)	2 tbsp	50	0
Softasilk (General Mills)	¼ cup	100	0
Soy (Arrowhead)	2 oz	250	11
Teff (Arrowhead)	2 oz	200	1
Unbleached (Gold Medal)	1 cup	400	1
Unbleached White (Arrowhead)	2 oz	200	1
Whole Wheat (Ceresota)	1 cup	400	2
Whole Wheat (Gold Medal)	1 cup	390	2
Whole Wheat (Heckers)	1 cup	400	2
Whole Wheat (Pillsbury Best)	1 cup	400	2
Whole Wheat (Red Band)	1 cup	400	2
Whole Wheat Blend (Gold Medal)	1 cup	370	2

FOOD	PORTION	CALORIES	FAT
Whole Wheat Stone Ground (Arrowhead)	2 oz	200	1
Wondra	1 cup	400	1
corn, masa	1 cup	416	4
corn, whole grain	1 cup	422	5
cottonseed lowfat	1 oz	94	tr
peanut, defatted	1 cup	196	tr
peanut, lowfat	1 cup	257	13
potato	1 cup	628	1
rice, brown	1 cup	574	4
rice, white	1 cup	578	2
rye, dark	1 cup	415	3
rye, light	1 cup	374	1
rye, medium	1 cup	361	2
sesame, lowfat	1 oz	95	tr
triticale whole grain	1 cup	440	2
white, all-purpose	1 cup	455	1
white, self-rising	1 cup	442	1
white bread	1 cup	495	2
white cake	1 cup	395	tr
whole wheat	1 cup	407	2

FRANKFURTER
(see HOT DOG)

FRENCH BEANS

DRIED
cooked	1 cup	228	1
raw	1 cup	631	4

FOOD	PORTION	CALORIES	FAT

FRENCH FRIES
(*see* POTATOES)

FRENCH TOAST

FROZEN

Cinnamon Swirl (Aunt Jemima)	3 oz	171	4
Cinnamon Swirl w/ Sausage (Great Starts)	5.5 oz	390	21
French Toast (Aunt Jemima)	3 oz	166	4
French Toast (Kid Cuisine)	4.11 oz	260	12
French Toast Sticks & Syrup (Quaker)	1 pkg (5.2 oz)	400	20
French Toast Wedges & Sausage (Quaker)	1 pkg (5.3 oz)	360	17
French Toast w/ Cinnamon (Weight Watchers)	2 slices	160	5
French Toast w/ Links (Weight Watchers)	4.5 oz	270	11
French Toast w/ LeanLinks (Healthy Starts)	6.5 oz	400	13
French Toast w/ Sausages (Great Starts)	5.5 oz	380	21
Mini French Toast w/ Sausage (Great Starts)	2.5 oz	190	9
Oatmeal French Toast w/ Lite Links (Great Starts)	4.65 oz	310	13

HOME RECIPE

french toast	1 slice	155	7

TAKE-OUT

w/ butter	2 slices	356	19

FROG'S LEGS

frog leg, as prep w/ seasoned flour & fried	1 (.8 oz)	70	5

FOOD	PORTION	CALORIES	FAT

FROSTING
(see CAKE)

FRUCTOSE
(see also SUGAR, SUGAR SUBSTITUTES)

Fructose (Estee)	1 tsp	12	0

FRUIT DRINKS

FROZEN

Seneca Cranberry Apple Juice Cocktail	6 oz	110	0
Seneca Grape Cranberry Juice Cocktail	6 oz	110	0
Seneca Raspberry Cranberry Juice Cocktail	6 oz	110	0
Tree Top Apple Citrus	6 oz	90	0
Tree Top Apple Grape	6 oz	100	0
Tree Top Apple Pear	6 oz	90	0
Tree Top Apple Raspberry	6 oz	80	0
citrus juice drink	1 cup	114	0
citrus juice drink, not prep	12 oz	684	tr
fruit punch	1 can (12 oz)	678	tr
fruit punch	1 cup	113	tr
lemonade	1 can (6 oz)	397	tr
lemonade	1 cup	100	tr
limeade	1 can (6 oz)	408	tr
limeade	1 cup	102	tr

MIX

Crystal Light Lemonade	8 oz	5	0
Crystal Light Lemon-Lime	8 oz	4	0
Kool-Aid Black Cherry	8 oz	98	0

FOOD	PORTION	CALORIES	FAT
Kool-Aid Cherry Sugar Free	8 oz	3	0
Kool-Aid Lemonade	8 oz	99	tr
Kool-Aid Lemonade Sugar Free	8 oz	4	tr
Kool-Aid Lemonade Sugar Sweetened	8 oz	78	tr
Kool-Aid Mountain Berry Punch Sugar Sweetened	8 oz	78	tr
Kool-Aid Orange	8 oz	98	0
Kool-Aid Rainbow Punch	8 oz	98	0
Kool-Aid Raspberry Sugar Sweetened	8 oz	79	tr
Kool-Aid Sunshine Punch	8 oz	99	0
Kool-Aid Tropical Punch Sugar Free	8 oz	3	tr
Kool-Aid Tropical Punch Sugar Sweetened	8 oz	84	tr
fruit punch	9 oz	97	0
lemonade	9 oz	113	tr
lemonade w/ Nutrasweet	1 pitcher (67 oz)	40	0
READY-TO-USE			
Bama Fruit Punch	8.45 oz	130	0
Dole Pineapple Grapefruit	6 oz	90	tr
Dole Pineapple Orange	6 oz	90	tr
Dole Pineapple Orange Banana	6 oz	90	tr
Dole Pineapple Pink Grapefruit	6 oz	100	tr
Hawaiian Punch Island Fruit Cocktail	6 oz	90	0
Hawaiian Punch Lite Fruit Juicy Red	6 oz	60	0
Hawaiian Punch Tropical Fruits	6 oz	90	0
Hawaiian Punch Very Berry	6 oz	90	0
Hawaiian Punch Wild Fruit	6 oz	90	0
Juice & More Apple Cherry	8 oz	120	0
Juice & More Apple Grape	8 oz	120	0

FOOD	PORTION	CALORIES	FAT
Juice & More Apple Raspberry	8 oz	120	0
Juice Works Appleberry	6 oz	100	0
Juicy Juice Apple Grape	6 oz	90	0
Kern's Apricot Orange Nectar	6 oz	112	0
Kern's Apricot Pineapple Nectar	6 oz	110	0
Kern's Coconut Pineapple Nectar	6 oz	120	0
Kern's Banana Pineapple Nectar	6 oz	120	0
Kern's Passionfruit Orange Nectar	6 oz	110	0
Kern's Strawberry Banana Nectar	6 oz	100	0
Kern's Tropical Nectar	6 oz	112	0
Libby's Passion Fruit Orange Nectar	8 oz	150	0
Libby's Strawberry Banana Nectar	8 oz	150	0
Mauna La'i Hawaiian Guava Fruit Drink	6 oz	100	0
Mauna La'i Hawaiian Guava Passion Fruit Drink	6 oz	100	0
Mott's Apple Cranberry	6 oz	83	0
Mott's Apple Cranberry	9.5 oz	167	0
Mott's Apple Grape	9.5 oz	139	0
Mott's Fruit Punch	9.5 oz	150	0
Mott's Grape Apple	9.5 oz	158	0
Ocean Spray Cranapple	6 oz	130	0
Ocean Spray Cranapple Low Calorie	6 oz	40	0
Ocean Spray Cran-Blueberry	6 oz	120	0
Ocean Spray Cran-Grape	6 oz	130	0
Ocean Spray Cranicot	6 oz	110	0
Ocean Spray Cran-Raspberry	6 oz	110	0
Ocean Spray Cran-Raspberry Low Calorie	6 oz	40	0
Ocean Spray Cran-Strawberry	6 oz	110	0
Ocean Spray Cran-Tastic	6 oz	110	0

FOOD	PORTION	CALORIES	FAT
Ocean Spray Pineapple Grapefruit Juice Cocktail	6 oz	110	0
S&W Apricot Pineapple Nectar	6 oz	120	0
Seneca Cranberry Apple Juice Cocktail	6 oz	110	0
Seneca Raspberry Cranberry Juice Cocktail	6 oz	110	0
Sipps Fruit Punch	8.45 oz	130	0
Sipps Lemonade	8.45 oz	85	0
Sipps Lemon Lime Cooler	8.45 oz	130	0
Sipps Mixed Berry	8.45 oz	130	0
Sipps Sunshine Punch	8.45 oz	130	0
Smucker's Apple Cranberry Juice	8 oz	120	0
Smucker's Orange Banana Juice	8 oz	120	0
Sunny Delight Florida Citrus Punch	6 oz	90	0
Tree Top Apple Citrus	6 oz	90	0
Tree Top Apple Cranberry	6 oz	100	0
Tree Top Apple Grape	6 oz	100	0
Tree Top Apple Pear	6 oz	90	0
Tree Top Apple Raspberry	6 oz	80	0
cranberry apple drink	6 oz	123	0
cranberry apricot drink	6 oz	118	0
fruit punch	6 oz	87	tr
orange & apricot	1 cup	128	tr
orange & grapefruit juice	1 cup	107	tr
pineapple & grapefruit	1 cup	117	tr
pineapple & orange drink	1 cup	125	0

FOOD	PORTION	CALORIES	FAT

FRUIT, MIXED
(see also individual names)

FOOD	PORTION	CALORIES	FAT
CANNED			
Chunky Mixed Fruit Diet (S&W)	½ cup	40	0
Chunky Mixed Fruit Natural Style (S&W)	½ cup	90	0
Chunky Mixed Fruit Unsweetened (S&W)	½ cup	40	0
Fruit Cocktail (Hunt's)	4 oz	90	tr
Fruit Cocktail Diet (S&W)	½ cup	40	0
Fruit Cocktail Heavy Syrup (S&W)	½ cup	90	0
Fruit Cocktail Natural Lite (S&W)	½ cup	60	0
Fruit Cocktail Natural Style (S&W)	½ cup	90	0
Fruit Cocktail Unsweetened (S&W)	½ cup	40	0
Tropical Fruit Salad (Dole)	½ cup	70	tr
fruit cocktail in heavy syrup	½ cup	93	tr
fruit cocktail juice pack	½ cup	56	tr
fruit cocktail water pack	½ cup	40	tr
fruit salad in heavy syrup	½ cup	94	tr
fruit salad in light syrup	½ cup	73	tr
fruit salad juice pack	½ cup	62	tr
fruit salad water pack	½ cup	37	tr
mixed fruit in heavy syrup	½ cup	92	tr
tropical fruit salad in heavy syrup	½ cup	110	tr
DRIED			
Fruit'n Nut Mix (Planters)	1 oz	150	9
mixed	11 oz pkg	712	1
FROZEN			
Mixed Fruit in Syrup (Birds Eye)	½ cup	123	tr
Tree Top Apple Cranberry, as prep	6 oz	100	0
mixed fruit sweetened	1 cup	245	tr

FOOD	PORTION	CALORIES	FAT

FRUIT SNACKS

Flavor Tree

FOOD	PORTION	CALORIES	FAT
Fruit Bears	1.05 oz	117	2
Fruit Circus	1.05 oz	117	2
Fruit Nibbles	½ pkg	118	2
Fruit Nibbles Cherry & Yogurt	½ pkg	133	4
Fruit Nibbles Orange & Yogurt	½ pkg	133	4
Fruit Nibbles Strawberry	½ pkg	135	5
Fruit People	1 oz	111	1
Fruit People Cherry	1 oz	111	2
Fruit People Lemon	1 oz	111	2
Fruit People Orange	1 oz	111	2
Fruit People Strawberry	1 oz	111	2
Fruit Roll Strawberry	1 roll	67	tr
Nibbles Cherry & Chocolate	1.05 oz	135	5

Health Valley

FOOD	PORTION	CALORIES	FAT
Bakes Apple	1 bar	100	3
Bakes Date	1 bar	100	3
Bakes Raisin	1 bar	100	3
Fat Free Fruit Bars 100% Organic Apple	1 bar	140	tr
Fat Free Fruit Bars 100% Organic Apricot	1 bar	140	tr
Fat Free Fruit Bars 100% Organic Date	1 bar	140	tr
Fat Free Fruit Bars 100% Organic Raisin	1 bar	140	tr
Fruit & Fitness Bars	2 bars	200	5
Oat Bran Bakes Apricot	1 bar	100	3
Oat Bran Bakes Fig & Nut	1 bar	110	3
Oat Bran Jumbo Fruit Bars Almond & Date	1 bar	170	5

FOOD	PORTION	CALORIES	FAT
Health Valley *(cont.)*			
Oat Bran Jumbo Fruit Bars Raisin & Cinnamon	1 bar	160	2
Rice Bran Jumbo Fruit Bars Almond & Date	1 bar	160	5
Sunkist Fun Fruit			
Alphabets	.9 oz	100	1
Animals	.9 oz	100	1
Berry Bunch	.9 oz	100	1
Cherry	.9 oz	100	1
Creme Supremes Cherry/ Chocolate Coated	½ pkg	135	5
Creme Supremes Cherry/Yogurt Coated	.9 oz	113	4
Dinosaurs Strawberry	.9 oz	100	1
Fantastic Fruit Punch	.9 oz	100	1
Grape	.9 oz	100	1
Numbers	.9 oz	100	1
Orange	.9 oz	100	1
Raspberry	.9 oz	100	1
Strawberry	.9 oz	100	1
Tropical Fruit	.9 oz	100	1
Weight Watchers Apple	½ oz	50	tr
Weight Watchers Cinnamon	½ oz	50	tr
Weight Watchers Peach	½ oz	50	tr
Weight Watchers Strawberry	½ oz	50	tr

GARBANZO
(*see* CHICKPEAS)

GARLIC

clove	1	4	tr
powder	1 tsp	9	tr

FOOD	PORTION	CALORIES	FAT

GEFILTE FISH

READY-TO-USE

FOOD	PORTION	CALORIES	FAT
Manischewitz	1 piece	107	4
Manischewitz Gefiltefish & Pike	1 piece	99	4
Manischewitz Gefiltefish & Pike Sweet	1 piece	129	4
Manischewitz Homestyle	1 piece	111	4
Manischewitz Sweet	1 piece	132	4
sweet	1 piece (1.5 oz)	35	1

GELATIN

DRINKS

FOOD	PORTION	CALORIES	FAT
Orange Flavored Drinking Gelatin w/ Nutrasweet (Knox)	1 envelope	39	tr

MIX

FOOD	PORTION	CALORIES	FAT
Apple (Royal)	½ cup	80	0
Apricot (Jell-O)	½ cup	80	tr
Blackberry (Jell-O)	½ cup	81	tr
Blackberry (Royal)	½ cup	80	0
Black Cherry (Jell-O)	½ cup	81	tr
Black Raspberry (Jell-O)	½ cup	81	tr
Cherry (Jell-O)	½ cup	81	tr
Cherry (Royal)	½ cup	80	0
Cherry Sugar Free (Diamond Crystal)	½ cup	8	tr
Cherry Sugar Free (Jell-O)	1 pop	9	tr
Cherry Sugar Free (Royal)	½ cup	8	0
Cherry w/ Nutrasweet (D-Zerta)	½ cup	8	tr
Concord Grape (Jell-O)	½ cup	81	tr
Concord Grape (Royal)	½ cup	80	0
Fruit Punch (Royal)	½ cup	80	0

FOOD	PORTION	CALORIES	FAT
Gelatin Desserts (Estee)	½ cup	8	0
Hawaiian Pineapple Sugar Free (Jell-O)	1 pop	8	tr
Lemon (Jell-O)	½ cup	81	tr
Lemon (Royal)	½ cup	80	0
Lemon Sugar Free (Diamond Crystal)	½ cup	8	tr
Lemon Sugar Free (Jell-O)	1 pop	8	tr
Lemon w/ Nutrasweet (D-Zerta)	½ cup	81	tr
Lemon-Lime (Royal)	½ cup	80	0
Lime (Jell-O)	½ cup	81	tr
Lime (Royal)	½ cup	80	0
Lime Sugar Free (Diamond Crystal)	½ cup	8	tr
Lime Sugar Free (Jell-O)	1 pop	8	tr
Lime Sugar Free (Royal)	½ cup	8	0
Lime w/ Nutrasweet (D-Zerta)	½ cup	9	tr
Mixed Berry (Royal)	½ cup	80	0
Mixed Fruit (Jell-O)	½ cup	81	tr
Mixed Fruit Sugar Free (Jell-O)	1 pop	8	tr
Orange (Jell-O)	½ cup	81	tr
Orange (Royal)	½ cup	80	0
Orange Pineapple (Jell-O)	½ cup	81	tr
Orange Sugar Free (Diamond Crystal)	½ cup	8	tr
Orange Sugar Free (Jell-O)	1 pop	8	tr
Orange Sugar Free (Royal)	½ cup	10	0
Orange w/ Nutrasweet (D-Zerta)	½ cup	8	tr
Peach (Jell-O)	½ cup	81	tr
Peach (Royal)	½ cup	80	0
Peach Sugar Free (Jell-O)	1 pop	8	tr
Pineapple (Royal)	½ cup	80	0

FOOD	PORTION	CALORIES	FAT
Raspberry (Jell-O)	½ cup	81	tr
Raspberry (Royal)	½ cup	80	0
Raspberry Sugar Free (Diamond Crystal)	½ cup	8	tr
Raspberry Sugar Free (Jell-O)	1 pop	8	tr
Raspberry Sugar Free (Royal)	½ cup	8	0
Raspberry w/ Nutrasweet (D-Zerta)	½ cup	8	tr
Strawberry (Jell-O)	½ cup	81	tr
Strawberry (Royal)	½ cup	80	0
Strawberry Sugar Free (Diamond Crystal)	½ cup	8	tr
Strawberry Sugar Free (Jell-O)	1 pop	8	tr
Strawberry Sugar Free (Royal)	½ cup	8	0
Strawberry w/ Nutrasweet (D-Zerta)	½ cup	8	tr
Strawberry Banana (Jell-O)	½ cup	81	tr
Strawberry Banana Sugar Free (Jell-O)	½ cup	8	0
Strawberry Banana Sugar Free (Royal)	½ cup	8	0
Strawberry-Orange (Royal)	½ cup	80	0
Triple Berry Sugar Free (Jell-O)	1 pop	8	tr
Tropical Fruit (Royal)	½ cup	80	0
Wild Strawberry (Jell-O)	½ cup	81	tr
fruit flavored	½ cup	70	0
low calorie	½ cup	8	0

GIBLETS

capon, simmered	1 cup (5 oz)	238	8
chicken, floured, fried	1 cup (5 oz)	402	19
chicken, simmered	1 cup (5 oz)	228	7
turkey, simmered	1 cup (5 oz)	243	7

FOOD	PORTION	CALORIES	FAT
GINGER			
ground	1 tsp	6	tr
root, fresh	¼ cup	17	tr
root, fresh	5 slices	8	tr
root, fresh, sliced	5 slices	8	tr
root, fresh, sliced	¼ cup	17	tr
GINKGO NUTS			
canned	1 oz	32	tr
dried	1 oz	99	tr
raw	1 oz	52	tr
GIZZARDS			
chicken, simmered	1 cup (5 oz)	222	5
turkey, simmered	1 cup (5 oz)	236	6
GOAT			
roasted	3 oz	122	3
GOOSE			
FRESH			
w/ skin, roasted	6.6 oz	574	41
w/ skin, roasted	½ goose (1.7 lbs)	2362	170
w/o skin, roasted	5 oz	340	18
w/o skin, roasted	½ goose (1.3 lbs)	1406	75
GOOSEBERRIES			
fresh	1 cup	67	1
CANNED			
in light syrup	½ cup	93	tr

FOOD	PORTION	CALORIES	FAT

GRANOLA
(see also CEREAL)

BARS

FOOD	PORTION	CALORIES	FAT
Fi-Bar Coconut	1	120	4
Fi-Bar Peanut Butter	1	130	4
Hershey Chocolate Covered Chocolate Chip	1 (1.2 oz)	170	8
Hershey Chocolate Covered Cocoa Creme	1 (1.2 oz)	180	9
Hershey Chocolate Covered Cookies & Creme	1 (1.2 oz)	170	8
Hershey Chocolate Covered Peanut Butter	1 (1.2 oz)	180	10
Kudos Chocolate Chip	1.2 oz	180	9
Kudos Nutty Fudge	1.3 oz	190	11
Kudos Peanut Butter	1.3 oz	190	11
New Trail Chocolate Covered Cookies & Creme	1	200	11
Quaker Chewy Chocolate Chip	1	128	5
Quaker Chewy Chunky Nut & Raisin	1	131	6
Quaker Chewy Cinnamon Raisin	1	128	5
Quaker Chewy Honey & Oats	1	125	4
Quaker Chewy Peanut Butter	1	128	5
Quaker Chewy Peanut Butter Chocolate Chip	1	131	6
Quaker Dipps Caramel Nut	1	148	6
Quaker Dipps Chocolate Chip	1	139	6
Quaker Dipps Chocolate Fudge	1	160	8
Quaker Dipps Peanut Butter	1	170	9
Quaker Dipps Peanut Butter Chocolate Chip	1	174	10
Quaker Dipps Rocky Road	1	140	7

FOOD	PORTION	CALORIES	FAT
Sunbelt Chewy Granola Chocolate Chip	1 bar (1.25 oz)	150	7
Sunbelt Chewy Granola Oats & Honey	1 bar (1 oz)	130	5
Sunbelt Chewy Granola w/ Almonds	1 bar (1 oz)	120	6
Sunbelt Chewy Granola w/ Raisins	1 bar (1.25 oz)	150	6
Sunbelt Fudge Dipped Chewy Granola Chocolate Chip	1 bar (1.5 oz)	210	10
Sunbelt Fudge Dipped Chewy Granola Macaroon	1 bar (1.4 oz)	200	11
Sunbelt Fudge Dipped Chewy Granola w/ Peanuts	1 bar (1.5 oz)	200	12
CEREAL			
Arrowhead Maple-Nut	2 oz	250	9
Erewhon Date Nut	1 oz	130	6
Erewhon Honey Almond	1 oz	130	6
Erewhon Maple	1 oz	130	5
Erewhon Spiced Apple	1 oz	130	6
Erewhon Sunflower Crunch	1 oz	130	4
Erewhon w/ Bran	1 oz	130	6
Nature Valley Cinnamon & Raisin	⅓ cup	120	4
Nature Valley Cinnamon & Raisin	⅓ cup + ½ cup milk	160	4
Nature Valley Coconut & Honey	⅓ cup	150	7
Nature Valley Coconut Honey	⅓ cup + ½ cup milk	190	7
Nature Valley Fruit & Nut	⅓ cup + ½ cup milk	170	5
Nature Valley Toasted Nut	⅓ cup	130	5
Nature Valley Toasted Nut	⅓ cup + ½ cup milk	170	5
Post Hearty	¼ cup	127	4

FOOD	PORTION	CALORIES	FAT
Post Hearty	¼ cup + ½ cup milk	203	8
Post Hearty w/ Raisins	¼ cup	123	4
Quaker Sun Country 100% Natural w/ Almonds	¼ cup	130	5
Quaker Sun Country 100% Natural w/ Raisins & Dates	¼ cup	123	5
Quaker Sun Country w/ Raisins	¼ cup	125	5
Sunbelt Banana Almond	1 oz	130	4
Sunbelt Fruit & Nut	1 oz	120	5

GRAPEFRUIT

FOOD	PORTION	CALORIES	FAT
CANNED			
Sections in Light Syrup (S&W)	½ cup	80	0
Sections Natural Style (S&W)	½ cup	40	0
Sections Unsweetened (S&W)	½ cup	40	0
juice pack	½ cup	46	tr
unsweetened	1 cup	93	tr
water pack	½ cup	44	tr
FRESH			
Chiquita Ruby Red	½	40	0
Dole	½	50	0
Ocean Spray Pink	½ med	50	0
Ocean Spray White	½ med	45	0
pink	½	37	tr
pink sections	1 cup	69	tr
red	½	37	tr
red sections	1 cup	69	tr
white	½	39	tr
white sections	1 cup	76	tr

FOOD	PORTION	CALORIES	FAT
JUICE			
Libby's	6 oz	70	0
Mott's	10 oz	124	0
Ocean Spray	6 oz	60	0
Ocean Spray Pink Grapefruit Juice Cocktail	6 oz	80	0
Ocean Spray Pink Premium Grapefruit Juice	6 oz	60	0
S&W Unsweetened	6 oz	80	0
Tree Top	6 oz	80	0
fresh	1 cup	96	tr
frzn	1 cup	102	tr
frzn, not prep	6 oz	302	1
sweetened	1 cup	116	tr

GRAPES

FOOD	PORTION	CALORIES	FAT
CANNED			
Thompson Seedless Premium (S&W)	½ cup	100	0
thompson seedless in heavy syrup	½ cup	94	tr
thompson seedless water pack	½ cup	48	tr
FRESH			
Dole	1½ cup	85	0
grapes	10	36	tr
JUICE			
Bama	8.45 oz	120	0
Crystal Light	8 oz	3	0
Hawaiian Punch	6 oz	90	0
Juice Works	6 oz	100	0
Kool-Aid	8 oz	98	0
Ocean Spray Concord Grape Concentrated, as prep	6 oz	100	0

FOOD	PORTION	CALORIES	FAT
S&W Concord Unsweetened	6 oz	100	0
Seneca	6 oz	115	0
Seneca Grape, frzn, as prep	6 oz	100	0
Seneca Natural, frzn, as prep	6 oz	115	0
Seneca White Grape Juice, frzn, as prep	6 oz	110	0
Sippin' Pak 100% Pure	8.45 oz	130	0
Sipps Grape	8.45 oz	130	0
Tree Top	6 oz	120	0
Tree Top Sparkling Juice	6 oz	120	0
bottled	1 cup	155	tr
frzn, sweetened, as prep	1 cup	128	tr
frzn, sweetened, not prep	6 oz	386	1
grape drink	6 oz	84	0

GRAVY
(*see also* SAUCE)

FOOD	PORTION	CALORIES	FAT
CANNED			
Au Jus (Franco-American)	2 oz	10	0
Beef (Franco-American)	2 oz	25	1
Bovril	1 heaping tsp	9	0
Chicken (Franco-American)	2 oz	45	4
Chicken Giblet (Franco-American)	2 oz	30	2
Cream (Franco-American)	2 oz	35	2
Marmite	1 heaping tsp	9	0
Mushroom (Franco-American)	2 oz	25	1
Pork (Franco-American)	2 oz	40	3
Turkey (Franco-American)	2 oz	30	2
au jus	1 cup	38	tr
beef	1 cup	124	6
beef	1 can (10 oz)	155	7

FOOD	PORTION	CALORIES	FAT
chicken	1 cup	189	14
mushroom	1 cup	120	6
turkey	1 cup	122	5
DRY			
Bournvita	2 heaping tsp	34	1
Brown (Pillsbury)	¼ cup	15	0
Chicken (Diamond Crystal)	2 oz	30	1
Chicken (Pillsbury)	¼ cup	25	1
Home Style (Pillsbury)	¼ cup	15	0
au jus	1 cup	32	1
brown	1 cup	75	2
chicken	1 cup	83	2
mushroom	1 cup	70	1
onion	1 cup	77	1
pork	1 cup	76	2
turkey	1 cup	87	2

GREAT NORTHERN BEANS

	PORTION	CALORIES	FAT
CANNED			
Great Northern (Green Giant)	½ cup	80	1
Great Northern (Hanover)	½ cup	110	0
Great Northern (Trappey's)	½ cup	80	1
Seasoned w/ Pork (Luck's)	7.25 oz	220	5
great northern	1 cup	300	1
DRIED			
Great Northern (Hurst Brand)	1 cup	277	1
cooked	1 cup	210	1
raw	1 cup	621	2

FOOD	PORTION	CALORIES	FAT

GREEN BEANS

FOOD	PORTION	CALORIES	FAT
CANNED			
Almondine (Green Giant)	½ cup	45	3
Cut (Green Giant)	½ cup	16	0
Cut (Libby)	½ cup	20	0
Cut (Owatonna)	½ cup	20	0
Cut (Seneca)	½ cup	20	0
Cut Natural Pack (Libby)	½ cup	20	1
Cut Premium Blue Lake (S&W)	½ cup	20	0
Cut Water Pack (S&W)	½ cup	20	0
Cuts Natural Pack (Seneca)	½ cup	20	0
Dilled (S&W)	½ cup	60	0
French (Green Giant)	½ cup	16	0
French (Libby)	½ cup	20	0
French (Owatonna)	½ cup	20	0
French (Seneca)	½ cup	20	0
French Natural Pack (Libby)	½ cup	20	1
French Natural Pack (Seneca)	½ cup	20	0
French Style Premium Blue Lake (S&W)	½ cup	20	0
Kitchen Sliced (Green Giant)	½ cup	16	0
Whole (Libby)	½ cup	20	0
Whole (Seneca)	½ cup	20	0
Whole Fancy Stringless (S&W)	½ cup	20	0
Whole Vertical Pack (S&W)	½ cup	20	0
FROZEN			
Bavarian Style Beans & Spaetzle (Birds Eye)	½ cup	98	5
Cut (Birds Eye)	½ cup	25	tr
Cut (Hanover)	½ cup	20	0

FOOD	PORTION	CALORIES	FAT
Cut (Southland)	3 oz	25	0
Cut in Butter Sauce (Green Giant)	½ cup	30	1
French (Birds Eye)	½ cup	26	tr
French (Southland)	3 oz	25	0
French Style Blue Lake (Hanover)	½ cup	25	0
French w/ Toasted Almonds (Birds Eye)	½ cup	52	2
Green Giant	½ cup	14	0
Harvest Fresh Cut (Green Giant)	½ cup	16	0
Italian (Birds Eye)	½ cup	31	tr
Italian Cut (Hanover)	½ cup	35	0
One Serve in Butter Sauce (Green Giant)	1 pkg	60	2
Whole (Birds Eye)	½ cup	23	tr
Whole Blue Lake (Hanover)	½ cup	30	0
SHELF STABLE Cut (Pantry Express)	½ cup	12	0

GROUNDCHERRIES

fresh	½ cup	37	tr

GROUPER

FRESH			
cooked	3 oz	100	1
cooked	1 fillet (7.1 oz)	238	3

GUAVA

guava sauce	½ cup	43	tr
fresh	1	45	1
JUICE Kern's Nectar	6 oz	110	0

FOOD	PORTION	CALORIES	FAT
Libby's Nectar	6 oz	110	0
Libby's Ripe Nectar	8 oz	140	0

GUINEA HEN

w/ skin, raw	½ hen (12.1 oz)	545	22
w/o skin, raw	½ hen (9.3 oz)	292	7

HADDOCK

cooked	3 oz	95	1
cooked	1 fillet (5.3 oz)	168	1
roe, raw	3½ oz	130	2
FROZEN			
Batter-Dipped (Van De Kamp's)	2 pieces	240	12
Breaded Fillets (Van De Kamp's)	1 fillet	180	13
Crunchy Batter Fillets (Mrs. Paul's)	2 fillets	190	5
Fishmarket Fresh (Gorton's)	5 oz	110	1
Light Fillets (Mrs. Paul's)	1 fillet	220	9
Lightly Breaded (Van De Kamp's)	5 oz	300	19
Microwave Lightly Breaded (Van De Kamp's)	5 oz	300	19
Microwave Entree in Lemon Butter (Gorton's)	1 pkg	360	21
Today's Catch (Van De Kamp's)	5 oz	110	0
SMOKED			
smoked	3 oz	99	1
smoked	1 oz	33	tr

HAKE

raw	3.5 oz	84	1

FOOD	PORTION	CALORIES	FAT

HALIBUT

FRESH

atlantic & pacific, cooked	½ fillet (5.6 oz)	223	5
atlantic & pacific, cooked	3 oz	119	2
greenland, baked	3 oz	203	15
greenland, baked	5.6 oz	380	28

FROZEN

Batter-Dipped (Van De Kamp's)	3 pieces	260	16
Lightly Breaded (Van De Kamp's)	4 oz	220	11
Microwave Lightly Breaded (Van De Kamp's)	4 oz	220	11

HAM

(*see also* HAM DISHES, LUNCHEON MEATS/COLD CUTS, PORK, TURKEY)

Armour Golden Star Boneless	1 oz	33	1
Armour Golden Star Canned	1 oz	32	tr
Armour Lower Salt 93% Fat Free	1 oz	35	1
Armour Lower Salt Boneless	1 oz	34	1
Armour Star Boneless	1 oz	41	2
Armour Star Canned	1 oz	34	1
Armour Star Speedy Cut	1 oz	44	3
Armour 1877 Boneless	1 oz	42	2
Carl Buddig	1 oz	50	3
Hansel 'n Gretel Baked Virginia	1 oz	34	1
Hansel 'n Gretel Black Forest	1 oz	32	1
Hansel 'n Gretel Cappy	1 oz	31	1
Hansel 'n Gretel Cooked Fresh	1 oz	33	1
Hansel 'n Gretel Deluxe	1 oz	31	1
Hansel 'n Gretel Honey Valley	1 oz	31	1
Hansel 'n Gretel Jalapeno	1 oz	25	1

FOOD	PORTION	CALORIES	FAT
Hansel 'n Gretel Lessalt	1 oz	30	1
Hansel 'n Gretel Lessalt Virginia	1 oz	32	1
Hansel 'n Gretel Light	1 oz	27	1
Hansel 'n Gretel Travane	1 oz	31	1
Krakus Polish Cooked	3.5 oz	193	12
Oscar Mayer Baked Cooked	1 slice (21 g)	21	tr
Oscar Mayer Boiled w/ Natural Juices	1 slice (21 g)	23	tr
Oscar Mayer Breakfast Ham Water Added	1 slice (43 g)	52	2
Oscar Mayer Chopped w/ Natural Juices	1 slice (28 g)	55	4
Oscar Mayer Cracked Black Pepper	1 slice (21 g)	24	tr
Oscar Mayer Ham & Cheese Loaf	1 slice (28 g)	76	6
Oscar Mayer Ham & Cheese Spread	1 oz	67	5
Oscar Mayer Ham Salad Spread w/ Natural Juice	1 oz	59	4
Oscar Mayer Honey w/ Natural Juices	1 slice (21 g)	26	1
Oscar Mayer Jubilee Boneless	1 oz	46	3
Oscar Mayer Jubilee Canned w/ Natural Juice	1 oz	31	1
Oscar Mayer Jubilee Slice w/ Water Added	1 oz	29	1
Oscar Mayer Jubilee Steak w/ Water Added	1 slice (2 oz)	59	2
Oscar Mayer Smoked Cooked	1 slice (21 g)	23	tr
Russer Lil' Salt Cooked	1 oz	30	1
Russer Lil' Salt Smoked	1 oz	30	1
The Spreadables Ham Salad	¼ can	100	6
Weight Watchers Deli Thin Oven Roasted	5 slices (⅓ oz)	12	tr

FOOD	PORTION	CALORIES	FAT
Weight Watchers Deli Thin Oven Roasted Honey Ham	5 slices (⅓ oz)	12	tr
Weight Watchers Deli Thin Premium Smoked	5 slices (⅓ oz)	12	tr
Weight Watchers Oven Roasted Honey Ham	2 slices (¾ oz)	25	1
Weight Watchers Oven Roasted Smoked	2 slices (¾ oz)	25	1
Weight Watchers Premium Cooked	2 slices (¾ oz)	25	1
boneless (11% fat), roasted	3 oz	151	8
boneless extra lean, roasted	3 oz	140	7
canned (13% fat), roasted	3 oz	192	13
canned (13% fat)	1 oz	54	4
canned extra lean	1 oz	41	2
canned extra lean	3 oz	142	7
canned extra lean (4% fat)	3 oz	116	4
center slice, lean & fat	4 oz	229	15
center slice, lean only	4 oz	220	9
chopped	1 oz	65	5
chopped, canned	1 oz	68	5
ham & cheese loaf	1 oz	73	6
ham & cheese spread	1 oz	69	5
ham & cheese spread	1 tbsp	37	3
ham salad spread	1 oz	61	4
ham salad spread	1 tbsp	32	2
minced	1 oz	75	6
patties, grilled	1 patty (2 oz)	203	18
patties, uncooked	1 (2.3 oz)	206	18
sliced, extra lean (5% fat)	1 oz	37	1
sliced, regular (11% fat)	1 oz	52	3
steak, boneless, extra lean	1 oz	35	1

FOOD	PORTION	CALORIES	FAT
whole, lean & fat, roasted	3 oz	207	14
whole, lean only, roasted	3 oz	133	5

HAM DISHES

FROZEN

Handy Pocket Cheese Sauce & Ham (Weight Watchers)	1 (4 oz)	200	6
Ovenstuffs Ham/Turkey Deli Melt	1 (4.75 oz)	360	15

HOME RECIPE

croquettes	1 (3.1)	217	14
salad	½ cup	287	23

TAKE-OUT

sandwich w/ cheese	1	353	15

HAMBURGER

(*see also* BEEF, FROZEN)

FROZEN

Kid Cuisine Beef Patty Sandwich w/ Cheese	6.25 oz	430	22
Kid Cuisine Mega Meal Double Beef Patty Sandwich w/ Cheese	9.1 oz	480	20
MicroMagic Cheeseburger	1 pkg (4.75 oz)	450	25
MicroMagic Hamburger	1 pkg (4 oz)	350	18

TAKE-OUT

double patty w/ bun	1 reg	544	28
double patty w/ bun, catsup, mayonnaise, mustard, pickle, onion, tomato	1 lg	540	27
double patty w/ bun, catsup, mustard, pickle, onion	1 reg	576	32
double patty w/ bun, cheese	1 reg	457	28

FOOD	PORTION	CALORIES	FAT
double patty w/ bun, cheese, catsup, mustard, mayonnaise, pickle, tomato	1 lg	706	44
double patty w/ bun, cheese, catsup, pickle, mayonnaise, onion, tomato	1 reg	416	21
double patty w/ double bun, catsup, pickle, mayonnaise, onion, tomato	1 reg	649	35
double patty w/ double bun, cheese	1 reg	461	22
single patty w/ bun	1 reg	275	12
single patty w/ bun	1 lg	400	23
single patty w/ bun, catsup, mayonnaise, mustard, pickle, onion, tomato	1 reg	279	13
single patty w/ bun, cheese	1 reg	320	15
single patty w/ bun, cheese	1 lg	608	33
single patty w/ bun, cheese, bacon, catsup, mustard, pickle, onion	1 lg	609	37
single patty w/ bun, cheese, ham, catsup, mayonnaise, pickle, tomato	1 lg	745	48
triple patty w/ bun, catsup, mustard, pickle	1 lg	693	41
triple patty w/ bun, cheese	1 lg	769	51

HEART

FOOD	PORTION	CALORIES	FAT
beef, simmered	3 oz	148	5
chicken, simmered	1 cup (5 oz)	268	11
lamb, braised	3 oz	158	7
pork, braised	1 (4.3 oz)	191	7
turkey, simmered	1 cup (5 oz)	257	9
veal, braised	3 oz	158	6

HERBAL TEA
(*see* TEA/HERBAL TEA)

FOOD	PORTION	CALORIES	FAT

HERBS/SPICES
(*see also individual names*)

FOOD	PORTION	CALORIES	FAT
All Purpose Seafood (Golden Dipt)	¼ tsp	2	0
Bar-B-Q Shaker (Diamond Crystal)	½ tsp	4	0
Blackened Redfish (Golden Dipt)	¼ tsp	2	0
Broiled Fish (Golden Dipt)	¼ tsp	2	0
Cajun Style Shrimp & Crab (Golden Dipt)	¼ tsp	2	0
Chef Seasoning (Diamond Crystal)	1 pkg (.45 oz)	2	0
Chef Shaker (Diamond Crystal)	½ tsp	4	0
Cleopatra's Secret (Nile Spice)	⅛ tsp	0	0
Desert Spice (Nile Spice)	⅛ tsp	0	0
French Shaker (Diamond Crystal)	½ tsp	4	0
Ginger Curry (Nile Spice)	⅛ tsp	0	0
Italian Shaker (Diamond Crystal)	½ tsp	4	0
Lemon Pepper Seafood (Golden Dipt)	¼ tsp	8	0
Maya Maize Popcorn Seasoning (Nile Spice)	½ tsp	0	tr
Mexican Shaker (Diamond Crystal)	½ tsp	4	0
Mrs. Dash Extra Spicy	1 tsp	12	tr
Mrs. Dash Garlic & Herb	1 tsp	12	tr
Mrs. Dash Lemon & Herb	1 tsp	12	tr
Mrs. Dash Low Pepper Blend	1 tsp	12	tr
Mrs. Dash Original	1 tsp	12	tr
Mrs. Dash Table Blend	1 tsp	12	tr
Nile Spice	⅛ tsp	0	0
curry powder	1 tsp	6	tr
poultry seasoning	1 tsp	5	tr
pumpkin pie spice	1 tsp	6	tr

FOOD	PORTION	CALORIES	FAT

HERRING

FRESH

atlantic, cooked	1 fillet (5 oz)	290	17
atlantic, cooked	3 oz	172	10
pacific, baked	3 oz	213	15
pacific fillet, baked	5.1 oz	360	26
roe, raw	3.5 oz	130	2

READY-TO-USE

atlantic, kippered	1 fillet (1.4 oz)	87	5
atlantic, pickled	½ oz	39	3

HICKORY NUTS

dried	1 oz	187	18

HOMINY

canned	½ cup	57	tr

HONEY

Burleson's Clover	1 tbsp	60	0
Burleson's Creamed	1 tbsp	60	0
Burleson's Natural	1 tbsp	60	0
Burleson's Pure	1 tbsp	60	0
Burleson's Raw	1 tbsp	60	0
Burleson's Rocky Mountain Clover	1 tbsp	60	0
Golden Blossom	1 tsp	20	0
Smucker's Single Serving	½ oz	45	0
honey	1 cup	1030	0
honey	1 tbsp	65	0

FOOD	PORTION	CALORIES	FAT

HONEYDEW

Chiquita	1 cup	70	0
Dole	1/10 melon	50	0
cubed	1 cup	60	tr
fresh	1/10 melon	46	tr

HORSE

roasted	3 oz	149	5

HORSERADISH

Gold's Hot	1 tsp	4	tr
Gold's Red	1 tsp	4	0
Gold's White	1 tsp	4	tr
Kraft Horseradish Mustard	1 tbsp	14	1
Kraft Cream Style Prepared	1 tbsp	12	1
Kraft Prepared	1 tbsp	10	1
Sauceworks Horseradish	1 tbsp	50	5

HOT CAKES
(see PANCAKES)

HOT DOG
(see also MEAT SUBSTITUTES, SAUSAGE, SAUSAGE SUBSTITUTES)

CHICKEN
Health Valley Wieners	1	96	8
Wampler Longacre	1 (2 oz)	144	44
Wampler Longacre	1 (1.6 oz)	115	35
Weaver	1 (1.6 oz)	115	10
chicken	1 (1.5 oz)	116	9

MEAT
Armour Lower Salt Jumbo	1	170	15

FOOD	PORTION	CALORIES	FAT
Armour Lower Salt Jumbo Beef	1	170	15
Armour Star Jumbo	1	190	18
Armour Star Jumbo Beef	1	190	18
Chefwich Chili Dog	5 oz	380	15
Hebrew National	1 (1.8 oz)	160	15
Hebrew National	1 (1.6 oz)	140	13
Hebrew National Deli Frankfurter	1 (2.3 oz)	200	19
Nathan's Famous Natural Casing Franks	1	158	14
Nathan's Famous Skinless Franks	1	176	16
Oscar Mayer Bacon & Cheddar Cheese	1 (1.6 oz)	143	13
Oscar Mayer Beef Franks	1 (1.6 oz)	144	13
Oscar Mayer Beef w/ Cheddar Franks	1 (1.6 oz)	130	11
Oscar Mayer Bun-Length Franks	1 (2 oz)	186	17
Oscar Mayer Bun-Length Wieners	1 (2 oz)	181	17
Oscar Mayer Cheese Hot Dogs	1 (1.6 oz)	145	13
Oscar Mayer German Blend Frankfurters	1 (2.7 oz)	230	21
Oscar Mayer Wieners	1 (1.6 oz)	144	13
Oscar Mayer Wieners Little	1 (.3 oz)	28	3
beef	1 (2 oz)	180	16
beef	1 (1.5)	142	13
beef & pork	1 (2 oz)	183	17
beef & pork	1 (1.5 oz)	144	13
pork cheesefurter smokie	1 (1.5 oz)	141	12
TAKE-OUT			
corndog	1	460	19
w/ bun, chili	1	297	13
w/ bun, plain	1	242	15

FOOD	PORTION	CALORIES	FAT
TURKEY			
Bil Mar Foods Cheese Franks	1 (1.6 oz)	109	9
Health Valley Wieners	1	96	8
Louis Rich	1 (1.6 oz)	103	9
Louis Rich Turkey Cheese Franks	1 (1.6 oz)	108	9
Mr. Turkey Franks	1 (2 oz)	132	11
Mr. Turkey Franks	1 (1.6 oz)	106	9
Mr. Turkey Franks	1 (½ oz)	79	7
Wampler Longacre	1 (1.6 oz)	102	31
turkey	1 (1.5 oz)	102	8

HUMMUS

hummus	⅓ cup	140	7
hummus	1 cup	420	21

HUSH PUPPY
(*see* CORNMEAL)

HYACINTH BEANS

dried, cooked	1 cup	228	1
dried, raw	1 cup	723	4

ICE CREAM AND FROZEN DESSERT

All Flavors Avari Creme Glace	1 oz	10	0
All Flavors Ice (Bresler's)	3.5 oz	120	0
All Flavors Ice Cream (Bresler's)	3.5 oz	230	12
All Flavors Royale Cremes (Bresler's)	4 oz	260	16
All Flavors Royale Lites (Bresler's)	4 oz	217	0
All Flavors Sherbet (Bresler's)	3.5 oz	140	2
Almond Praline Light (Edy's)	4 oz	140	5
Banana Cream (Fi-Bar)	1 bar	93	tr

FOOD	PORTION	CALORIES	FAT
Banana Fruit & Cream (Chiquita)	1 bar	80	2
Banana-Politan Light (Edy's)	4 oz	110	4
Berry Berry Berry (Mocha Mix)	3.5 oz	209	9
Berry Blend Pops (Crystal Light)	1 bar	14	tr
Berry Punch (Jell-O)	1 pop	31	tr
Black Cherry (Sealtest Free)	½ cup	100	0
Blueberry Sorbet & Cream (Haagen-Dazs)	4 oz	190	8
Blueberry Fruit & Cream (Chiquita)	1 bar	80	1
Bordeaux Cherry (Healthy Choice)	4 oz	120	1
Bubble Crazy (Good Humor)	3 oz	74	1
Bubble O Bill (Good Humor)	3.5 oz	149	8
Butter Almond (Breyers)	½ cup	170	10
Butter Crunch (Sealtest)	½ cup	150	7
Butter Pecan (Breyers)	½ cup	180	12
Butter Pecan (Frusen Gladje)	½ cup	280	21
Butter Pecan (Haagen-Dazs)	4 oz	390	24
Butter Pecan (Sealtest)	½ cup	160	9
Butter Pecan Light (Edy's)	4 oz	140	5
Buttered Pecan (Lady Borden)	½ cup	180	12
Cafe Au Lait Light (Edy's)	4 oz	110	4
Candy Bar Light (Edy's)	4 oz	140	5
Caramel Almond Crunch Bar (Haagen-Dazs)	1	240	18
Caramel Nut Ice Milk (Light N'Lively)	½ cup	120	4
Caramel Nut Sundae (Haagen-Dazs)	4 oz	310	21
Cherry (Jell-O)	1 pop	32	tr
Cherry & Ice Cream Swirl (Chiquita)	1 bar	80	3
Cherry Cola Kick (Good Humor)	4.5 oz	106	1
Cherry Fruit & Juice Bars (Chiquita)	1 bar (2 oz)	50	0

FOOD	PORTION	CALORIES	FAT
Cherry Fruit Bars (Jell-O)	1 bar (1.8 oz)	39	tr
Cherry Garcia (Ben & Jerry's)	4 oz	280	17
Cherry Italian Ice (Good Humor)	6 oz	138	tr
Cherry/Orange Ice Stripes (Good Humor)	1.5 oz	35	0
Cherry Pop (Ben & Jerry's)	1	330	24
Cherry Vanilla (Breyers)	½ cup	150	7
Chip Candy Crunch (Good Humor)	3 oz	347	24
Chocolate (Ben & Jerry's)	4 oz	260	16
Chocolate (Breyers)	½ cup	160	8
Chocolate (Frusen Gladje)	½ cup	240	17
Chocolate (Haagen-Dazs)	4 oz	270	17
Chocolate (Healthy Choice)	4 oz	130	2
Chocolate (Sealtest)	½ cup	140	6
Chocolate (Sealtest Free)	½ cup	100	0
Chocolate (Simple Pleasures)	4 oz	140	tr
Chocolate (Ultra Slim-Fast)	4 oz	100	tr
Chocolate American Dream (Edy's)	3 oz	90	1
Chocolate Brownie Bar (Ben & Jerry's)	1	360	18
Chocolate Brownie Light (Ben & Jerry's)	4 oz	230	10
Chocolate Caramel Sundae Light (Simple Pleasures)	4 oz	90	tr
Chocolate Chip (Sealtest)	½ cup	150	8
Chocolate Chip (Simple Pleasures)	4 oz	150	3
Chocolate Chip American Dream (Edy's)	3 oz	100	1
Chocolate Chip Ice Milk (Light N'Lively)	½ cup	120	4
Chocolate Chip Ice Milk (Weight Watchers)	½ cup	120	4

FOOD	PORTION	CALORIES	FAT
Chocolate Chip Light (Edy's)	4 oz	120	4
Chocolate Chocolate Chip (Frusen Gladje)	½ cup	270	18
Chocolate Chocolate Chip (Haagen-Dazs)	4 oz	290	20
Chocolate Chocolate Mint (Haagen-Dazs)	4 oz	300	20
Chocolate Creamy Lites Bar (Carnation)	1	50	2
Chocolate Dark Chocolate Bar (Haagen-Dazs)	1	390	27
Chocolate Dip Bar (Weight Watchers)	1 (2 oz)	110	7
Chocolate Eclair (Good Humor)	3 oz	187	10
Chocolate Fat Free Frozen Dessert (Weight Watchers)	½ cup	80	0
Chocolate Flavor Coated Vanilla Ice Cream (Good Humor)	3 oz	198	14
Chocolate Fudge (Ultra Slim-Fast)	4 oz	120	tr
Chocolate Fudge Brownie (Ben & Jerry's)	4 oz	280	16
Chocolate Fudge Cake (Good Humor)	6.3 oz	214	15
Chocolate Fudge Heaven Sundae Bar (Carnation)	1	150	9
Chocolate Fudge Mousse Light (Edy's)	4 oz	130	5
Chocolate Fudge Swirl Dessert Bar (Sealtest Free)	1	90	0
Chocolate Fudge Twirl Ice Milk (Breyers Light)	½ cup	130	4
Chocolate Ice Milk (Borden)	½ cup	100	2
Chocolate Ice Milk (Breyers Light)	½ cup	120	4
Chocolate Light (Simple Pleasures)	4 oz	80	tr

FOOD	PORTION	CALORIES	FAT
Chocolate Malt (Good Humor)	3 oz	187	13
Chocolate Malted Bars (Carnation)	1	70	3
Chocolate Marshmallow Sundae (Sealtest)	½ cup	150	6
Chocolate Mousse Bar Sugar Free (Weight Watchers)	1 (1.75 oz)	35	tr
Chocolate Swirl (Borden)	½ cup	130	6
Chocolate Swirl Fat Free Frozen Dessert (Weight Watchers)	½ cup	90	0
Chocolate Treat Bar Sugar Free (Weight Watchers)	1 (2.75 oz)	90	0
Chocolate/Vanilla Cool 'N Creamy Bars (Crystal Light)	1 bar	55	2
Chunky Monkey (Ben & Jerry's)	4 oz	290	18
Cocoa-Fudge 'N Cream (Fi-Bar)	1 bar	93	tr
Coconut Bar (Good Humor)	3 oz	207	14
Coffee (Breyers)	½ cup	150	8
Coffee (Haagen-Dazs)	4 oz	270	17
Coffee (Sealtest)	½ cup	140	7
Coffee (Simple Pleasures)	4 oz	120	tr
Coffee Almond Fudge Light (Ben & Jerry's)	4 oz	230	10
Coffee Heath Bar Crunch (Ben & Jerry's)	4 oz	290	19
Coffee Ice Milk (Light N'Lively)	½ cup	100	3
Combo Cup Vanilla/Chocolate (Good Humor)	6 oz	201	9
Cookies N' Cream (Breyers)	½ cup	170	9
Cookies N' Cream (Healthy Choice)	4 oz	130	2
Cookies N' Cream (Simple Pleasures)	4 oz	150	2
Cookies 'N' Cream American Dream (Edy's)	3 oz	100	1

FOOD	PORTION	CALORIES	FAT
Cookies N' Cream Ice Milk (Light N'Lively)	½ cup	110	3
Cookies 'N' Cream Light (Edy's)	4 oz	120	5
Deep Chocolate (Haagen-Dazs)	4 oz	290	14
Deep Chocolate Fudge (Haagen-Dazs)	4 oz	290	14
Deluxe Sundae (Good Humor)	6 oz	300	11
Double Chcoloate Fudge Cool 'N Creamy Bars (Crystal Light)	1 bar	55	2
Double Fudge Bar (Weight Watchers)	1 (1.75 oz)	60	1
Dreamy Caramel Cream Light (Edy's)	4 oz	140	4
Dutch Chocolate (American Glace)	4 oz	48	0
Dutch Chocolate (Mocha Mix)	3.5 oz	210	12
Dutch Chocolate Olde Fashioned Recipe (Borden)	½ cup	130	6
English Toffee Crunch Bar (Weight Watchers)	1 (2 oz)	120	11
Fat Frog (Good Humor)	3 oz	154	9
French Vanilla (Sealtest)	½ cup	140	7
Fresh Lites Cherry (Dole)	1 bar	25	tr
Fresh Lites Chocolate Chip (Dole)	1 bar	60	1
Fresh Lites Lemon (Dole)	1 bar	25	tr
Fresh Lites Pineapple Orange (Dole)	1 bar	25	tr
Fresh Lites Raspberry (Dole)	1 bar	25	tr
Fruit Flavored Sherbet (Land O'Lakes)	4 oz	130	2
Fruit N' Cream Bar Peach (Dole)	1 bar	90	1
Fruit N' Cream Bar Raspberry (Dole)	1 bar	90	1
Fruit N' Cream Bar Strawberry (Dole)	1 bar	90	1
Fruit N' Juice Bar Peach Passion Fruit (Dole)	1 bar	70	tr

FOOD	PORTION	CALORIES	FAT
Fruit N' Juice Bar Pineapple (Dole)	1 bar	70	tr
Fruit N' Juice Bar Pineapple Orange Banana (Dole)	1 bar	70	tr
Fruit N' Juice Bar Raspberry (Dole)	1 bar	70	tr
Fruit N' Juice Bar Strawberry (Dole)	1 bar	70	tr
Fruit Punch Fruit Slush (Wyler's)	4 oz	140	0
Fruit Punch Pops (Crystal Light)	1 bar	14	tr
Fudge Bar (Good Humor)	2.5 oz	127	tr
Fudge Bar (Ultra Slim-Fast)	1	90	tr
Fudge Pop Bar (Haagen-Dazs)	1	210	14
Fudge Royale (Sealtest)	½ cup	140	7
Full O'Chocolate (Good Humor)	3 oz	245	18
Grape (Jell-O)	1 pop	31	tr
Grape/Lemon Ice Stripes (Good Humor)	1.5 oz	35	0
Grape/Lemon Italian Ice (Good Humor)	6 oz	138	tr
Gummy Dinosaur Colossal Fossil Lemon/Cherry (Good Humor)	3 oz	75	tr
Gummy Dinosaur Colossal Fossil Lemon/Grape (Good Humor)	3 oz	75	tr
Heath Bar (Ben & Jerry's)	4 oz	300	17
Heath Bar Crunch Light (Ben & Jerry's)	4 oz	230	10
Heath Bar Crunch Pop (Ben & Jerry's)	1	350	24
Heavenly Hash (Mocha Mix)	3.5 oz	244	13
Heavenly Hash (Sealtest)	½ cup	150	7
Heavenly Hash Ice Milk (Breyers Light)	½ cup	150	5
Heavenly Hash Ice Milk (Light N'Lively)	½ cup	120	4
Honey Vanilla (Haagen Dazs)	4 oz	250	16

FOOD	PORTION	CALORIES	FAT
Ice Cream Sandwich Chocolate Chip Cookie Chocolate (Good Humor)	4 oz	268	11
Ice Cream Sandwich Chocolate Chip Cookie Vanilla (Good Humor)	4 oz	246	11
Ice Cream Sandwich Vanilla (Good Humor)	2.5 oz	162	5
Jumbo Jet Star (Good Humor)	4.5 oz	85	tr
Keylime Sorbet & Cream (Haagen-Dazs)	4 oz	190	7
King Cone (Good Humor)	5.5 oz	315	19
Lemon Calippo (Good Humor)	4.5 oz	112	tr
Lemon Ice (Ben & Jerry's)	4 oz	105	0
Lemon/Lime Swirl (Jell-O)	1 pop	33	tr
Lemon White Italian Ice (Good Humor)	6 oz	138	tr
Lemonade SunTops (Dole)	1 bar	40	tr
Lemoney-Lime Juice Bar (Fi-Bar)	1 bar	63	tr
Life Savers Ice Pops	1	35	0
Life Savers Ice Pops Sugar Free	1	12	0
Lime Sherbet (Sealtest)	½ cup	130	1
Macadamia Brittle (Haagen-Dazs)	4 oz	280	18
Malt Ball 'N' Fudge Light (Edy's)	4 oz	140	5
Mandarin Orange Sorbet (Dole)	4 oz	110	tr
Maple Walnut (Sealtest)	½ cup	160	9
Marble Fudge Light (Edy's)	4 oz	120	4
Mint Chocolate (Breyers)	½ cup	170	10
Mint Chocolate Chocolate Chip (Simple Pleasures)	4 oz	150	2
Mixed Berry (Jell-O)	1 pop	31	tr
Mixed Berry & Ice Cream Swirl (Chiquita)	1 bar	80	3
Mixed Berry Bars (Jell-O)	1 bar (1.8 oz)	42	tr

FOOD	PORTION	CALORIES	FAT
Mocha Almond Fudge (Mocha Mix)	3.5 oz	229	11
Mocha Almond Fudge American Dream (Edy's)	3 oz	110	1
Mocha Almond Fudge Light (Edy's)	4 oz	140	5
Neapolitan (Healthy Choice)	4 oz	120	2
Neapolitan (Mocha Mix)	3.5 oz	208	11
Neapolitan Fat Free Frozen Dessert (Weight Watchers)	½ cup	80	0
New York Super Fudge Chocolate (Ben & Jerry's)	4 oz	310	20
New York Super Fudge Chocolate Pop (Ben & Jerry's)	1	340	26
ONE-ders Brownies 'N Creme (Weight Watchers)	4 oz	130	4
ONE-ders Chocolate Chip (Weight Watchers)	4 oz	120	4
ONE-ders Heavenly Hash (Weight Watchers)	4 oz	130	3
ONE-ders Pralines 'N Creme (Weight Watchers)	4 oz	130	4
ONE-ders Strawberry (Weight Watchers)	4 oz	110	3
Orange (Jell-O)	1 pop	31	tr
Orange & Ice Cream Swirl (Chiquita)	1 bar	80	3
Orange & Cream Pop (Haagen-Dazs)	1	130	6
Orange Bars (Jell-O)	1 (1.8 oz)	42	tr
Orange Calippo (Good Humor)	4.5 oz	110	tr
Orange/Pineapple Swirl (Jell-O)	1 pop	31	tr
Orange Pops (Crystal Light)	1	13	tr
Orange/Raspberry Italian Ice (Good Humor)	6 oz	138	tr
Orange Sherbet (Borden)	½ cup	110	1
Orange Sherbet (Sealtest)	½ cup	130	1

FOOD	PORTION	CALORIES	FAT
Orange Sherbet Push-Up (Good Humor)	3 oz	56	tr
Orange Sorbet & Cream (Haagen-Dazs)	4 oz	190	8
Orange/Vanilla Cool 'N Creamy Bars	1	31	tr
Orange Vanilla Treat Bar Sugar Free Fat Free (Weight Watchers)	1 (1.75 oz)	30	0
Oreo Mint (Ben & Jerry's)	4 oz	280	17
Original Cheesecake Bar (Carnation)	1	120	6
Passion-fruit (Vitari)	4 oz	80	0
Peach (Breyers)	½ cup	130	6
Peach (Mocha Mix)	3.5 oz	198	9
Peach (Sealtest Free)	½ cup	100	0
Peach (Simple Pleasures)	4 oz	120	tr
Peach (Ultra Slim-Fast)	4 oz	100	tr
Peach (Vitari)	4 oz	80	0
Peach Sorbet (Dole)	4 oz	110	tr
Peach Fruit & Cream (Chiquita)	1 bar	80	1
Peach Light (Ben & Jerry's)	4 oz	200	8
Peanut Butter & Chocolate Light (Edy's)	4 oz	130	5
Peanut Butter Crunch Bar (Haagen-Dazs)	1	270	21
Peanut Fudge Sundae (Sealtest)	½ cup	140	7
Pecan Praline (Simple Pleasures)	4 oz	140	2
Pecan Pralines 'N Creme Ice Milk (Weight Watchers)	½ cup	130	4
Pineapple Sorbet (Dole)	4 oz	110	tr
Pineapple Pops (Crystal Light)	1	13	tr
Pink Lemonade Pops (Crystal Light)	1	14	tr
Praline Almond Ice Milk (Breyers Light)	½ cup	130	5

FOOD	PORTION	CALORIES	FAT
Praline & Caramel (Healthy Choice)	4 oz	130	2
Pralines & Caramel (Ultra Slim-Fast)	4 oz	120	tr
Punch SunTops (Dole)	1 bar	40	tr
Rain Forest (Ben & Jerry's)	4 oz	300	20
Rainbow Sherbet (Sealtest)	½ cup	130	1
Raspberries 'N Cream (Fi-Bar)	1 bar	93	tr
Raspberry (Jell-O)	1 pop	29	tr
Raspberry & Ice Cream Swirl (Chiquita)	1 bar	80	3
Raspberry Banana Fruit & Juice Bars (Chiquita)	1 (2 oz)	50	0
Raspberry Bars (Jell-O)	1 (1.8 oz)	41	tr
Raspberry Berry Swirl Bars (Carnation)	1	70	3
Raspberry Fruit & Cream (Chiquita)	1 bar	80	1
Raspberry Fruit & Juice Bars (Chiquita)	1 (2 oz)	50	0
Raspberry Ice (Ben & Jerry's)	4 oz	105	0
Raspberry Peach Bars (Jell-O)	1 (1.8 oz)	40	tr
Raspberry/Peach Swirl (Jell-O)	1 pop	29	tr
Raspberry Pops (Crystal Light)	1	14	tr
Raspberry Sorbet (Dole)	4 oz	110	tr
Raspberry Sorbet (Frusen Gladje)	½ cup	140	0
Raspberry Sorbet & Cream (Haagen-Dazs)	4 oz	180	8
Raspberry Truffle Light (Edy's)	4 oz	110	5
Red Raspberry Sherbet (Sealtest)	½ cup	130	1
Rocky Road (Healthy Choice)	4 oz	140	1
Rocky Road American Dream (Edy's)	3 oz	110	1
Rocky Road Light (Edy's)	4 oz	130	5
Rum Raisin (Haagen-Dazs)	4 oz	250	17

FOOD	PORTION	CALORIES	FAT
Rum Raisin (Simple Pleasures)	4 oz	130	tr
Scribbler (Good Humor)	3 oz	120	1
Shark Bar (Good Humor)	3 oz	63	tr
Skinny Dip	4 oz	36	0
Strawberries 'N Cream Olde Fashioned Recipe (Borden)	½ cup	130	5
Strawberries and Cream (Good Humor)	3 oz	96	2
Strawberry (Borden)	½ cup	130	6
Strawberry (Breyers)	½ cup	130	6
Strawberry (Frusen Gladje)	½ cup	230	15
Strawberry (Haagen-Dazs)	4 oz	250	15
Strawberry (Healthy Choice)	4 oz	110	1
Strawberry (Jell-O)	1 pop	31	tr
Strawberry (Sealtest)	½ cup	130	5
Strawberry (Sealtest Free)	½ cup	100	0
Strawberry (Simple Pleasures)	4 oz	120	tr
Strawberry American Dream (Edy's)	3 oz	70	tr
Strawberry & Ice Cream Swirl (Chiquita)	1 bar	80	3
Strawberry Banana (Jell-O)	1 pop	31	tr
Strawberry Berry Swirl Bar (Carnation)	1	70	3
Strawberry Banana Bars (Jell-O)	1 (1.8 oz)	39	tr
Strawberry Banana Fruit & Cream (Chiquita)	1 bar	80	2
Strawberry Banana Fruit & Juice Bars (Chiquita)	1 (2 oz)	50	0
Strawberry Banana Swirl (Jell-O)	1 pop	31	tr
Strawberry Bars (Jell-O)	1 (1.8 oz)	41	tr
Strawberry Cheesecake Bars (Carnation)	1	125	6

FOOD	PORTION	CALORIES	FAT
Strawberry Creamy Lites Bar (Carnation)	1	50	2
Strawberry Finger Bar (Good Humor)	2.5 oz	49	tr
Strawberry Fruit & Cream (Chiquita)	1 bar	80	1
Strawberry Fruit & Juice Bars (Chiquita)	1 (2 oz)	50	0
Strawberry Ice (Ben & Jerry's)	4 oz	77	0
Strawberry Ice Milk (Borden)	½ cup	90	2
Strawberry Ice Milk (Breyers Light)	½ cup	110	3
Strawberry Light (Edy's)	4 oz	110	4
Strawberry Nectar Juice Bar (Fi-Bar)	1	63	tr
Strawberry Pops (Crystal Light)	1	13	tr
Strawberry Shortcake (Good Humor)	3 oz	186	12
Strawberry Sorbet (Dole)	4 oz	100	tr
Strawberry Swirl (Mocha Mix)	3.5 oz	209	9
Strawberry Tropical Mix (Jell-O)	1 bar (1.8 oz)	40	tr
Sundae Cone (Borden)	1	210	12
Sundae Cone (Meadow Gold)	1	210	12
SunTops Grape (Dole)	1 bar	40	tr
SunTops Orange (Dole)	1 bar	40	tr
Supreme (Good Humor)	3.5 oz	342	23
Swiss Chocolate Candy Almond (Frusen Gladje)	½ cup	270	19
Tahitian Vanilla (American Glace)	4 oz	48	0
Tasti D-Lite	4 oz	40	1
Toasted Almond (Good Humor)	3 oz	193	10
Toasted Almond (Mocha Mix)	3.5 oz	229	13
Toasted Almond American Dream (Edy's)	3 oz	110	1
Toffee Crunch (Simple Pleasures)	4 oz	130	tr

FOOD	PORTION	CALORIES	FAT
Toffee Fudge Parfait Ice Milk (Breyers Light)	½ cup	140	5
Tofulite	4 oz	150	7
Tofutti Cappuccino Love Drops	4 oz	230	12
Tofutti Chocolate Cuties	4 oz	140	5
Tofutti Chocolate Love Drops	4 oz	220	13
Tofutti Chocolate Supreme	4 oz	210	13
Tofutti Lite, Lite Applejack Vanilla Twirl	4 oz	90	tr
Tofutti Lite, Lite Cappuccino Vanilla Twirl	4 oz	90	tr
Tofutti Lite, Lite Chocolate Strawberry Twirl	4 oz	90	tr
Tofutti Lite, Lite Chocolate Vanilla Twirl	4 oz	90	tr
Tofutti Lite, Lite Strawberry Vanilla Twirl	4 oz	90	tr
Tofutti Lite, Lite Vanilla Chocolate Strawberry Twirl	4 oz	90	tr
Tofutti Soft Serve Hi-Lite Chocolate	4 oz	100	1
Tofutti Soft Serve Hi-Lite Vanilla	4 oz	90	1
Tofutti Soft Serve Regular	4 oz	158	8
Tofutti Vanilla	4 oz	200	11
Tofutti Vanilla Almond Bark	4 oz	230	14
Tofutti Vanilla Cuties	4 oz	130	5
Tofutti Vanilla Love Drops	4 oz	220	12
Tofutti Wildberry	4 oz	210	12
Triple Chocolate Stripes (Sealtest)	½ cup	140	7
Tropical Delite Juice Bar (Fi-Bar)	1	63	tr
Twister (Good Humor)	3 oz	131	7
Vanilla (Ben & Jerry's)	4 oz	250	17
Vanilla (Breyers)	½ cup	150	8

FOOD	PORTION	CALORIES	FAT
Vanilla (Eagle Brand)	½ cup	150	9
Vanilla (Frusen Gladje)	½ cup	230	17
Vanilla (Haagen-Dazs)	4 oz	260	17
Vanilla (Healthy Choice)	4 oz	120	2
Vanilla (Land O'Lakes)	4 oz	140	7
Vanilla (Mocha Mix)	3.5 oz	209	11
Vanilla (Sealtest)	½ cup	140	7
Vanilla (Sealtest Free)	½ cup	100	0
Vanilla (Simple Pleasures)	4 oz	120	tr
Vanilla (Ultra Slim-Fast)	4 oz	90	tr
Vanilla American Dream (Edy's)	3 oz	80	tr
Vanilla Brownie Bar (Ben & Jerry's)	1	350	18
Vanilla Caramel Nut, Heaven Bar (Carnation)	1	225	15
Vanilla Chocolate Chip (Ben & Jerry's)	4 oz	290	19
Vanilla Chocolate Sandwich (Ultra Slim-Fast)	1	140	2
Vanilla-Chocolate-Strawberry (Edy's)	4 oz	110	4
Vanilla Chocolate Strawberry American Dream (Edy's)	3 oz	80	1
Vanilla Cookie Crunch Bar (Ultra Slim-Fast)	1	90	4
Vanilla Crunch Bar (Haagen-Dazs)	1	220	16
Vanilla Cup (Good Humor)	3 oz	98	5
Vanilla Fat Free Frozen Dessert (Weight Watchers)	½ cup	80	0
Vanilla Fosters Freeze	1 oz	43	1
Vanilla Fudge (Haagen-Dazs)	4 oz	270	17
Vanilla Fudge Cookie (Ultra Slim-Fast)	4 oz	110	tr
Vanilla Fudge Heaven Sundae Bars (Carnation)	1	150	9

FOOD	PORTION	CALORIES	FAT
Vanilla Fudge Light (Ben & Jerry's)	4 oz	230	9
Vanilla Fudge Nut (Carnation)	1 bar	222	15
Vanilla Fudge Royale (Sealtest Free)	½ cup	100	0
Vanilla Fudge Swirl Dessert Bar (Sealtest Free)	1	80	0
Vanilla Fudge Swirl Light (Simple Pleasures)	4 oz	90	tr
Vanilla Fudge Twirl (Breyers)	½ cup	160	8
Vanilla Fudge Twirl Ice Milk (Light N'Lively)	½ cup	110	3
Vanilla Ice Milk (Borden)	½ cup	90	2
Vanilla Ice Milk (Breyers Light)	½ cup	120	4
Vanilla Ice Milk (Land O'Lakes)	4 oz	90	3
Vanilla Ice Milk (Light N'Lively)	½ cup	100	3
Vanilla Light (Ben & Jerry's)	4 oz	190	7
Vanilla Light (Edy's)	4 oz	100	4
Vanilla Light (Simple Pleasures)	4 oz	80	tr
Vanilla Milk Chocolate Almond Bar	1	370	27
Vanilla Milk Chocolate Bar (Haagen-Dazs)	1	360	27
Vanilla Milk Chocolate Brittle Bar (Haagen-Dazs)	1	370	25
Vanilla Oatmeal Sandwich (Ultra Slim-Fast)	1	150	3
Vanilla Old Fashioned (Healthy Choice)	4 oz	120	2
Vanilla Olde Fashioned Recipe (Borden)	½ cup	130	7
Vanilla Peanut Butter Swirl (Haagen-Dazs)	4 oz	280	21
Vanilla Red Raspberry Parfait Ice Milk (Breyers Light)	½ cup	130	3
Vanilla Sandwich (Ultra Slim-Fast)	1	140	2

FOOD	PORTION	CALORIES	FAT
Vanilla Sandwich Bar Fat free (Weight Watchers)	1 (2.5 oz)	130	0
Vanilla Strawberry Royale (Sealtest Free)	½ cup	100	0
Vanilla Strawberry Swirl Dessert Bar (Sealtest Free)	1	80	0
Vanilla Swiss Almond (Frusen Gladje)	½ cup	270	19
Vanilla Swiss Almond (Haagen-Dazs)	4 oz	290	19
Vanilla w/ Chocolate Covered Almonds Ice Milk (Light N'Lively)	½ cup	120	4
Vanilla w/ Orange Sherbet (Sealtest)	½ cup	130	4
Vanilla w/ Raspberry Twirl Ice Milk (Light N'Lively)	½ cup	110	3
Vanilla w/ Red Raspberry Sherbet (Sealtest)	½ cup	130	4
Viennetta Petites Chocolate Mint (Good Humor)	5 oz	236	14
Viennetta Petites Vanilla (Good Humor)	5 oz	236	14
Viennetta Regular Chocolate (Good Humor)	5 oz	225	14
Viennetta Regular Vanilla (Good Humor)	5 oz	225	14
Watermelon Italian Ice (Good Humor)	6 oz	138	tr
Whammy (Good Humor)	1.6 oz	95	7
Wild Berry Swirl (Healthy Choice)	4 oz	120	2
Wildberry Cream (Fi-Bar)	1 bar	93	tr
Wild Cherry Pops (Crystal Light)	1	13	tr
french vanilla, soft serve	1 cup	377	23
french vanilla, soft serve	½ gal	3014	180
orange sherbet	1 cup	270	4
orange sherbet	½ gal	2158	31

FOOD	PORTION	CALORIES	FAT
orange sherbet (home recipe)	½ cup	120	2
vanilla, 10% fat	1 cup	269	14
vanilla, 10% fat	½ gal	2153	115
vanilla, 16% fat	1 cup	349	24
vanilla, 16% fat	½ gal	2805	190
vanilla ice milk	1 cup	184	6
vanilla ice milk	½ gal	1469	45
vanilla ice milk, soft serve	1 cup	223	5
vanilla ice milk, soft serve	½ gal	1787	37
TAKE-OUT			
cone, vanilla ice milk, soft serve	1 (4.6 oz)	164	6
sundae, caramel	1 (5.4 oz)	303	9
sundae, hot fudge	1 (5.4 oz)	284	9
sundae, strawberry	1 (5.4 oz)	269	8

ICE CREAM CONES AND CUPS

Comet Cups	1	18	tr
Comet Sugar Cone	1	50	tr
Comet Waffle Cone	1	70	tr
Keebler Sugar Cones	1	45	tr
Keebler Vanilla Cups	1	15	tr

ICE CREAM TOPPINGS
(*see also* SYRUP)

Butterscotch (Kraft)	1 tbsp	60	1
Butterscotch (Smucker's)	2 tbsp	140	1
Butterscotch Special Recipe (Smucker's)	2 tbsp	160	3
Caramel (Kraft)	1 tbsp	60	0
Caramel (Smucker's)	2 tbsp	140	1

FOOD	PORTION	CALORIES	FAT
Chocolate (Kraft)	1 tbsp	50	0
Chocolate Fudge (Hershey)	2 tbsp	100	4
Chocolate Fudge (Smucker's)	2 tbsp	130	1
Chocolate Fudge Magic Shell (Smucker's)	2 tbsp	190	15
Chocolate Magic Shell (Smucker's)	2 tbsp	190	15
Chocolate Nut Magic Shell (Smucker's)	2 tbsp	200	16
Chocolate Syrup (Smucker's)	2 tbsp	130	0
Dark Chocolate Special Recipe (Smucker's)	2 tbsp	130	1
Hot Caramel (Smucker's)	2 tbsp	150	4
Hot Fudge (Kraft)	1 tbsp	70	0
Hot Fudge (Smucker's)	2 tbsp	110	4
Hot Fudge Light (Smucker's)	2 tbsp	70	tr
Hot Fudge Special Recipe (Smucker's)	2 tbsp	150	5
Hot Toffee Fudge (Smucker's)	2 tbsp	110	4
Marshmallow (Smucker's)	2 tbsp	120	0
Marshmallow Creme (Kraft)	1 oz	90	0
Peanut Butter Caramel (Smucker's)	2 tbsp	150	2
Pecans in Syrup (Smucker's)	2 tbsp	130	1
Pineapple (Kraft)	1 tbsp	50	0
Pineapple (Smucker's)	2 tbsp	130	0
Strawberry (Kraft)	1 tbsp	50	0
Strawberry (Smucker's)	2 tbsp	120	0
Swiss Milk Chocolate Fudge (Smucker's)	2 tbsp	140	1
Walnuts in Syrup (Smucker's)	2 tbsp	130	1

ICED TEA
(see TEA/HERBAL TEA)

FOOD	PORTION	CALORIES	FAT

ICING
(*see* CAKE)

INSTANT BREAKFAST
(*see* BREAKFAST DRINKS)

ITALIAN FOOD
(*see* DINNER, PASTA, PASTA DINNERS, PASTA SALADS)

JACKFRUIT

FOOD	PORTION	CALORIES	FAT
fresh	3.5 oz	70	tr

JAM/JELLY/PRESERVES

FOOD	PORTION	CALORIES	FAT
ALL FRUIT			
Apple Butter Simply Fruit (Smucker's)	1 tsp	12	0
Blueberry Fruit Spread (Pritikin)	1 tsp	14	0
Peach Fruit Spread (Pritikin)	1 tsp	14	0
Red Raspberry Fruit Spread (Pritikin)	1 tsp	14	0
Simply Fruit Spread, All Flavors (Smucker's)	1 tsp	16	0
Strawberry Fruit Spread (Pritikin)	1 tsp	14	0
REDUCED CALORIE			
Apricot Pineapple Preserves (S&W)	1 tsp	4	0
Blueberry Jam (S&W)	1 tsp	4	0
Concord Grape Jelly (S&W)	1 tsp	4	0
Grape Jelly Reduced Calorie (Kraft)	1 tsp	6	0
Grape Spread (Weight Watchers)	1 tsp	8	0
Imitation Blackberry Jelly Single Serving (Smucker's)	⅜ oz pkg	4	0
Imitation Cherry Jelly Single Serving (Smucker's)	⅜ oz pkg	4	0

FOOD	PORTION	CALORIES	FAT
Imitation Grape Jelly Single Serving (Smucker's)	⅜ oz pkg	4	0
Jelly, All Flavors (Estee)	1 tsp	2	0
Low Sugar Spread, All Flavors (Smucker's)	1 tsp	8	0
Orange Marmalade (S&W)	1 tsp	4	0
Preserves, All Flavors (Louis Sherry)	1 tsp	2	0
Raspberry Spread (Weight Watchers)	1 tsp	8	0
Red Raspberry Jam (S&W)	1 tsp	4	0
Red Tart Cherry Preserves (S&W)	1 tsp	4	0
Slenderella Reduced Calorie Fruit Spread, All Flavors	1 tsp	7	0
Strawberry Jam (S&W)	1 tsp	4	0
Strawberry Preserves Reduced Calorie (Kraft)	1 tsp	6	0
Strawberry Spread (Weight Watchers)	1 tsp	8	0
diet jelly (artificially sweetened)	1 tbsp	6	tr
REGULAR			
Apple Butter (BAMA)	2 tsp	25	0
Apple Butter (White House)	1 oz	50	0
Apple Butter Autumn Harvest (Smucker's)	1 tsp	12	0
Apple Butter Natural (Smucker's)	1 tsp	12	0
Apple Cider Butter (Smucker's)	1 tsp	12	0
Apple Jelly (BAMA)	2 tsp	30	0
Grape Jelly (BAMA)	2 tsp	30	0
Jam, All Flavors (Smucker's)	1 tsp	18	0
Jelly, All Flavors (Home Brands)	2 tsp	35	0
Jelly, All Flavors (Smucker's)	1 tsp	18	0

FOOD	PORTION	CALORIES	FAT
Jelly, All Varieties (Kraft)	1 tsp	17	0
Orange Marmalade (Smucker's)	1 tsp	18	0
Peach Butter (Smucker's)	1 tsp	15	0
Peach Preserves (BAMA)	2 tsp	30	0
Preserves, All Flavors (Home Brands)	2 tsp	35	0
Preserves, All Flavors (Smucker's)	1 tsp	18	0
Preserves, All Varieties (Kraft)	1 tsp	17	0
Pumpkin Butter Autumn Harvest (Smucker's)	1 tsp	12	0
Red Plum Jam (BAMA)	2 tsp	30	0
Single Serving Jelly, All Flavors (Smucker's)	½ oz	38	0
Single Serving Preserves, All Flavors (Smucker's)	½ oz	38	0
Strawberry Preserves (BAMA)	2 tsp	30	0
apple jelly	3.5 oz	259	0
apricot jam	3.5 oz	250	0
blackberry jam	3.5 oz	237	0
cherry jam	3.5 oz	250	0
orange jam	3.5 oz	243	0
plum jam	3.5 oz	241	0
quince jam	3.5 oz	236	0
raspberry jam	3.5 oz	248	0
raspberry jelly	3.5 oz	259	0
red currant jam	3.5 oz	237	0
red currant jelly	3.5 oz	265	0
rose hip jam	3.5 oz	250	0
strawberry jam	3.5 oz	234	0

JAPANESE FOOD
(*see* ORIENTAL FOOD)

FOOD	PORTION	CALORIES	FAT

JAVA PLUM

fresh	1 cup	82	tr
fresh	1	5	tr

JELLY
(*see* JAM/JELLY/PRESERVES)

JERUSALEM ARTICHOKE
(*see* ARTICHOKE)

JEW'S EAR

pepeao, dried	½ cup	36	tr
pepeao, raw, sliced	1 cup	25	tr

JUJUBE

fresh	3.5 oz	105	tr

KALE

FRESH

Dole, chopped	½ cup	17	1
chopped, cooked	½ cup	21	tr
raw, chopped	½ cup	21	tr
scotch, chopped, cooked	½ cup	18	tr

FROZEN

chopped, cooked	½ cup	20	tr

KEFIR

kefir	3.5 oz	66	4

KIDNEY

beef, simmered	3 oz	122	3
lamb, braised	3 oz	117	3

FOOD	PORTION	CALORIES	FAT
pork, braised	3 oz	128	4
veal, braised	3 oz	139	5

KIDNEY BEANS

CANNED

FOOD	PORTION	CALORIES	FAT
Dark Red (Green Giant)	½ cup	90	0
Dark Red (Hanover)	½ cup	110	0
Dark Red (Ranch Style)	7.5 oz	170	1
Dark Red (Trappey's)	½ cup	90	0
Dark Red (Van Camp's)	1 cup	182	1
Dark Red Lite 50% Less Salt (S&W)	½ cup	120	0
Dark Red Premium (S&W)	½ cup	120	1
Jalapeno Light Red (Trappey's)	½ cup	90	0
Light Red (Green Giant)	½ cup	90	0
Light Red (Trappey's)	½ cup	90	0
Light Red (Van Camp's)	1 cup	184	1
Light Red in Sauce (Hanover)	½ cup	120	0
New Orleans Style (Trappey's)	½ cup	100	2
New Orleans Style Red (Van Camp's)	1 cup	178	1
Red (Hunt's)	4 oz	100	tr
Red Kidney Baked Beans (B&M)	⅞ cup	290	7
Red Kidney Beans Spanish Style (Goya)	7.5 oz	140	1
Red w/ Chili Gravy (Trappey's)	½ cup	100	1
Seasoned w/ Pork (Luck's)	7.5 oz	220	6
Special Cook Red Kidney Beans (Luck's)	7.5 oz	190	4
Water Pack (S&W)	½ cup	90	0
kidney beans	1 cup	208	1
red	1 cup	216	1

FOOD	PORTION	CALORIES	FAT
DRIED			
Arrowhead Red	2 oz	190	1
Hurst Brand	1 cup	254	1
california red, cooked	1 cup	219	tr
california red, raw	1 cup	609	tr
kidney beans, cooked	1 cup	225	1
kidney beans, raw	1 cup	613	2
red, cooked	1 cup	225	1
red, raw	1 cup	619	2
royal red, cooked	1 cup	218	tr
royal red, raw	1 cup	605	1
SPROUTS			
cooked	1 lb	152	3
raw	½ cup	27	tr

KIWI

FOOD	PORTION	CALORIES	FAT
Dole	2	90	1
fresh	1 med	46	tr

KOHLRABI

FOOD	PORTION	CALORIES	FAT
raw, sliced	½ cup	19	tr
sliced, cooked	½ cup	24	tr

KUMQUATS

FOOD	PORTION	CALORIES	FAT
fresh	1	12	tr

LAMB
(*see also* LAMB DISHES)

FOOD	PORTION	CALORIES	FAT
FRESH			
cubed, lean only, braised	3 oz	190	7
cubed, lean only, broiled	3 oz	158	6

FOOD	PORTION	CALORIES	FAT
ground, broiled	3 oz	240	17
leg, lean & fat, Choice, roasted	3 oz	219	14
loin chop w/ bone lean & fat, Choice broiled	1 chop (2.3 oz)	201	15
loin chop w/ bone, lean only, Choice, broiled	1 chop (1.6 oz)	100	5
rib chop, lean & fat, Choice, broiled	3 oz	307	25
rib chop, lean only, Choice, broiled	3 oz	200	11
shank, lean & fat, Choice, braised	3 oz	206	11
shank, lean & fat, Choice, roasted	3 oz	191	11
shoulder chop, w/ bone, lean & fat, Choice, braised	1 chop (2.5 oz)	244	17
shoulder chop, w/ bone, lean only, Choice, braised	1 chop (1.9 oz)	152	8
sirloin, lean & fat, Choice, roasted	3 oz	248	21
FROZEN			
new zealand, lean & fat, cooked	3 oz	259	19
new zealand, lean only, cooked	3 oz	175	8

LAMB DISHES

TAKE-OUT			
curry	¾ cup	345	17
moussaka	5.6 oz	312	21
stew	¾ cup	124	5

LAMB'S-QUARTERS

FRESH			
chopped, cooked	½ cup	29	1

LECITHIN
(*see* SOY)

FOOD	PORTION	CALORIES	FAT

LEEKS

freeze dried	1 tbsp	1	0
FRESH			
chopped, cooked	¼ cup	8	tr
cooked	1 (4.4 oz)	38	tr
raw	1 (4.4 oz)	76	tr
raw, chopped	¼ cup	16	tr

LEMON

Dole	1	18	0
lemon	1 med	22	tr
peel	1 tbsp	0	tr
wedge	1	5	tr
JUICE			
Realemon	1 oz	6	0
Seneca	1 tbsp	6	0
bottled	1 tbsp	3	tr
fresh	1 tbsp	4	0
frzn	1 tbsp	3	tr

LEMONADE
(*see* FRUIT DRINKS)

LEMON CURD

lemon curd made w/ egg	2 tsp	29	1

LEMON EXTRACT

Virginia Dare	1 tsp	22	0

FOOD	PORTION	CALORIES	FAT

LENTILS

CANNED
Fast Menu Hearty Lentils & Garden Vegetables (Health Valley)	7.5 oz	150	4
Fast Menu Organic Lentils w/ Tofu Wieners (Health Valley)	7.5 oz	170	5

DRIED
Arrowhead Green	2 oz	190	1
Arrowhead Red	2 oz	195	1
Hurst Brand, cooked	1 cup	258	tr
cooked	1 cup	231	1
raw	1 cup	649	2

SPROUTS
raw	½ cup	40	tr

LETTUCE

Dole Butter Lettuce	1 head	21	tr
Dole Iceberg	⅙ med head	20	0
Dole Leaf, shredded	1½ cup	12	0
Dole Romaine, shredded	1½ cup	18	1
bibb	1 head (6 oz)	21	tr
boston	1 head (6 oz)	21	tr
boston	2 leaves	2	tr
iceberg	1 leaf	1	tr
iceberg	1 head (19 oz)	70	1
looseleaf, shredded	½ cup	5	tr
romaine, shredded	½ cup	4	tr

LIMA BEANS

CANNED
Baby Green (Trappey's)	½ cup	90	1

FOOD	PORTION	CALORIES	FAT
Baby White (Trappey's)	½ cup	90	1
Giant Seasoned w/ Pork (Luck's)	7.5 oz	230	7
Lima Beans (Libby)	½ cup	80	0
Lima Beans (Seneca)	½ cup	80	0
Lima Beans w/ Ham (Dennison's)	7.5 oz	250	7
Small Fancy (S&W)	½ cup	80	0
Small Seasoned w/ Pork (Luck's)	7.5 oz	220	7
large	1 cup	191	tr
lima beans	½ cup	93	tr
DRIED			
Baby Lima (Hurst Brand)	1 cup	262	1
baby, cooked	1 cup	229	1
baby, raw	1 cup	677	2
cooked	½ cup	104	tr
large, cooked	1 cup	217	1
large, raw	1 cup	602	1
FROZEN			
Baby (Birds Eye)	½ cup	127	tr
Baby (Hanover)	½ cup	110	0
Fordhook (Birds Eye)	½ cup	100	tr
Fordhook (Hanover)	½ cup	100	0
Harvest Fresh (Green Giant)	½ cup	80	0
In Butter Sauce (Green Giant)	½ cup	100	3
cooked	½ cup	94	tr
fordhook, cooked	½ cup	85	tr

LIME

fresh lime	1	20	tr
JUICE			
Realime	1 oz	6	0

FOOD	PORTION	CALORIES	FAT
bottled	1 tbsp	3	tr
fresh	1 tbsp	4	tr

LINCOD
fresh blue, raw	3.5 oz	83	1

LING
baked	3 oz	95	1
fillet, baked	5.3 oz	168	1

LINGCOD
baked	3 oz	93	1
fillet, baked	5.3 oz	164	2

LIQUOR/LIQUEUR
(*see also* BEER AND ALE, DRINK MIXERS, MALT, WINE, WINE COOLERS)

anisette	⅔ oz	74	0
apricot brandy	⅔ oz	64	0
benedictine	⅔ oz	69	0
bloody mary	5 oz	116	tr
bourbon & soda	4 oz	105	0
coffee liqueur	1.5 oz	174	tr
coffee liqueur w/ cream	1.5 oz	154	7
creme de menthe	1.5 oz	186	tr
curacao liqueur	⅔ oz	54	0
daiquiri	2 oz	111	0
gin	1.5 oz	110	0
gin & tonic	7.5 oz	171	0
manhattan	2 oz	128	0
martini	2.5 oz	156	0
mint julep	10 oz	210	0

FOOD	PORTION	CALORIES	FAT
old-fashioned	2.5 oz	127	0
pina colada	4.5 oz	262	3
rum	1.5 oz	97	0
screwdriver	7 oz	174	tr
sloe gin fizz	2.5 oz	132	0
tequila sunrise	5.5 oz	189	tr
tom collins	7.5 oz	121	0
vodka	1.5 oz	97	0
whiskey	1.5 oz	105	0
whiskey sour	3 oz	123	tr
whiskey sour mix, as prep	3.6 oz	169	0
whiskey sour mix, not prep	1 pkg (.6 oz)	64	0

LIVER
(*see also* PÂTÉ)

FOOD	PORTION	CALORIES	FAT
Beef, raw (Dakota Lean)	3 oz	100	1
beef, braised	3 oz	137	4
beef, pan-fried	3 oz	184	7
chicken, stewed	1 cup (5 oz)	219	8
duck, raw	1 (1.5 oz)	60	2
goose, raw	1 (3.3 oz)	125	4
lamb, braised	3 oz	187	7
lamb, fried	3 oz	202	11
pork, braised	3 oz	141	4
sheep, raw	3.5 oz	131	4
turkey, simmered	1 cup (5 oz)	237	8
veal, braised	3 oz	140	6
veal, fried	3 oz	208	10

FOOD	PORTION	CALORIES	FAT
LOBSTER			
FRESH			
northern, cooked	1 cup	142	1
northern, cooked	3 oz	83	1
spiny, steamed	1 (5.7 oz)	233	3
spiny, steamed	3 oz	122	2
FROZEN			
Gulfstream Tails (King & Prince)	8 oz	227	2
Gulfstream Tails (King & Prince)	6 oz	170	1
TAKE-OUT			
newburg	1 cup	485	27
LOGANBERRIES			
frzn	1 cup	80	tr
LONGANS			
fresh	1	2	0
LOQUATS			
fresh	1	5	tr
LOTUS			
root, raw, sliced	10 slices	45	tr
root, sliced, cooked	10 slices	59	tr
seeds dried	1 oz	94	1

LOX
 (*see* SALMON)

LUNCHEON MEATS/COLD CUTS
 (*see also* CHICKEN, HAM, MEAT SUBSTITUTES, TURKEY)

Armour Beef Bologna Lower Salt	1 oz	90	8

FOOD	PORTION	CALORIES	FAT
Armour Salami Lower Salt	1 oz	80	7
Carl Buddig Corned Beef	1 oz	40	2
Carl Buddig Beef	1 oz	40	2
Carl Buddig Pastrami	1 oz	40	2
Hansel 'N Gretel Healthy Deli			
Bologna, Beef & Pork	1 oz	41	2
Cooked Corn Beef	1 oz	35	1
Italian Roast Beef	1 oz	31	1
Pastrami Round	1 oz	34	1
Regular Roast Beef	1 oz	30	tr
St. Paddy's Corned Beef	1 oz	24	tr
Hebrew National Bologna Midget	1 oz	60	5
Hebrew National Salami Midget	1 oz	57	4
Oscar Mayer			
Bar-B-Q Loaf	1 slice (28 g)	48	3
Bologna	1 slice (28 g)	90	8
Bologna Beef	1 slice (28 g)	90	8
Bologna Beef Garlic Flavored	1 slice (28 g)	89	8
Bologna Beef Lebanon	1 slice	49	3
Bologna w/ Cheese	1 slice (23 g)	74	7
Braunschweiger German Brand	1 oz	94	9
Braunschweiger Sliced	1 slice (28 g)	96	9
Braunschweiger Tube	1 oz	96	9
Corned Beef	1 slice (17 g)	16	tr
Cotto Salami	1 slice (23 g)	54	4
Cotto Salami Beef	1 slice (23 g)	46	3
Genoa Salami Beef	1 slice (9 g)	34	3
Hard Salami	1 slice (9 g)	34	3
Head Cheese	1 slice (28 g)	55	4
Honey Loaf	1 slice (28 g)	35	1

FOOD	PORTION	CALORIES	FAT
Oscar Mayer *(cont.)*			
Jalapeno	1 slice (28 g)	72	6
Liver Cheese Pork Fat Wrap	1 slice (38 g)	116	10
Luncheon Meat	1 slice (28 g)	98	9
Luxury Loaf	1 slice (28 g)	38	1
New England Brand Sausage	1 slice (23 g)	31	2
Old Fashioned Loaf	1 slice (28 g)	64	4
Olive Loaf	1 slice (28 g)	62	4
Pastrami	1 slice (17 g)	16	tr
Peppered Loaf	1 slice (28 g)	43	2
Pickle & Pimiento Loaf	1 slice (28 g)	63	4
Picnic Loaf	1 slice (28 g)	62	4
Salami for Beer	1 slice (23 g)	55	5
Salami for Beer Beef	1 slice (23 g)	66	6
Sandwich Spread	1 oz	67	5
Smoked Beef	1 slice (14 g)	14	tr
Summer Sausage Thuringer Cervelat	1 slice (23 g)	73	7
Summer Sausage Thuringer Cervelat Beef	1 slice (23 g)	72	6
Russer Lil' Salt			
Bologna	1 oz	70	5
Bologna, Beef	1 oz	80	5
Braunschweiger	1 oz	70	5
Cooked Salami	1 oz	60	4
Old Fashioned Loaf	1 oz	60	4
P & P Loaf	1 oz	60	4
Weight Watchers Bologna	2 slices (¾ oz)	35	2
barbecue loaf, pork & beef	1 oz	49	3
beerwurst, beef	1 slice (4 oz)	75	7
beerwurst, pork	1 slice (4 oz)	55	4

FOOD	PORTION	CALORIES	FAT
berliner, pork & beef	1 oz	65	4
blood sausage	1 oz	95	9
bologna, beef	1 oz	88	8
bologna, beef & pork	1 oz	89	8
bologna, pork	1 oz	70	6
braunschweiger, pork	1 oz	102	9
corned beef loaf	1 oz	43	2
dried beef	1 oz	47	1
dried beef	5 slices (21 g)	35	tr
dutch brand loaf, pork & beef	1 oz	68	5
headcheese, pork	1 oz	60	5
honey loaf, pork & beef	1 oz	36	1
honey roll sausage, beef	1 oz	42	2
lebanon bologna, beef	1 oz	60	4
liver cheese, pork	1 oz	86	7
liverwurst, pork	1 oz	92	8
luncheon meat, beef loaf	1 oz	87	7
luncheon meat, pork & beef	1 oz	100	9
luncheon meat, pork, canned	1 oz	95	9
luncheon sausage, pork & beef	1 oz	74	6
luxury loaf, pork	1 oz	40	1
mortadella, beef & pork	1 oz	88	7
mother's loaf, pork	1 oz	80	6
new england brand sausage, pork & beef	1 oz	46	2
olive loaf, pork	1 oz	67	5
peppered loaf, pork & beef	1 oz	42	2
pepperoni, pork & beef	1 (9 oz)	1248	110
pepperoni, pork & beef	1 slice (.2 oz)	27	2
pickle & pimiento loaf, pork	1 oz	74	6

FOOD	PORTION	CALORIES	FAT
picnic loaf, pork & beef	1 oz	66	5
salami, cooked, beef & pork	1 oz	71	6
salami, hard, pork & beef	1 pkg (4 oz)	472	39
salami, hard, pork & beef	1 slice (⅓ oz)	42	3
salami, hard, pork	1 pkg (4 oz)	460	38
salami, hard, pork	1 slice (⅓ oz)	41	4
sandwich spread pork & beef	1 tbsp	35	3
sandwich spread pork & beef	1 oz	67	5
summer sausage thuringer cervelat	1 oz	98	8
TAKE-OUT			
submarine w/ salami, ham, cheese, lettuce, tomato, onion, oil	1	456	19

LUPINES

dried, cooked	1 cup	197	5
dried, raw	1 cup	668	17

LYCHEES

fresh	1 cup	6	tr

MACADAMIA NUTS

Candy Glazed (Mauna Loa)	1 oz	170	14
Chocolate Covered (Mauna Loa)	1 oz	170	13
Honey Roasted (Mauna Loa)	1 oz	200	17
Macadamia Nut Brittle (Mauna Loa)	1 oz	150	8
Roasted & Salted (Mauna Loa)	1 oz	210	21
dried	1 oz	199	21
oil roasted	1 oz	204	22

MACARONI
(*see* PASTA)

FOOD	PORTION	CALORIES	FAT
MACE			
ground	1 tsp	8	1
MACKEREL			
CANNED			
Jack (Empress)	4 oz	140	8
jack	1 cup	296	12
jack	1 can (12.7 oz)	563	23
FRESH			
atlantic, cooked	3 oz	223	15
jack, baked	3 oz	171	9
jack fillet, baked	6.2 oz	354	18
king, baked	3 oz	114	2
king fillet, baked	5.4 oz	207	4
pacific, baked	3 oz	171	9
pacific fillet, baked	6.2 oz	354	18
spanish, cooked	3 oz	134	5
spanish, cooked	1 fillet (5.1 oz)	230	9
MALT			
Olde English	12 oz	163	0
Schaefer	12 oz	165	0
Schlitz	12 oz	177	0
nonalcoholic	12 oz	32	0
MALTED MILK			
Carnation Chocolate	3 heaping tsp (21 g)	79	tr
Carnation Original	3 heaping tsp (21 g)	90	2
Kraft Malted Milk Instant Chocolate	3 tsp	90	1

FOOD	PORTION	CALORIES	FAT
Kraft Malted Milk Instant Natural	3 tsp	90	2
chocolate flavor powder	3 heaping tsp (¾ oz)	79	1
chocolate, as prep w/ milk	1 cup	229	9
natural flavor powder	3 heaping tsp (¾ oz)	87	2
natural flavor, as prep w/ milk	1 cup	237	10

MAMMY APPLE

fresh	1	431	4

MANGO

fresh	1	135	1

JUICE
Kern's Nectar	6 oz	110	0
Libby's Nectar	6 oz	110	0

MARGARINE
(*see also* BUTTER BLENDS, BUTTER SUBSTITUTES)

REDUCED CALORIE
Fleischmann's Diet	1 tbsp	50	6
Fleischmann's Extra Light Corn Oil Spread	1 tbsp	50	6
Mazola Diet	1 tbsp	50	6
Mazola Diet	1 cup	815	93
Mazola Light Corn Oil Spread	1 tbsp	50	6
Mazola Light Corn Oil Spread	1 cup	835	94
Parkay Diet Soft	1 tbsp	50	6
Smart Beat	1 tbsp	25	3
Smart Beat Unsalted	1 tbsp	25	3
Weight Watchers Extra Light Sweet Unsalted Tub	1 tbsp	50	6

FOOD	PORTION	CALORIES	FAT
Weight Watchers Extra Light Tub	1 tbsp	50	6
Weight Watchers Light Stick	1 tbsp	60	7
diet	1 tsp	17	2
diet	1 cup	800	90
REGULAR			
Blue Bonnet	1 tbsp	100	11
Fleischmann's	1 tbsp	100	11
Fleischmann's Light Corn Oil Stick	1 tbsp	80	8
Fleischmann's Sweet Unsalted	1 tbsp	100	11
Krona	1 tbsp	100	11
Land O'Lakes	1 tsp	35	4
Land O'Lakes Premium Corn Oil	1 tsp	35	4
Land O'Lakes Premium Corn Oil Stick	1 tbsp	100	11
Land O'Lakes Regular Stick	1 tbsp	100	11
Mazola	1 cup	1650	184
Mazola	1 tbsp	100	11
Mazola Unsalted	1 cup	1635	184
Mazola Unsalted	1 tbsp	100	11
Mother's	1 tbsp	100	11
Mother's Unsalted	1 tbsp	100	11
Nucanola	1 tbsp	90	10
Parkay	1 tbsp	100	11
Promise	1tbsp	90	10
Spread w/ Sweet Cream	1 tsp	30	4
Spread w/ Sweet Cream Unsalted	1 tsp	30	4
corn	1 stick (4 oz)	815	91
corn	1 tsp	34	4
salted	1 stick (4 oz)	815	91
salted	1 tsp	39	4

FOOD	PORTION	CALORIES	FAT
unsalted	1 stick (4 oz)	809	91
unsalted	1 tsp	34	4
SOFT			
Blue Bonnet	1 tbsp	100	11
Chiffon	1 tbsp	90	10
Chiffon Stick	1 tbsp	100	11
Chiffon Unsalted	1 tbsp	90	10
Fleischmann's	1 tbsp	100	11
Fleischmann's Light Corn Oil Spread	1 tbsp	80	8
Fleischmann's Sweet Unsalted	1 tbsp	100	11
I Can't Believe It's Not Butter!	1 tbsp	90	10
Land O'Lakes Regular Soft Tub	1 tbsp	100	11
Land O'Lakes Tub	1 tsp	35	4
Mother's Salted	1 tbsp	100	11
Mother's Unsalted	1 tbsp	100	11
Parkay Soft	1 tbsp	100	11
Parkay Spread	1 tbsp	60	7
Promise	1 tbsp	90	10
Spread w/ Sweet Cream	1 tsp	25	3
corn	1 tsp	34	4
corn	1 cup	1626	183
safflower	1 tsp	34	4
safflower	1 cup	1626	183
soybean, salted	1 tsp	34	4
soybean, salted	1 cup	1626	183
soybean, unsalted	1 tsp	34	4
soybean, unsalted	1 cup	1626	182
tub, salted	1 tsp	34	4
tub, salted	1 cup	1626	183

FOOD	PORTION	CALORIES	FAT
tub, unsalted	1 tsp	34	4
tub, unsalted	1 cup	1626	182
SQUEEZE			
Parkay Squeeze	1 tbsp	90	10
soybean & cottonseed	1 tsp	34	4
WHIPPED			
Blue Bonnet Whipped Spread	1 tbsp	80	9
Chiffon	1 tbsp	70	8
Fleischmann's Lightly Salted	1 tbsp	70	7
Fleischmann's Unsalted	1 tbsp	70	7
Miracle Brand	1 tbsp	60	7
Miracle Brand Stick	1 tbsp	70	7
Parkay	1 tbsp	70	7
Parkay Stick	1 tbsp	70	7

MARJORAM

FOOD	PORTION	CALORIES	FAT
dried	1 tsp	2	tr

MARSHMALLOW

FOOD	PORTION	CALORIES	FAT
Campfire (Borden)	2 lg	40	0
Campfire Miniature (Borden)	24	40	0
Funmallows (Kraft)	1	30	0
Funmallows Miniature (Kraft)	10	18	0
Jet-Puffed (Kraft)	1	25	0
Miniature (Kraft)	10	18	0

MATZO

FOOD	PORTION	CALORIES	FAT
Manischewitz			
American Matzo	1	115	2
Daily Thin Tea	1	103	tr
Dietetic Thins	1	91	tr

FOOD	PORTION	CALORIES	FAT
Manischewitz *(cont.)*			
Egg N' Onion	1	112	tr
Matzo Cracker Miniatures	10	90	tr
Matzo Farfel	1 cup	180	1
Matzo Meal	1 cup	514	1
Passover	1	129	tr
Passover Egg	1	132	2
Passover Egg Matzo Crackers	10	108	2
Salted Thin	1	100	tr
Unsalted	1	110	tr
Wheat Matzo Crackers	10	90	1
Whole Wheat w/ Bran	1	110	1

MAYONNAISE
(*see also* MAYONNAISE TYPE SALAD DRESSING, RELISH)

FOOD	PORTION	CALORIES	FAT
REDUCED CALORIE			
Best Foods Cholesterol Free Reduced Calorie	1 cup	760	75
Best Foods Cholesterol Free Reduced Calorie	1 tbsp	50	5
Best Foods Light	1 cup	760	78
Best Foods Light	1 tbsp	50	5
Diamond Crystal	1 tbsp	50	5
Estee	1 tbsp	50	5
Hellmann's Light Reduced Calorie	1 cup	760	78
Hellmann's Light Reduced Calorie	1 tbsp	50	5
Hellmann's Cholesterol Free Reduced Calorie	1 cup	760	75
Hellmann's Cholesterol Free Reduced Calorie	1 tbsp	50	5
Kraft Free	1 tbsp	12	0

FOOD	PORTION	CALORIES	FAT
Kraft Light	1 tbsp	50	5
Smart Beat Canola Oil	1 tbsp	40	4
Smart Beat Corn Oil	1 tbsp	40	4
Weight Watchers Fat Free	1 tbsp	12	0
Weight Watchers Light	1 tbsp	50	5
Weight Watchers Low Sodium	1 tbsp	50	1
reduced calorie	1 cup	556	46
reduced calorie	1 tbsp	34	3
REGULAR			
Best Foods Real	1 cup	1570	175
Best Foods Real	1 tbsp	100	11
Hellmann's	1 cup	1570	173
Hellmann's Real	1 tbsp	100	11
Kraft Real Mayonnaise	1 tbsp	100	12
Kraft Sandwich Spread	1 tbsp	50	5
Mother's	1 tbsp	100	11
mayonnaise	1 cup	1577	175
mayonnaise	1 tbsp	99	11
sandwich spread	1 tbsp	60	5

MAYONNAISE TYPE SALAD DRESSING
(*see also* MAYONNAISE, RELISH)

FOOD	PORTION	CALORIES	FAT
REDUCED CALORIE			
Miracle Whip Free	1 tbsp	20	0
Miracle Whip Light	1 tbsp	45	4
Smart Beat	1 tbsp	12	0
Weight Watchers Fat Free Whipped Dressing	1 tbsp	16	0
reduced calorie w/o cholesterol	1 cup	1084	107
reduced calorie w/o cholesterol	1 tbsp	68	7

FOOD	PORTION	CALORIES	FAT
REGULAR			
Bright Day Dressing	1 tbsp	60	6
Miracle Whip	1 tbsp	70	7
Miracle Whip Coleslaw Dressing	1 tbsp	70	6
Spin Blend	1 tbsp	60	5
Spin Blend Cholesterol Free	1 tbsp	40	4
home recipe	1 cup	400	24
home recipe	1 tbsp	25	2
mayonnaise type salad dressing	1 cup	916	78
mayonnaise type salad dressing	1 tbsp	57	5

MEAT SUBSTITUTES

(*see also* CHICKEN SUBSTITUTES, SAUSAGE SUBSTITUTES, TURKEY SUBSTITUTES)

FOOD	PORTION	CALORIES	FAT
Bolono, frzn (Worthington)	3.5 oz	138	5
Corn Dogs (Loma Linda)	1 (2.5 oz)	250	19
Dinner Cuts (Loma Linda)	2 (3.5 oz)	110	1
Dinner Cuts No Salt Added (Loma Linda)	2 (3.5 oz)	110	1
Fripats, frzn (Worthington)	3.5 oz	294	19
Griddle Steaks (Loma Linda)	1 (2 oz)	190	13
Griddle Steaks (Loma Linda)	1 (1.7 oz)	160	11
Leanies, frzn (Worthington)	3.5 oz	252	17
Meatless Big Franks (Loma Linda)	1 (1.8 oz)	100	5
Meatless Bologna (Loma Linda)	2 slices (2 oz)	150	9
Meatless Redi-Burger (Loma Linda)	½ (2.4 oz)	130	6
Meatless Roast Beef (Loma Linda)	2 slices (2 oz)	107	3
Meatless Salami (Loma Linda)	2 slices (2 oz)	98	2
Meatless Salami, frzn (Worthington)	3.5 oz	198	11
Meatless Savory Meatballs (Loma Linda)	7 meatballs (2.5 oz)	190	8

FOOD	PORTION	CALORIES	FAT
Meatless Sizzle Burger (Loma Linda)	1 (2.5 oz)	210	11
Meatless Sizzle Franks (Loma Linda)	2 (2.4 oz)	170	13
Meatless Swiss Steak w/ Gravy (Loma Linda)	1 steak (2.6 oz)	140	8
Meatless Vita-Burger Chunks (Loma Linda)	¼ cup	70	tr
Meatless Vita-Burger Granules (Loma Linda)	3 tbsp	70	tr
Nuteena (Loma Linda)	½ (2.4 oz)	160	12
Okara Pattie, frzn (Natural Touch)	3.5 oz	208	16
Olive Loaf (Loma Linda)	2 slices (2 oz)	119	6
Patties, frzn (Morningstar Farms)	3.5 oz	240	17
Patty Mix (Loma Linda)	¼ cup	50	1
Prime Stakes, canned (Worthington)	3.5 oz	182	12
Prosage Chub, frzn (Worthington)	3.5 oz	245	17
Prosage Links, frzn (Worthington)	3.5 oz	280	20
Prosage Patties, frzn (Worthington)	3.5 oz	279	18
Proteena (Loma Linda)	½ (2.5 oz)	140	6
Salisbury Steak Style Dinner (Jaclyn's)	11 oz	260	8
Salsa Chicken Style Dinner (Jaclyn's)	11.5 oz	325	9
Saucettes, canned (Worthington)	3.5 oz	210	14
Savory Dinner Loaf, mix not prep (Loma Linda)	¼ cup	50	1
Sesame Chicken Style Dinner (Jaclyn's)	11.5 oz	345	8
Sirloin Strips Style Dinner (Jaclyn's)	12 oz	290	6
Soysage (Spring Creek)	1 patty (1.6 oz)	63	tr
Stakelets, frzn (Worthington)	3.5 oz	178	12
Stew Pac (Loma Linda)	2 oz	70	2
Tastee Cuts (Loma Linda)	2 pieces (2.5 oz)	70	1

FOOD	PORTION	CALORIES	FAT
Tender Bits (Loma Linda)	4 pieces (2 oz)	80	3
Tender Rounds w/ Gravy (Loma Linda)	6 pieces (2.6 oz)	120	4
Tofu Pups (Lightlife)	1 (1.5 oz)	92	5
Vege-Burger (Loma Linda)	½ cup	110	1
Vege-Burger NSA (Loma Linda)	½ cup	140	2
Vegelona (Loma Linda)	½	100	1
Wham, frzn (Worthington)	3.5 oz	184	11
simulated sausage	1 patty (38 g)	97	7
simulated sausage	1 link (25 g)	64	5
simulated meat product	1 oz	88	1

MELON
(*see also individual names*)

FRESH
Cantalene (Chiquita)	1 cup	60	0
Honey Mist (Chiquita)	1 cup	80	0

FROZEN
melon balls	1 cup	55	tr

MEXICAN FOOD
(*see also* CHIPS, DINNER, PEPPERS, SNACKS)

CANNED
Enchilada Sauce Hot (El Molino)	2 tbsp	16	1
Enchilada Sauce Mild (Rosarita)	2.5 oz	25	1
Enchiladas (Gebhardt)	2	310	24
Green Chili Sauce Hot (El Molino)	2 tbsp	10	0
Jalapeno Sliced (Trappey's)	1 oz	6	0
Mexican Sauce (Pritikin)	4 oz	50	1
Picante Chunky Hot (Rosarita)	3 tbsp	18	tr
Picante Chunky Medium (Rosarita)	3 tbsp	16	tr

FOOD	PORTION	CALORIES	FAT
Picante Chunky Mild (Rosarita)	3 tbsp	25	tr
Picante Hot (Chi Chi's)	1 oz	11	tr
Picante Mild (Chi Chi's)	1 oz	11	tr
Taco Sauce Red Mild (El Molino)	2 tbsp	10	0
Taco Sauce Thick & Smooth Hot (Ortega)	1 tbsp	8	0
Taco Sauce Thick & Smooth Mild (Ortega)	1 tbsp	8	0
Taco Sauce Western Style (Ortega)	1 oz	8	0
Taco Sauce Hot (Chi Chi's)	1 oz	17	tr
Taco Sauce Mild (Chi Chi's)	1 oz	18	tr
Tamales (Derby)	2	160	7
Tamales (Gebhardt)	2	290	22
Tamales (Wolf Brand)	7.5 oz	328	25
Tamales Jumbo (Gebhardt)	2	400	30
Tamales w/ Sauce (Van Camp's)	1 cup	293	16
Tamalitos in Chili Gravy (Dennison's)	7.5 oz	310	16

FROZEN
Banquet

FOOD	PORTION	CALORIES	FAT
Beef Enchilada & Tamale w/ Chili Gravy	10 oz	300	10
Chimichanga	9.5 oz	480	21
Enchilada Chicken	11 oz	340	9
Enchilada Beef	11 oz	370	12
Enchilada Cheese	11 oz	340	9
Enchiladas Beef w/ Chili Sauce	7 oz	270	13
Tamale Beef	11 oz	420	18

El Charrito

FOOD	PORTION	CALORIES	FAT
Burrito Grande B&B	1 pkg (6 oz)	430	16
Burrito Grande Green Chili B&B	1 pkg (6 oz)	410	14
Burrito Grande Jalapeno	1 pkg (6 oz)	410	15

FOOD	PORTION	CALORIES	FAT
El Charrito *(cont.)*			
Burrito Grande Red Chili B&B	1 pkg (6 oz)	410	15
Burrito Green Chili B&B	1 pkg (5 oz)	370	16
Burrito Red Chili B&B	1 pkg (5 oz)	380	18
Burrito Red Hot B&B	1 pkg (5 oz)	540	18
Burrito Red Hot Beef	1 pkg (5 oz)	340	17
Enchilada Beef Dinner	1 pkg (13.75 oz)	620	31
Enchilada Cheese Dinner	1 pkg (13.75 oz)	570	24
Enchilada Chicken Dinner	1 pkg (13.75 oz)	510	17
Enchilada Grande Beef Dinner	1 pkg (21 oz)	950	49
Enchiladas, 3 Beef	1 pkg (11 oz)	560	31
Enchiladas, 3 Cheese	1 pkg (11 oz)	470	20
Enchiladas, 3 Chicken	1 pkg (11 oz)	440	13
Enchiladas, 6 Beef	1 pkg (16.25 oz)	880	49
Enchiladas, 6 Beef & Cheese	1 pkg (16.25 oz)	880	42
Enchiladas, 6 Cheese	1 pkg (16.25 oz)	780	30
Enchiladas, 4 Grande Beef	1 pkg (16.5 oz)	890	47
Grande Mexican Dinner	1 pkg (20 oz)	850	47
Mexican Dinner	1 pkg (14.25 oz)	690	35
Queso Dinner	1 pkg (13.25 oz)	490	16
Satillo Dinner	1 pkg (13.5 oz)	570	24
Satillo Grande Dinner	1 pkg (20.75 oz)	820	34
Tortillas Corn	2	95	1
Tortillas Flour	2	170	4
Healthy Choice			
Enchilada Beef	12.75 oz	350	5
Enchilada Chicken	12.75 oz	330	5
Enchilada Chicken	9.5 oz	280	6
Fajitas Beef	7 oz	210	4
Fajitas Chicken	7 oz	200	3

FOOD	PORTION	CALORIES	FAT
Le Menu Entree Lightstyle Enchilada Chicken	8 oz	280	8
Lean Cuisine Enchanadas Beef & Bean	9.25 oz	240	6
Lean Cuisine Enchanadas Chicken	9.86 oz	290	9
Patio Britos			
Beef & Bean	1 (3 oz)	210	9
Nacho Beef	1 (3 oz)	220	11
Nacho Cheese	1 (3.63 oz)	250	10
Spicy Chicken & Cheese	1 (3 oz)	210	9
Patio Burritos			
Hot Beef & Bean Red Chili	1 (5 oz)	340	13
Medium Beef & Bean	1 (5 oz)	370	16
Mild Beef & Bean Green Chili	1 (5 oz)	330	12
Red Hot Beef & Bean Red Chili	1 (5 oz)	360	15
Patio Enchilada Beef Dinner	13.25 oz	520	24
Patio Enchilada Cheese Dinner	12 oz	370	10
Patio Fiesta Dinner	12 oz	460	20
Patio Mexican Dinner	13.25	540	25
Patio Tamale Dinner	13 oz	470	21
Swanson Enchiladas Beef	13.75 oz	480	21
Swanson Mexican Style Combination	14.25 oz	490	18
Swanson Mexican Style Hungry Man	20.25 oz	820	41
Van De Kamp's			
Burrito Beef & Bean	5 oz	320	9
Burrito Beef & Cheese	5 oz	320	11
Burrito Beef/Bean Green Chile	5 oz	330	11
Burrito Beef/Bean Red Chile	5 oz	320	12
Van De Kamp's Mexican Classic			
Burrito Crispy Fried	6 oz	365	15
Burrito Grande Sirloin	11 oz	440	15
Burrito Grande w/ Rice & Corn	14.75 oz	530	20

FOOD	PORTION	CALORIES	FAT
Van De Kamp's Mexican Classic *(cont.)*			
Chicken Suiza w/ Rice & Beans	14.75 oz	550	20
Enchilada Beef/Cheese w/ Rice & Beans	14.75 oz	540	20
Enchilada Cheese Ranchero	5.5 oz	250	15
Enchilada Cheese w/ Rice & Beans	14.75 oz	620	30
Enchilada Shredded Beef	5.5 oz	180	10
Enchilada Shredded Beef w/ Rice & Corn	14.75 oz	490	15
Enchilada Suiza Chicken	5.5 oz	220	10
Taquitos Shredded Beef w/ Guacamole	8 oz	490	25
Tostada Beef Supreme	8.5 oz	530	30
Van De Kamp's Mexican Holiday			
Enchilada Beef	7.5 oz	250	15
Enchilada Cheese	7.5 oz	270	15
Enchilada Chicken	7.5 oz	250	10
Enchilada Dinner Beef	12 oz	390	15
Enchilada Dinner Cheese	12 oz	450	20
Enchiladas, 4 Beef	8.5 oz	340	15
Enchiladas, 4 Cheese	8.5 oz	370	20
Mexican Dinner	11.5 oz	420	20
Weight Watchers			
Enchiladas Ranchero Beef	9.12 oz	190	5
Enchiladas Ranchero Cheese	8.87 oz	260	10
Enchiladas Suiza Chicken	9 oz	230	7
Fajitas Chicken	6.75 oz	210	5
MIX			
Masa Harina de Maiz (Quaker)	2 tortillas	137	2
Masa Trigo (Quaker)	2 tortillas	149	4
Menudo Mix (Gebhardt)	1 tsp	5	tr

FOOD	PORTION	CALORIES	FAT
Taco Meat Seasoning Mix Mild, as prep (Ortega)	1 filled taco	90	1
READY-TO-USE			
Taco Shells (Gebhardt)	1	50	2
Taco Shells (Rosarita)	1	50	2
Tostada Shells (Rosarita)	1	60	3
tortilla corn	1 (1 oz)	65	1
TAKE-OUT			
burrito w/ apple	1 sm (2.6 oz)	231	10
burrito w/ apple	1 lg (5.4 oz)	484	20
burrito w/ beans, cheese & beef	2 (7.1 oz)	331	13
burrito w/ beans, cheese & chili peppers	2 (11.8 oz)	663	23
burrito w/ cherry	1 sm (2.6 oz)	231	10
burrito w/ cherry	1 lg (5.4 oz)	484	20
burrito w/ beans	2 (7.6 oz)	448	14
burrito w/ beans & cheese	2 (6.5 oz)	377	12
burrito w/ beans & chili peppers	2 (7.2 oz)	413	15
burrito w/ beans & meat	2 (8.1 oz)	508	18
burrito w/ beef	2 (7.7 oz)	523	21
burrito w/ beef & chili peppers	2 (7.1 oz)	426	17
chimichanga w/ beef	1 (6.1 oz)	425	20
chimichanga w/ beef & cheese	1 (6.4 oz)	443	23
chimichanga w/ beef & red chili peppers	1 (6.7 oz)	424	19
chimichanga w/ beef, cheese & red chili peppers	1 (6.3 oz)	364	18
enchilada w/ cheese	1 (5.7 oz)	320	19
enchilada w/ cheese & beef	1 (6.7 oz)	324	18
enchilada w/ eggplant	1	142	5
enchirito w/ cheese, beef & beans	1 (6.8 oz)	344	16

FOOD	PORTION	CALORIES	FAT
frijoles w/ cheese	1 cup (5.9 oz)	226	8
nachos w/ cheese	6–8 (4 oz)	345	19
nachos w/ cheese & jalapeno peppers	6–8 (7.2 oz)	607	34
nachos w/ cheese, beans, ground beef & peppers	6–8 (8.9 oz)	568	31
nachos w/ cinnamon & sugar	6–8 (3.8 oz)	592	36
taco	1 sm (6 oz)	370	21
taco salad	1½ cups	279	15
taco salad w/ chili con carne	1½ cups	288	13
tostada w/ beans & cheese	1 (5.1 oz)	223	10
tostada w/ beans, beef & cheese	1 (7.9 oz)	334	17
tostada w/ beef & cheese	1 (5.7 oz)	315	16
tostada w/ guacamole	2 (9.2 oz)	360	23

MILK
(*see also* CHOCOLATE, COCOA, MILK DRINKS)

CANNED

FOOD	PORTION	CALORIES	FAT
Carnation Evaporated	½ cup	170	10
Carnation Evaporated Lowfat	½ cup	110	3
Carnation Evaporated Skim	½ cup	100	tr
Carnation Sweetened Condensed	1 oz	123	3
Carnation Sweetened Condensed	⅓ cup	318	9
Eagle Sweetened Condensed	⅓ cup	320	9
Pet 99 Evaporated Skim	½ cup	100	0
Pet Evaporated	½ cup	170	10
condensed, sweetened	1 oz	123	3
condensed, sweetened	1 cup	982	27
evaporated	½ cup	169	10
evaporated, skim	½ cup	99	tr

FOOD	PORTION	CALORIES	FAT
DRIED			
Carnation, as prep	8 oz	80	tr
Carnation, as prep	1 qt	320	tr
Flash Instant, as prep	8 oz	80	tr
Nutra/Balance Lactose Reduced, as prep	8 oz	80	tr
Sanalac, as prep	8 oz	80	tr
buttermilk	1 tbsp	25	tr
nonfat instantized	1 pkg (3.2 oz)	244	tr
LIQUID, LOWFAT			
1%	1 cup	102	3
1%	1 qt	409	10
1% protein fortified	1 cup	119	3
2%	1 cup	121	5
2%	1 qt	485	19
CalciMilk	1 cup	102	3
Friendship Buttermilk	8 oz	120	4
Lactaid 1%	1 cup	102	3
Land O'Lakes 1%	8 oz	100	3
Land O'Lakes 2%	8 oz	120	5
buttermilk	1 cup	99	2
buttermilk	1 qt	396	9
LIQUID, REGULAR			
Borden	1 cup	150	8
Borden Hi-Calcium	1 cup	150	8
Farmland 75% Cholesterol Reduced	8 oz	150	8
Land O'Lakes	8 oz	150	8
buffalo	3.5 oz	112	8
camel	3.5 oz	80	4
donkey	3.5 oz	43	1

FOOD	PORTION	CALORIES	FAT
goat	1 cup	168	10
goat	1 qt	672	40
human	1 cup	171	11
indian buffalo	1 cup	236	17
low sodium	1 cup	149	8
mare	3.5 oz	49	2
sheep	1 cup	264	17
whole	1 cup	150	8
LIQUID, SKIM			
Borden	1 cup	90	1
Farmland Skim Plus	8 oz	100	tr
Lactaid Nonfat	1 cup	86	tr
Land O'Lakes	8 oz	90	tr
Weight Watchers	1 cup	90	tr
skim	1 cup	86	tr
skim	1 qt	342	2
skim, protein fortified	1 cup	100	1
skim, protein fortified	1 qt	400	2

MILK DRINKS
(see also BREAKFAST DRINKS, CHOCOLATE, COCOA)

FOOD	PORTION	CALORIES	FAT
Chocolate Milk (Land O'Lakes)	8 oz	210	8
Chocolate Milk (Meadow Gold)	1 cup	210	8
Chocolate Milk 1% (Land O'Lakes)	8 oz	160	3
Chocolate Milk 1% (Lactaid)	1 cup	158	3
Chocolate Milk 2% (Hershey)	1 cup	190	5
Chocolate Skim Milk (Land O'Lakes)	8 oz	140	tr
Dutch Brand Chocolate Lowfat (Borden)	1 cup	180	5
Quik Banana Lowfat Milk (Nestle)	8 oz	190	4

FOOD	PORTION	CALORIES	FAT
Quik Chocolate (Nestle)	¾ oz	90	1
Quik Chocolate, as prep w/ 2% milk (Nestle)	8 oz	210	5
Quik Chocolate, as prep w/ skim milk (Nestle)	8 oz	170	1
Quik Chocolate, as prep w/ whole milk (Nestle)	8 oz	230	9
Quik Chocolate Lowfat Milk (Nestle)	8 oz	200	5
Quik Strawberry (Nestle)	¾ oz	80	0
Quik Strawberry, as prep w/ 2% milk (Nestle)	8 oz	200	5
Quik Strawberry, as prep w/ skim milk (Nestle)	8 oz	160	0
Quik Strawberry, as prep w/ whole milk (Nestle)	8 oz	220	8
Quik Strawberry Lowfat Milk (Nestle)	8 oz	200	4
Quik Lite Ready to Drink Chocolate Lowfat (Nestle)	8 oz	130	5
Quik Ready to Drink Chocolate (Nestle)	8 oz	230	9
Quik Ready to Drink Strawberry (Nestle)	8 oz	230	8
Quik Sugar Free Chocolate (Nestle)	1 heaping tsp	18	tr
Quik Sugar Free Chocolate, as prep w/ 2% milk (Nestle)	8 oz	140	5
Quik Syrup Chocolate (Nestle)	1⅔ tbsp	100	1
Quik Syrup Chocolate, as prep w/ 2% milk (Nestle)	8 oz	220	5
Quik Syrup Chocolate, as prep w/ skim milk (Nestle)	8 oz	220	9
Quik Syrup Chocolate, as prep w/ whole milk (Nestle)	8 oz	240	9
Quik Syrup Strawberry (Nestle)	1⅔ tbsp	100	0
Quik Syrup Strawberry, as prep w/ 2% milk (Nestle)	8 oz	220	5

FOOD	PORTION	CALORIES	FAT
Quik Syrup Strawberry, as prep w/ skim milk (Nestle)	8 oz	180	0
Quik Syrup Strawberry, as prep w/ whole milk (Nestle)	8 oz	240	8
Quik Vanilla Lowfat Milk (Nestle)	8 oz	200	4
Whole Chocolate Milk (Hershey)	8 oz	210	9
chocolate milk	1 cup	208	8
chocolate milk	1 qt	833	34
chocolate milk 1%	1 cup	158	3
chocolate milk 1%	1 qt	630	10
chocolate milk 2%	1 cup	179	5
strawberry flavor mix, as prep w/ whole milk	9 oz	234	8

MILK SUBSTITUTES
(*see also* COFFEE WHITENERS)

FOOD	PORTION	CALORIES	FAT
Honey Vanilla (Spring Creek)	1 oz	23	5
Original (Spring Creek)	1 oz	21	5
Plain (Spring Creek)	1 oz	15	5
Vitamite (Deihl)	8 oz	100	5
imitation milk	1 cup	150	8
imitation milk	1 qt	600	33

MILKFISH

FOOD	PORTION	CALORIES	FAT
baked	3 oz	162	7

MILKSHAKE

FOOD	PORTION	CALORIES	FAT
Chocolate (Frostee)	1 cup	200	8
Chocolate (MicroMagic)	1 (10.5 oz)	290	8
Chocolate Fudge (Weight Watchers)	1 pkg	70	tr
Orange Sherbet (Weight Watchers)	1 pkg	70	tr
Strawberry (Frostee)	1 cup	180	7

FOOD	PORTION	CALORIES	FAT
chocolate	10 oz	360	11
chocolate thick shake	10.6 oz	356	8
strawberry	10 oz	319	8
vanilla	10 oz	314	8
vanilla thick shake	11 oz	350	10

MILLET

Millet Hulled (Arrowhead)	1 oz	90	1
cooked	½ cup	143	1
raw	½ cup	378	4

MINERAL/BOTTLED WATER

Artesia	7 oz	0	0
Artesia Almund	7 oz	0	0
Artesia Cranberi	7 oz	0	0
Artesia Lemin	7 oz	0	0
Artesia Orange	7 oz	0	0
Crystal Geyser Sparkling Cola Berry	6 oz	0	0
Crystal Geyser Sparkling Lemon	6 oz	0	0
Crystal Geyser Sparkling Lime	6 oz	0	0
Crystal Geyser Sparkling Mineral	6 oz	0	0
Crystal Geyser Sparkling Natural Wild Cherry	6 oz	0	0
Crystal Geyser Sparkling Orange	6 oz	0	0
Diamond Spring	1 qt (liter)	0	0
Evian	1 liter	0	0
Glenpatrick Spring Pure Irish	8 oz	0	0
Mountain Valley	1 qt (liter)	0	0
San Pellegrino	1 liter (33.8 oz)	0	0
Saratoga Sparkling	8 oz	0	0
Schweppes Vichy	6 oz	0	0

FOOD	PORTION	CALORIES	FAT

MISO

miso	½ cup	284	8

MOCHA

Bavarian Mint Mocha, as prep (Hills Bros.)	6 oz	50	1
Bavarian Mint Mocha Sugar Free, as prep (Hills Bros.)	6 oz	35	1
Cafe Mocha, as prep (Hills Bros.)	6 oz	50	1
Cafe Mocha, as prep (MJB Co.)	6 oz	50	1
Cherry Mocha, as prep (MJB Co.)	6 oz	50	1
Fudge Mocha Sugar Free, as prep (MJB Co.)	6 oz	40	2
Mint Mocha, as prep (MJB Co.)	6 oz	50	1
Mint Mocha Sugar Free, as prep (MJB Co.)	6 oz	35	1
Swiss Mocha, as prep (Hills Bros.)	6 oz	40	2
Vanilla Mocha Sugar Free, as prep (MJB Co.)	6 oz	40	2

MOLASSES

Brer Rabbit Dark	2 tbsp	110	0
Brer Rabbit Light	2 tbsp	110	0
Grandma's Gold Label	1 tbsp	70	0
Grandma's Green Label	1 tbsp	70	0
blackstrap	2 tbsp	85	0
molasses	2 tbsp	85	0

MONKFISH

baked	3 oz	82	2

FOOD	PORTION	CALORIES	FAT

MOOSE

roasted	3 oz	114	1

MOTH BEANS

dried, cooked	1 cup	207	1
dried, raw	1 cup	673	3

MOUSSE

FROZEN

Chocolate (Sara Lee)	1 Slice (2.7 oz)	260	17
Chocolate (Weight Watchers)	1 (2.5 oz)	160	3
Chocolate Light (Sara Lee)	1 (3 oz)	170	8
Light Classics Strawberry (Sara Lee)	1 slice (53.8 g)	180	11
Praline Pecan (Weight Watchers)	1 (2.71 oz)	180	4
San Francisco Chocolate (Pepperidge Farm)	1	490	34

HOME RECIPE

crab	¼ cup	364	20
orange	½ cup	87	5

MIX

Amaretto, as prep (Estee)	½ cup	70	3
Black Forest Mousse Tiarra Dessert, as prep (Duncan Hines)	1/12 cake	260	13
Cherries & Cream Mousse Tiarra Dessert, as prep (Duncan Hines)	1/12 cake	250	11
Chocolate Amaretto Mousse Tiarra Dessert, as prep (Duncan Hines)	1/12 cake	270	16
Chocolate Fudge Mousse No Bake Dessert, as prep (Jell-O)	½ cup	138	6
Chocolate Mousse (Weight Watchers)	½ cup	70	3

FOOD	PORTION	CALORIES	FAT
Chocolate Mousse No Bake Dessert, as prep (Jell-O)	½ cup	141	5
Chocolate Mousse Tiarra Dessert, as prep (Duncan Hines)	1/12 cake	270	16
Dark Chocolate Mousse Mix, as prep (Knorr)	½ cup	90	5
Milk Chocolate Mousse Mix, as prep (Knorr)	½ cup	90	5
Orange Chocolate, as prep (Estee)	½ cup	70	3
Unflavored Mousse Mix, as prep (Knorr)	½ cup	80	5
White Chocolate Almond Mousse, as prep (Weight Watchers)	½ cup	70	3
White Chocolate Mousse Mix, as prep (Knorr)	½ cup	80	4

MUFFIN

FROZEN

FOOD	PORTION	CALORIES	FAT
Almond & Date Oat Bran Fancy Fruit (Health Valley)	1	180	4
Apple Oat Bran (Sara Lee)	1	190	6
Apple Spice (Healthy Choice)	1 (2.5 oz)	190	4
Apple Spice (Sara Lee)	1	220	8
Apple Spice Fat Free (Health Valley)	1	140	tr
Banana Fat Free (Health Valley)	1	130	tr
Banana Nut (Healthy Choice)	1 (2.5 oz)	180	6
Banana Nut (Pepperidge Farm)	1	170	6
Banana Nut (Weight Watchers)	1 (2.5 oz)	170	5
Blueberry (Healthy Choice)	1 (2.5 oz)	190	4
Blueberry (Pepperidge Farm)	1	170	7
Blueberry (Sara Lee)	1	200	8
Blueberry (Weight Watchers)	1 (2.5 oz)	170	5

FOOD	PORTION	CALORIES	FAT
Blueberry Free & Light (Sara Lee)	1	120	0
Cheese Streusel (Sara Lee)	1	220	11
Chocolate Chunk (Sara Lee)	1	220	8
Cholesterol Free Multi-Grain Muesli (Pepperidge Farm)	1	200	8
Cholesterol Free Oat Bran w/ Apple (Pepperidge Farm)	1	190	7
Cholesterol Free Raisin Bran (Pepperidge Farm)	1	170	6
Cinnamon Swirl (Pepperidge Farm)	1	190	6
Corn (Pepperidge Farm)	1	180	7
Egg, Canadian Bacon & Cheese (Great Starts)	4.1 oz	290	15
Golden Corn (Sara Lee)	1	240	13
Oat Bran (Sara Lee)	1	210	8
Oat Bran Fancy Fruit Blueberry (Health Valley)	1	140	4
Oat Bran Fancy Fruit Raisin (Health Valley)	1	180	5
Raisin Bran (Sara Lee)	1	220	7
Raisin Spice Fat Free (Health Valley)	1	140	tr
Rice Bran Fancy Fruit Raisin (Health Valley)	1	210	7
HOME RECIPE			
blueberry	1 (1.5 oz)	135	5
bran	1 (1.5 oz)	125	6
MIX			
Blue Corn (Arrowhead)	1	110	4
Blueberry Bakery Style (Duncan Hines)	1	190	6
Bran & Honey (Duncan Hines)	1	120	4
Bran & Honey Nut Bakery Style (Duncan Hines)	1	200	7

FOOD	PORTION	CALORIES	FAT
Cinnamon Swirl Bakery Style (Duncan Hines)	1	200	7
Corn Muffin (Dromedary)	1	120	4
Corn Muffin Mix (Flako)	1	120	4
Cranberry Orange Nut Bakery Style (Duncan Hines)	1	200	8
Oat Bran (Estee)	1	100	4
Oat Bran Apple Spice (Arrowhead)	1	120	4
Oat Bran Wheat Free (Arrowhead)	1	100	5
Pecan Nut Bakery Style (Duncan Hines)	1	220	11
Wheat Bran (Arrowhead)	2	270	7
Wild Blueberry (Duncan Hines)	1	110	3
blueberry	1 (1.5 oz)	140	5
bran	1 (1.5 oz)	140	4
corn	1 (1.5 oz)	145	6

MULBERRIES

fresh	1 cup	61	1

MULLET

striped, cooked	3 oz	127	4

MUNG BEANS

DRIED

Arrowhead Red	2 oz	50	1
cooked	1 cup	213	1
raw	1 cup	719	2

SPROUTS

canned	½ cup	8	tr
cooked	½ cup	13	tr

FOOD	PORTION	CALORIES	FAT
raw	½ cup	16	tr
stir-fried	½ cup	31	tr

MUNGO BEANS

dried, cooked	1 cup	190	1
dried, raw	1 cup	726	4

MUSHROOMS

CANNED

Button (Empress)	2 oz	14	0
Button Sliced (Empress)	2 oz	14	0
Mushrooms (B In B)	¼ cup	12	0
Mushrooms (Libby)	¼ cup	35	0
Mushrooms (Seneca)	¼ cup	35	0
Mushrooms w/ Garlic (B In B)	¼ cup	12	0
Oriental Straw Mushrooms (Green Giant)	¼ cup	12	0
Pieces & Stems (Empress)	2 oz	14	0
Pieces & Stems (Green Giant)	¼ cup	12	0
Sliced (Green Giant)	¼ cup	12	0
Straw Mushrooms Broken (Empress)	2 oz	10	0
Whole (Green Giant)	¼ cup	12	0
chanterelle	3.5 oz	12	1
pieces	½ cup	19	tr
whole	1 (.4 oz)	3	tr

DRIED

chanterelle	3.5 oz	89	2
shiitake	4 (½ oz)	44	tr

FRESH

chanterelle	3½ oz	11	tr

FOOD	PORTION	CALORIES	FAT
enoki, raw	1	2	tr
morel	3.5 oz	9	tr
raw	1 (½ oz)	5	tr
raw, sliced	½ cup	9	tr
shitake, cooked	4 (2.5 oz)	40	tr
sliced, cooked	½ cup	21	tr
whole, cooked	1 (.4 oz)	3	tr
FROZEN			
Breaded Mushrooms (Ore Ida)	2.67 oz	120	7

MUSKRAT

FOOD	PORTION	CALORIES	FAT
roasted	3 oz	199	10

MUSSELS

FOOD	PORTION	CALORIES	FAT
FRESH			
blue, cooked	3 oz	147	4
blue, raw	1 cup	129	3
blue, raw	3 oz	73	2

MUSTARD

FOOD	PORTION	CALORIES	FAT
DRY			
mustard seed, yellow	1 tsp	15	1
READY-TO-USE			
Grey Poupon Country Dijon	1 tsp	6	0
Grey Poupon Dijon	1 tsp	6	0
Grey Poupon Parisian	1 tsp	6	0
Gulden's Diablo	1 tsp	8	0
Gulden's Mild	1 tsp	6	0
Gulden's Spicy Brown	1 tsp	8	0
Heinz Mild Yellow	1 tbsp	8	tr

FOOD	PORTION	CALORIES	FAT
Heinz Spicy Brown	1 tbsp	14	1
Kosciuszko	1 tbsp	11	1
Kraft Horseradish	1 tbsp	14	1
Kraft Pure Prepared	1 tbsp	4	1
Plochman's Dijon	1 tbsp	11	1
Plochman's Spicy Brown	1 tbsp	11	1
Plochman's Stone Ground	1 tbsp	11	1
Plochman's Yellow	1 tbsp	11	1
yellow	1 tsp	5	tr

MUSTARD GREENS

FRESH
| chopped, cooked | ½ cup | 11 | tr |
| raw, chopped | ½ cup | 7 | tr |

FROZEN
| chopped, cooked | ½ cup | 14 | tr |

NATTO

| natto | ½ cup | 187 | 10 |

NAVY BEANS

CANNED
Jalapeno (Trappey's)	½ cup	90	1
Navy Beans (Hanover)	½ cup	100	0
Ole Fashion Navies (Ranch Style)	7.5 oz	160	2
Seasoned w/ Pork (Luck's)	7.5 oz	230	7
Trappey's	½ cup	90	1
navy	1 cup	296	1

DRIED
| Hurst Brand | 1 cup | 277 | 1 |

FOOD	PORTION	CALORIES	FAT
cooked	1 cup	259	1
raw	1 cup	697	3
SPROUTS			
cooked	3.5 oz	78	1
raw	½ cup	35	tr

NECTARINE

Dole	1	70	1
fresh	1	67	1

NEUFCHATEL CHEESE
(*see* CREAM CHEESE)

NON-DAIRY CREAMERS
(*see* COFFEE WHITENERS)

NON-DAIRY WHIPPED TOPPINGS
(*see* WHIPPED TOPPINGS)

NOODLES
(*see also* PASTA DINNERS)

CANNED			
Van Camp's Noodle Weenee	1 cup	245	9
DRY			
Chinese (Azumaya)	4 oz	293	1
Chow Mein Narrow (La Choy)	½ cup	150	8
Chow Mein Wide (La Choy)	½ cup	150	8
Egg (Creamette)	2 oz	221	3
Egg (Golden Grain)	2 oz	210	2
Egg (Mueller's)	2 oz	220	3
Egg (Ronzoni)	2 oz	211	2
Egg (Skinner)	2 oz	220	3

FOOD	PORTION	CALORIES	FAT
Fine, Medium, Wide & Extra Wide (P&R)	2 oz	220	3
Japanese (Azumaya)	4 oz	289	1
Noodle Trio (Mueller's)	2 oz	220	2
Rice (La Choy)	½ cup	130	5
Spinach Egg (Ronzoni)	2 oz	209	2
Spinach Egg Light'N Fluffy (Skinner)	2 oz	220	3
cellophane	1 cup	492	tr
chow mein	1 cup	237	14
egg, cooked	1 cup	212	2
japanese soba, cooked	½ cup	56	tr
japanese somen, cooked	½ cup	115	tr
spinach/egg, cooked	1 cup	211	3
DRY MIX Kraft Egg Noodle w/ Chicken Dinner, as prep	¾ cup	240	9
La Choy Ramen Noodles Beef, as prep	1 cup	200	8
La Choy Ramen Noodles Chicken, as prep	1 cup	200	7
La Choy Ramen Noodles Oriental, as prep	½ pkg	190	7
Lipton Noodles & Sauce			
Alfredo, as prep	¼ pkg	146	4
Beef, as prep	¼ pkg	128	2
Butter, as prep	¼ pkg	148	4
Butter & Herb, as prep	¼ pkg	140	3
Cheese, as prep	¼ pkg	141	2
Chicken, as prep	¼ pkg	130	2
Parmesan, as prep	¼ pkg	143	4
Sour Cream & Chive, as prep	¼ pkg	144	3
Stroganoff, as prep	¼ pkg	131	3

FOOD	PORTION	CALORIES	FAT
Noodle Roni			
Chicken & Mushroom, as prep	½ cup	160	4
Fettuccini, as prep	½ cup	300	18
Herb & Butter, as prep	½ cup	160	7
Parmesano, as prep	½ cup	240	13
Romanoff, as prep	½ cup	240	11
Stroganoff, as prep	½ cup	350	17
Ultra Slim-Fast			
Noodles & Alfredo Sauce	2.3 oz	240	4
Noodles & Beef	2.3 oz	230	3
Noodles & Cheese	2.3 oz	230	4
Noodles & Chicken Sauce	2.3 oz	220	3
Noodles &Tomato Herb Sauce	2.3 oz	220	3
TAKE-OUT			
noodle pudding	½ cup	132	7

NUTMEG

ground	1 tsp	12	1

NUTRITIONAL SUPPLEMENTS

(*see also* BREAKFAST BAR, BREAKFAST DRINKS, FIBER, PECTIN, OIL, FISH OIL)

FOOD	PORTION	CALORIES	FAT
DIET			
Dynatrim Dutch Chocolate, as prep w/ 1% milk	8 oz	220	4
Dynatrim Strawberry Royale, as prep w/ 1% milk	8 oz	220	4
Dynatrim Vanilla, as prep w/ 1% milk	8 oz	220	4
Figurines Chocolate	1 bar	100	5
Figurines Chocolate Caramel	1 bar	100	6
Figurines Chocolate Peanut Butter	1 bar	100	6

FOOD	PORTION	CALORIES	FAT
Figurines S'Mores	1 bar	100	5
Figurines Vanilla	1 bar	100	5
Slender Chocolate	10 oz	220	4
Slender Chocolate Fudge	10 oz	220	4
Slender Chocolate Malt	10 oz	220	4
Slender Milk Chocolate	10 oz	220	4
Slender Vanilla	10 oz	220	4
Slender Bars Chocolate	2 bars	270	14
Slender Bars Chocolate Chip	2 bars	270	14
Slender Bars Chocolate Peanut Butter	2 bars	270	15
Slender Bars Vanilla	2 bars	270	15
Slender Instant Chocolate	1 pkg (1.06 oz)	110	1
Slender Instant Chocolate, as prep w/ 2% milk	1 pkg + 6 oz milk	200	5
Slender Instant Dutch Chocolate	1 pkg	110	1
Slender Instant Dutch Chocolate, as prep w/ 2% milk	1 pkg + 6 oz milk	200	5
Slender Instant French Vanilla	1 pkg (1.04 oz)	110	tr
Slender Instant French Vanilla, as prep w/ 2% milk	1 pkg + 6 oz milk	200	4
Slim-Fast Nutrition Bar Dutch Chocolate	1	130	4
Slim-Fast Nutrition Bar Peanut Butter	1	140	6
Slim-Fast Powder Chocolate, as prep w/ skim milk	8 oz	190	1
Slim-Fast Powder Chocolate Malt, as prep w/ skim milk	8 oz	190	tr
Slim-Fast Powder Strawberry, as prep w/ skim milk	8 oz	190	1
Slim-Fast Powder Vanilla, as prep w/ skim milk	8 oz	190	1

FOOD	PORTION	CALORIES	FAT
Ultra Slim-Fast Cafe Mocha, as prep w/ skim milk	8 oz	200	tr
Ultra Slim-Fast Chocolate Royale, as prep w/ skim milk	8 oz	200	1
Ultra Slim-Fast Crunch Bar Cocoa Almond	1	110	3
Ultra Slim-Fast Crunch Bar Cocoa Raspberry	1	100	3
Ultra Slim-Fast Crunch Bar Vanilla Almond	1	110	4
Ultra Slim-Fast Dutch Chocolate, as prep w/ water	8 oz	220	tr
Ultra Slim-Fast French Vanilla, as prep w/ skim milk	8 oz	190	tr
Ultra Slim-Fast French Vanilla, as prep w/ water	8 oz	220	tr
Ultra Slim-Fast Fruit Juice Mix, as prep w/ fruit juice	8 oz	200	tr
Ultra Slim-Fast Hot Cocoa, as prep w/ water	8 oz	190	tr
Ultra Slim-Fast Pina Colada, as prep w/ skim milk	8 oz	180	tr
Ultra Slim-Fast Ready-to-Drink Chocolate Royale	12 oz	250	1
Ultra Slim-Fast Ready-to-Drink French Vanilla	12 oz	220	tr
Ultra Slim-Fast Ready-to-Drink Strawberry Supreme	12 oz	220	1
Ultra Slim-Fast Strawberry, as prep w/ skim milk	8 oz	190	1
Ultra Slim-Fast Strawberry Supreme, as prep w/ water	8 oz	220	tr
REGULAR			
EggPro	4 oz	220	4
Fi-Bar Apple	1 (1 oz)	90	3

FOOD	PORTION	CALORIES	FAT
Fi-Bar Cocoa Almond	1	130	4
Fi-Bar Cocoa Peanut	1	130	4
Fi-Bar Cranberry & Wild Berries	1 (1 oz)	100	3
Fi-Bar Lemon	1 (1 oz)	90	3
Fi-Bar Mandarin Orange	1 (1 oz)	99	4
Fi-Bar Raspberry	1 (1 oz)	100	3
Fi-Bar Strawberry	1 (1 oz)	100	3
Fi-Bar Treat Yourself Right Almond	1	152	6
Fi-Bar Treat Yourself Right Peanutty Butter	1	152	5
Fi-Bar Vanilla Almond	1	130	4
Fi-Bar Vanilla Peanut	1	130	4
Fi-Bar Nuggets Almond Cappuccino Crunch	1 pkg	136	6
Fi-Bar Nuggets Almond Butter Crunch	1 pkg	163	11
Fi-Bar Nuggets Coconut Almond Crunch	1 pkg	136	6
Fi-Bar Nuggets Peanut Butter Crunch	1 pkg	160	10
Gookinaid Lemonade, as prep	1 cup	45	0
Malsovit Mealwafers	2	152	8
Meal on the Go Apple	1 bar (3 oz)	294	5
Meal on the Go Banana w/ Pecans	1 bar (3 oz)	289	10
Meal on the Go Original	1 bar (3 oz)	286	9
Nutra/Balance Frozen Pudding Butterscotch	4 oz	225	8
Nutra/Balance Frozen Pudding Chocolate	4 oz	225	8
Nutra/Balance Frozen Pudding Tapioca	4 oz	225	8
Nutra/Balance Frozen Pudding Vanilla	4 oz	225	8
NutraShake Chocolate	4 oz	200	6

FOOD	PORTION	CALORIES	FAT
NutraShake Strawberry	4 oz	200	6
NutraShake Vanilla	4 oz	200	6
NutraShake w/ Fibre Strawberry	6 oz	300	2
NutraShake w/ Fibre Vanilla	6 oz	300	2
Nutri-Care Strawberry	1 pkg (1.13 oz)	120	1
Nutri-Care, Strawberry, as prep w/ 1 cup 2% milk	1 pkg (1.13 oz)	260	5
Nutri-Care Strawberry, as prep w/ 1 cup whole milk	1 pkg (1.13 oz)	280	9

NUTS, MIXED
(see also individual names)

FOOD	PORTION	CALORIES	FAT
Cashews & Peanuts, Honey Roasted (Planters)	1 oz	170	12
Mixed Nuts Lightly Salted (Planters)	1 oz	170	15
Mixed Nuts w/ Peanuts (Guy's)	1 oz	180	16
Peanuts & Cashews Honey Roasted	1 oz	170	12
Tasty Mix (Guy's)	1 oz	130	7
dry roasted w/ peanuts	1 oz	169	15
dry roasted w/ peanuts, salted	1 oz	169	15
oil roasted w/ peanuts	1 oz	175	16
oil roasted w/ peanuts, salted	1 oz	175	16
oil roasted w/o peanuts	1 oz	175	16
oil roasted w/o peanuts, salted	1 oz	175	16

OCTOBER BEANS

CANNED

FOOD	PORTION	CALORIES	FAT
Seasoned w/ Pork (Luck's)	7.25 oz	230	6

OCTOPUS

FOOD	PORTION	CALORIES	FAT
fresh, steamed	3 oz	140	2
fresh	1 cup	39	tr

FOOD	PORTION	CALORIES	FAT
OIL			
(*see also* FAT)			
Bertolli Classico	1 tbsp	120	14
Bertolli Extra Light	1 tbsp	120	14
Bertolli Extra Virgin	1 tbsp	120	14
Crisco	1 tbsp	120	14
Crisco Corn Oil	1 tbsp	120	14
Italica	1 tbsp	120	9
Mazola	1 tbsp	120	14
Mazola	1 cup	1955	221
Mazola No Stick	2.5-second spray	2	tr
Orville Redenbacher's	1 tbsp	120	14
Planters Peanut	1 tbsp	120	14
Planters Popcorn	1 tbsp	120	13
Pompeian	1 tbsp	130	14
Puritan	1 tbsp	120	14
Smart Beat	1 tbsp	120	14
Smart Beat Canola	1 tbsp	120	14
Weight Watchers Butter Spray	1-second spray	2	tr
Weight Watchers Cooking Spray	1-second spray	2	tr
Wesson Canola	1 tbsp	120	14
Wesson Corn	1 tbsp	120	14
Wesson Lite Cooking Spray	.5-second spray	0	0
Wesson Olive	1 tbsp	120	14
Wesson Sunflower	1 tbsp	120	14
Wesson Vegetable	1 tbsp	120	14
almond	1 tbsp	120	14
almond	1 cup	1927	218
apricot kernel	1 tbsp	120	14

FOOD	PORTION	CALORIES	FAT
apricot kernel	1 cup	1927	218
avocado	1 tbsp	124	14
avocado	1 cup	1927	218
babassu (palm)	1 tbsp	120	14
canola	1 tbsp	124	14
canola	1 cup	1927	218
coconut	1 tbsp	117	14
corn	1 tbsp	120	14
corn	1 cup	1927	218
cottonseed	1 tbsp	120	14
cottonseed	1 cup	1927	218
cupu assu	1 tbsp	120	14
grapeseed	1 tbsp	120	14
hazelnut	1 tbsp	120	14
hazelnut	1 cup	1927	218
mustard	1 tbsp	124	14
mustard	1 cup	1927	218
oat	1 tbsp	120	14
olive	1 tbsp	119	14
olive	1 cup	1909	216
palm	1 tbsp	120	14
palm	1 cup	1927	218
palm kernel	1 tbsp	117	14
palm kernel	1 cup	1879	218
peanut	1 tbsp	119	14
peanut	1 cup	1909	216
poppyseed	1 tbsp	120	14
pumpkin seed	3.5 oz	925	100
rice bran	1 tbsp	120	14
safflower	1 tbsp	120	14

FOOD	PORTION	CALORIES	FAT
safflower	1 cup	1927	218
sesame	1 tbsp	120	14
sheanut	1 tbsp	120	14
soybean	1 tbsp	120	14
soybean	1 cup	1927	218
sunflower	1 tbsp	120	14
sunflower	1 cup	1927	218
teaseed	1 tbsp	120	14
tomatoseed	1 tbsp	120	14
vegetable	1 tbsp	120	14
vegetable	1 cup	1927	218
walnut	1 tbsp	120	14
walnut	1 cup	1927	218
wheat germ	1 tbsp	120	14
FISH OIL			
cod	1 tbsp	123	14
herring	1 tbsp	123	14
menhaden	1 tbsp	123	14
salmon	1 tbsp	123	14
sardine	1 tbsp	123	14
shark	3.5 oz	945	100
whale	3.5 oz	945	100

OKRA

FOOD	PORTION	CALORIES	FAT
CANNED			
Creole Cumbo (Trappey's)	½ cup	25	0
Cut (Trappey's)	½ cup	25	0
FRESH			
raw	8 pods	36	tr
raw, sliced	½ cup	19	tr

FOOD	PORTION	CALORIES	FAT
sliced, cooked	8 pods	27	tr
sliced, cooked	½ cup	25	tr
FROZEN Breaded (Ore Ida)	3 oz	170	10
Cut (Hanover)	½ cup	25	0
Whole (Hanover)	½ cup	35	0
sliced, cooked	½ cup	34	tr
sliced, cooked	1 pkg (10 oz)	94	1

OLIVES

FOOD	PORTION	CALORIES	FAT
California Ripe	2 jumbo	188	9
California Ripe	3 sm	4	tr
Ripe Extra Large (S&W)	3.5 oz	163	18
Ripe Pitted Large (S&W)	3.5 oz	163	18
Spanish Green (Tee Pee)	2 oz	98	10
green	3 extra lg	15	2
green	4 med	15	2
ripe	1 sm	4	tr
ripe	1 lg	5	tr
ripe	1 jumbo	7	1
ripe	1 colossal	12	1

ONION

FOOD	PORTION	CALORIES	FAT
CANNED Lightly Spiced Cocktail Onions (Vlasic)	1 oz	4	0
Whole Small (S&W)	½ cup	35	0
DRIED flakes	1 tbsp	16	tr
powder	1 tsp	7	tr

FOOD	PORTION	CALORIES	FAT
FRESH			
Dole	1 med	60	0
Dole Green, chopped	1 tbsp	2	tr
Vidalia (Antioch Farms)	1 med	60	0
chopped, cooked	½ cup	47	tr
raw, chopped	1 tbsp	4	tr
raw, chopped	½ cup	30	tr
scallions, raw, chopped	1 tbsp	2	tr
scallions, raw, sliced	½ cup	16	tr
welsh, raw	3½ oz	34	tr
FROZEN			
Chopped (Ore Ida)	2 oz	20	tr
Chopped (Southland)	2 oz	15	0
Crispy Onion Rings (Mrs. Paul's)	2.5 oz	190	12
Onion Ringers (Ore Ida)	2 oz	150	9
Onions Small Whole (Birds Eye)	½ cup	40	tr
Onions Small w/ Cream Sauce (Birds Eye)	½ cup	100	6
chopped, cooked	1 tbsp	4	tr
chopped, cooked	½ cup	30	tr
rings	7 (2.5 oz)	285	19
rings, cooked	2 (.7 oz)	81	5
whole, cooked	3.5 oz	28	tr
TAKE-OUT			
rings, breaded & fried	8–9	275	16

OPOSSUM

roasted	3 oz	188	9

FOOD	PORTION	CALORIES	FAT

ORANGE

CANNED

FOOD	PORTION	CALORIES	FAT
Mandarin Natural Style (S&W)	½ cup	60	0
Mandarin Oranges (Empress)	5.5 oz	100	0
Mandarin Oranges From Japan (Empress)	5.5 oz	35	0
Mandarin Segments (Dole)	½ cup	70	tr
Mandarin Selected Sections in Heavy Syrup (S&W)	½ cup	76	0
Mandarin Unsweetened (S&W)	½ cup	28	0
Pineapple Mandarin Orange Segments (Dole)	½ cup	60	tr

FRESH

FOOD	PORTION	CALORIES	FAT
Dole	1	50	0
california valencia	1	59	tr
california navel	1	65	tr
florida	1	69	tr
peel	1 tbsp	6	tr
sections	1 cup	85	tr

JUICE

FOOD	PORTION	CALORIES	FAT
Bama	8.45 oz	120	0
Crystal Light	8 oz	4	tr
Hawaiian Punch	6 oz	100	0
Juice Works	6 oz	90	0
Libby's	6 oz	80	0
Mott's Orange Fruit Juice Blend	9.5 oz	139	0
Ocean Spray	6 oz	80	0
S&W 100% Unsweetened	6 oz	83	0
Sippin' Pak 100% Pure	8.45 oz	110	0
SIPPS Orange	8.45 oz	130	0

FOOD	PORTION	CALORIES	FAT
Tang	8 oz	87	tr
Tang Sugar Free	8 oz	5	tr
Tree Top	6 oz	90	0
canned	1 cup	104	tr
chilled	1 cup	110	1
fresh	1 cup	111	tr
frzn, as prep	1 cup	112	tr
frzn, not prep	6 oz	339	tr
mandarin orange	3.5 oz	47	tr
orange drink	6 oz	94	0

ORANGE EXTRACT

Virginia Dare	1 tsp	22	0

OREGANO

ground	1 tsp	5	tr

ORGAN MEATS
(see BRAINS, GIBLETS, GIZZARD, HEART, KIDNEY, LIVER)

ORIENTAL FOOD
(see also DINNER, NOODLES, RICE)

CANNED
Chun King Divider Pak

Beef Chow Mein	8 oz	110	2
Beef Chow Mein	7 oz	100	2
Beef Pepper Oriental	7 oz	110	4
Chicken Chow Mein	7 oz	110	4
Chicken Chow Mein	8 oz	120	4
Pork Chow Mein Mein	7 oz	120	4
Shrimp Chow Mein	7 oz	100	2

FOOD	PORTION	CALORIES	FAT
Chun King Stir-Fry Entree			
Chow Mein w/ Beef	6 oz	290	19
Chow Mein w/ Chicken	6 oz	220	11
Egg Foo Yung	5 oz	140	8
Pepper Steak	6 oz	250	17
Sukiyaki	6 oz	290	19
La Choy Bi-Pack Beef Pepper	¾ cup	80	2
La Choy Bi-Pack Chow Mein Shrimp	¾ cup	70	1
La Choy Dinner Chow Mein Chicken	½ pkg	300	17
La Choy Entree			
Beef Pepper Oriental	¾ cup	100	4
Chow Mein Beef	¾ cup	40	2
Chow Mein Chicken	¾ cup	70	4
Chow Mein Meatless	¾ cup	25	tr
Chow Mein Shrimp	¾ cup	35	1
Sweet & Sour Chicken	¾ cup	240	2
Sweet & Sour Pork	¾ cup	250	4
chow mein chicken	1 cup	95	tr
FRESH			
Won Ton Wraps (Azumaya)	1	23	tr
FROZEN			
Benihana Oriental Lites Chicken in Spicy Garlic Sauce	9 oz	270	4
Birds Eye			
Chinese Style International Recipe	½ cup	68	4
Chinese Style Stir Fry Vegetable	½ cup	36	tr
Chow Mein Style International Recipe	½ cup	89	4
Japanese Style International Recipe	½ cup	88	4
Japanese Style Stir Fry Vegetable	½ cup	29	tr

FOOD	PORTION	CALORIES	FAT
Mandarin Style International Recipe	½ cup	86	4
Chun King			
Beef Pepper Oriental	13 oz	319	3
Chicken Chow Mein	13 oz	370	6
Crunchy Walnut Chicken	13 oz	310	5
Egg Rolls, Chicken	1 (3.6 oz)	220	8
Egg Rolls, Meat & Shrimp	1 (3.6 oz)	220	8
Egg Rolls, Shrimp	1 (3.6 oz)	200	6
Fried Rice w/ Chicken	8 oz	260	4
Fried Rice w/ Pork	8 oz	270	6
Imperial Chicken	13 oz	300	1
Restaurant Style Egg Rolls, Pork	1 (3 oz)	180	6
Sweet & Sour Pork	13 oz	400	5
Dining Light Chicken Chow Mein	9 oz	180	2
Healthy Choice Chicken Chow Mein	8.5 oz	220	3
La Choy			
Almond Chicken Egg Roll Restaurant Style	1 (3 oz)	120	3
Chicken Snack Egg Roll	2	90	3
Lobster Snack Egg Roll	1 (1.45 oz)	75	2
Meat & Shrimp Snack Egg Roll	1 (1.45 oz)	80	3
Pork Egg Roll Restaurant Style	1 (3 oz)	150	5
Shrimp Egg Roll Restaurant Style	1 (3 oz)	130	4
Shrimp Snack Egg Roll	1 (1.45 oz)	75	2
Sweet & Sour Chicken Egg Roll Restaurant Style	1 (3 oz)	150	4
Lean Cuisine Chicken Chow Mein w/ Rice	9 oz	240	5
HOME RECIPE			
chop suey w/ beef & pork	1 cup	300	17
chow mein chicken	1 cup	255	10

FOOD	PORTION	CALORIES	FAT
MIX			
Kikkoman Chow Mein Seasoning	1⅛-oz pkg	98	tr
Kikkoman Teriyaki Baste & Glaze	1 tbsp	24	tr
La Choy Dinner Classics Egg Foo Yung	2 patties + 3 oz sauce	170	7
La Choy Dinner Classics Pepper Steak	¾ cup	180	9
La Choy Dinner Classics Sweet & Sour	¾ cup	310	6
TAKE-OUT			
chicken teriyaki	¾ cup	399	27
chop suey w/ pork	1 cup	375	29
chow mein pork	1 cup	425	24
chow mein shrimp	1 cup	221	10
fried rice	6.6 oz	249	6
fried rice w/ egg	6.7	395	20
wonton	1 cup	205	3
wonton, fried	½ cup (1 oz)	111	8

OYSTERS

FOOD	PORTION	CALORIES	FAT
CANNED			
Fancy Whole (S&W)	2 oz	95	3
Whole (Bumble Bee)	½ cup (3.5 oz)	100	4
Whole (Empress)	4 oz	100	4
eastern	1 cup	170	6
eastern	3 oz	58	2
FRESH			
eastern, raw	6 med	58	2
eastern, raw	1 cup	170	6
eastern, cooked	6 med	58	2
eastern, cooked	3 oz	117	4

FOOD	PORTION	CALORIES	FAT
pacific, raw	1 med	41	1
pacific, raw	3 oz	69	2
steamed	1 med	41	1
steamed	3 oz	138	4
FROZEN			
Carnation Jumbo or Extra Select Breaded Oysters (King & Prince)	3.5 oz	130	2
TAKE-OUT			
battered & fried	6 (4.9 oz)	368	18
breaded & fried	6 (4.9 oz)	368	18
eastern, breaded & fried	6 med	173	11
eastern, breaded & fried	3 oz	167	11
oysters rockefeller	3	66	2
stew	1 cup	278	18

PANCAKE/WAFFLE SYRUP
(*see also* SYRUP)

FOOD	PORTION	CALORIES	FAT
Alaga Breakfast	2 tbsp	108	0
Alaga Butter Lite	2 tbsp	54	0
Alaga Honey Flavor	2 tbsp	124	0
Alaga Lite	2 tbsp	54	0
Aunt Jemima	2 tbsp	110	0
Aunt Jemima Butter Lite	2 tbsp	50	0
Aunt Jemima Lite	2 tbsp	50	0
Brer Rabbit Dark	2 tbsp	120	0
Brer Rabbit Light	2 tbsp	120	0
Estee	1 tbsp	8	0
Golden Griddle	1 tbsp	50	0
Golden Griddle	1 cup	885	0
Karo	1 tbsp	60	0

FOOD	PORTION	CALORIES	FAT
Log Cabin Buttered	1 oz	106	tr
Log Cabin Country Kitchen	1 oz	101	0
Log Cabin Lite	1 oz	61	tr
Log Cabin Maple Honey	1 oz	106	0
Log Cabin Regular	1 oz	99	tr
Tastee	2 tbsp	121	0
Tastee Maple	2 tbsp	113	0
Weight Watchers	1 tbsp	25	0
Whitfield White Label	2 tbsp	121	0
Whitfield Yellow Label	2 tbsp	125	0
Whitfield Yellow Label Butter Flavor	2 tbsp	117	0
Whitfield Yellow Label Maple Flavor	2 tbsp	117	0
low calorie	1 tbsp	12	0
maple	2 tbsp	122	0

PANCAKES

FROZEN
Blueberry (Aunt Jemima)	3.48 oz	220	4
Blueberry (Kid Cuisine)	3.47 oz	210	9
Buttermilk (Aunt Jemima)	3.48 oz	210	3
Buttermilk (Kid Cuisine)	4.17 oz	180	4
Buttermilk (Weight Watchers)	2 (2.5 oz)	140	3
Buttermilk Batter, as prep (Aunt Jemima)	3.6 oz	180	2
Lite Pancakes & Lite Links (Quaker)	1 pkg (6 oz)	310	10
Lite Pancakes & Lite Syrup (Quaker)	1 pkg (6 oz)	260	3
Original (Aunt Jemima)	3.48 oz	211	4
Original Batter, as prep (Aunt Jemima)	3.6 oz	183	2
Pancake (Morningstar Farms)	3.5 oz	232	5
Pancakes & Sausages (Great Starts)	6 oz	460	22

FOOD	PORTION	CALORIES	FAT
Pancakes & Sausages (Quaker)	1 pkg (6 oz)	420	16
Pancakes w/ Bacon (Great Starts)	4.5 oz	400	20
Pancakes w/ Lean Links (Healthy Starts)	6 oz	360	8
Pancakes w/ Links (Weight Watchers)	4 oz	220	10
Rolled Pancakes w/ Apples (Kid Cuisine)	3.85 oz	210	7
Silver Dollar Pancakes & Sausage (Great Starts)	3.75 oz	310	4
Whole Wheat Pancakes & Lite Links (Great Starts)	5.5 oz	350	16
HOME RECIPE			
plain	1 (4" diam)	60	2
MIX			
Blueberry (Hungry Jack)	3 (4" diam)	320	15
Blue Corn Pancake & Waffle Mix (Arrowhead)	½ cup	330	5
Buckwheat Pancake & Waffle Mix (Arrowhead)	½ cup	270	2
Buckwheat Pancake & Waffle Mix (Aunt Jemima)	3 (4" diam)	230	8
Buttermilk (Hungry Jack)	3 (4" diam)	240	11
Buttermilk Complete (Hungry Jack)	3 (4" diam)	180	1
Buttermilk Complete Packets (Hungry Jack)	3 (4" diam)	180	3
Buttermilk Complete Pancake & Waffle Mix (Aunt Jemima)	3 (4" diam)	230	3
Buttermilk Pancake & Waffle Mix (Aunt Jemima)	3 (4" diam)	220	8
Complete Pancake & Waffle Mix (Aunt Jemima)	3 (4" diam)	250	4
Extra Lights (Hungry Jack)	3 (4" diam)	210	7
Extra Lights Complete (Hungry Jack)	3 (4" diam)	190	2

FOOD	PORTION	CALORIES	FAT
Griddle Lite Pancake Mix (Arrowhead)	½ cup	260	3
Multigrain Pancake & Waffle Mix (Arrowhead)	½ cup	350	2
Oat Bran Pancake & Waffle Mix (Arrowhead)	½ cup	200	2
Original Pancake & Waffle Mix (Aunt Jemima)	3 (4" diam)	200	7
Pancake Mix (Estee)	3 (3" diam)	100	0
Pancake Mix, not prep (Health Valley)	1 oz	100	1
Panshakes (Hungry Jack)	3 (4" diam)	250	6
Whole Wheat Pancake & Waffle Mix (Aunt Jemima)	3 (4" diam)	270	9
TAKE-OUT			
buckwheat	1 (4" diam)	55	2
potato	1 (4" diam)	78	6
w/ butter & syrup	3	519	14

PANCREAS
(see SWEETBREADS)

PAPAYA

FRESH			
Papaya (Produce Marketing Assoc)	½	80	0
cubed	1 cup	54	tr
papaya	1	117	tr
JUICE			
Goya Nectar	6 oz	110	0
Kern's Nectar	6 oz	110	0
Libby's Nectar	6 oz	110	0
nectar	1 cup	142	tr

FOOD	PORTION	CALORIES	FAT

PAPRIKA

paprika	1 tsp	6	tr

PARSLEY

Dole, chopped	1 tbsp	10	tr
dry	1 tsp	1	tr
dry	1 tbsp	1	tr
fresh, chopped	½ cup	11	tr

PARSNIPS

FRESH

cooked	1 (5.6 oz)	130	tr
cooked, sliced	½ cup	63	tr
raw, sliced	½ cup	50	tr

PASSION FRUIT

purple	1	18	tr
purple juice	1 cup	126	tr
yellow juice	1 cup	149	tr

PASTA

(*see also* NOODLES, PASTA DINNERS, PASTA SALAD)

DRY

Acini de Pepe (San Giorgio)	2 oz	210	1
Alphabets (P&R)	2 oz	210	1
Alphabets (San Giorgio)	2 oz	210	1
Alphabets (Skinner)	2 oz	210	1
Baby Pastina (San Giorgio)	2 oz	210	1
Bows, Medium & Small (P&R)	2 oz	220	3
Capellini (Delmonico)	2 oz	210	1
Capellini (P&R)	2 oz	210	1

FOOD	PORTION	CALORIES	FAT
Capellini (San Giorgio)	2 oz	210	1
Dinosaurs (Mueller's)	2 oz	210	1
Ditalini (San Giorgio)	2 oz	210	1
Elbow Macaroni (Delmonico)	2 oz	210	1
Elbow Macaroni (San Giorgio)	2 oz	210	1
Elbow Macaroni (Skinner)	2 oz	210	1
Elbow Macaroni, Regular & Large (P&R)	2 oz	210	1
Elbow Spaghetti (Delmonico)	2 oz	210	1
Elbow Style (Weight Watchers)	2 oz	160	1
Fettuccini (P&R)	2 oz	210	1
Fettuccini, Egg (P&R)	2 oz	210	1
Fettuccini (Skinner)	2 oz	210	1
Fideo Enrollacio (Skinner)	2 oz	210	1
Flakes (San Giorgio)	2 oz	210	1
Fusili Cut (San Giorgio)	2 oz	210	1
Fusili Cut (P&R)	2 oz	210	1
Jungle Animals (Mueller's)	2 oz	210	1
Kluski (San Giorgio)	2 oz	220	3
Lasagna (Delmonico)	2 oz	210	1
Lasagna (Skinner)	2 oz	210	1
Lasagna Jumbo (P&R)	2 oz	210	1
Lasagna No Boil (DeFino)	1 oz	102	tr
Lasagna Spinach Whole Wheat (Health Valley)	2 oz	170	1
Lasagna Whole Wheat (Health Valley)	2 oz	170	1
Lasagne (Mueller's)	2 oz	210	1
Linguini (P&R)	2 oz	210	1
Linguini (San Giorgio)	2 oz	210	1
Linguini (Skinner)	2 oz	210	1

FOOD	PORTION	CALORIES	FAT
Linguini, Egg (Creamette)	2 oz	221	3
Macaroni (Ronzoni)	2 oz	209	tr
Manicotti (P&R)	2 oz	210	1
Manicotti (San Giorgio)	2 oz	210	1
Manicotti (Skinner)	2 oz	210	1
Monsters (Mueller's)	2 oz	210	1
Mostaccioli (Delmonico)	2 oz	210	1
Mostaccioli (Skinner)	2 oz	210	1
Mostaccioli Rigati (San Giorgio)	2 oz	210	1
Orzo (San Giorgio)	2 oz	210	1
Outer Space (Mueller's)	2 oz	210	1
Pasta (Golden Grain)	2 oz	203	1
Perciatelli (P&R)	2 oz	210	1
Perciatelli (San Giorgio)	2 oz	210	1
Pot Pie Bows (San Giorgio)	2 oz	220	3
Pot Pie Squares (San Giorgio)	2 oz	220	3
Racing Wheels (San Giorgio)	2 oz	210	1
Ribbon Pasta Whole Wheat (Pritikin)	2 oz	220	2
Ribbons No Boil (DeFino)	2 oz	204	2
Rigatoni (Delmonico)	2 oz	210	1
Rigatoni (San Giorgio)	2 oz	210	1
Rigatoni (Skinner)	2 oz	210	1
Rings (P&R)	2 oz	210	1
Rippled Lasagne (San Giorgio)	2 oz	210	1
Ripplets (Skinner)	2 oz	210	1
Rotelle (Creamette)	2 oz	210	1
Rotini (Delmonico)	2 oz	210	1
Rotini (San Giorgio)	2 oz	210	1
Rotini, Rainbow (Creamette)	2 oz	210	1
Shell Macaroni (Skinner)	2 oz	210	1

FOOD	PORTION	CALORIES	FAT
Shells, Jumbo (P&R)	2 oz	210	1
Shells, Large, Medium & Small (P&R)	2 oz	210	1
Shells, Large, Medium, Small & Jumbo (San Giorgio)	2 oz	210	1
Shells, Regular & Jumbo (Delmonico)	2 oz	210	1
Spaghetti (Delmonico)	2 oz	210	1
Spaghetti (Mueller's)	2 oz	210	1
Spaghetti (San Giorgio)	2 oz	210	1
Spaghetti (Skinner)	2 oz	210	1
Spaghetti, Amaranth (Health Valley)	2 oz	170	1
Spaghetti, Egg (Creamette)	2 oz	221	3
Spaghetti, Oat Bran (Health Valley)	2 oz	120	1
Spaghetti, Regular & Thin (P&R)	2 oz	210	1
Spaghetti, Spinach Whole Wheat (Health Valley)	2 oz	170	1
Spaghetti, Thin (Creamette)	2 oz	210	1
Spaghetti, Whole Wheat (Health Valley)	2 oz	170	1
Spaghetti Wheels (Hanover)	½ cup	90	0
Spaghetti, Whole Wheat (Pritikin)	2 oz	220	2
Spaghettini (Delmonico)	2 oz	210	1
Spaghettini (San Giorgio)	2 oz	210	1
Spaghettini (Weight Watchers)	2 oz	160	1
Spinach Macaroni (Ronzoni)	2 oz	203	tr
Teddy Bears (Mueller's)	2 oz	210	1
Tubettini (San Giorgio)	2 oz	210	1
Twirls (Skinner)	2 oz	210	1
Twists Tri Color (Mueller's)	2 oz	210	1
Vermicelli (Delmonico)	2 oz	210	1

FOOD	PORTION	CALORIES	FAT
Vermicelli (P&R)	2 oz	210	1
Vermicelli (San Giorgio)	2 oz	210	1
Vermicelli (Skinner)	2 oz	210	1
Ziti (Creamette)	2 oz	210	1
Ziti Cut (Delmonico)	2 oz	210	1
Ziti Cut (San Giorgio)	2 oz	210	1
corn, cooked	1 cup	176	1
elbows, cooked	1 cup	197	tr
protein-fortified, cooked	1 cup	188	tr
shells, cooked	1 cup	197	tr
spaghetti, cooked	1 cup	197	tr
spaghetti, protein-fortified, cooked	1 cup	229	tr
spinach spaghetti, cooked	1 cup	183	tr
spirals, cooked	1 cup	197	tr
vegetable, cooked	1 cup	171	tr
whole wheat, cooked	1 cup	174	tr
whole wheat, cooked	1 cup	174	tr
FRESH			
plain made w/ egg	4.5 oz	368	3
plain made w/ egg, cooked	2 oz	75	tr
spinach made w/ egg	4.5 oz	370	3
spinach made w/ egg, cooked	2 oz	74	tr
HOME RECIPE			
made w/ egg, cooked	2 oz	74	tr
made w/o egg, cooked	2 oz	71	tr

FOOD	PORTION	CALORIES	FAT

PASTA DINNERS
(see also DINNER, PASTA SALAD)

CANNED
Chef Boyardee

FOOD	PORTION	CALORIES	FAT
ABC's & 1, 2, 3's in Sauce	7.5 oz	160	1
ABC's & 1, 2, 3's w/ Mini Meatballs	7.5 oz	240	9
Beef Ravioli	7 oz	180	5
Beef Ravioli in Sauce	8.7 oz	240	6
Beef Ravioli in Tomato & Meat Sauce	7.5 oz	210	5
Beef-O-Getti	7.5 oz	220	9
Beefaroni	7.5 oz	220	8
Cheese Ravioli in Beef & Tomato Sauce	7.5 oz	200	3
Cheese Ravioli in Tomato Sauce	7.5 oz	200	5
Chicken Ravioli	7.5 oz	180	4
Dinosaurs in Spaghetti Sauce w/ Cheese Flavor	7.5 oz	155	1
Dinosaurs w/ Mini Meatballs	7.5 oz	235	8
Lasagna	7.5 oz	230	8
Macaroni Shells in Tomato Sauce	7.5 oz	150	1
Microwave Bowl ABC's & 1, 2, 3's w/ Mini Meatballs	7.5 oz	260	11
Microwave Bowl Beef Ravioli	7.5 oz	190	4
Microwave Bowl Beefaroni	7.5 oz	220	7
Microwave Bowl Lasagna	7.5 oz	230	9
Microwave Bowl Spaghetti w/ Meatballs	7.5 oz	240	10
Microwave Bowl Tic Tac Toes w/ Meatballs	7.5 oz	260	11
Mini Bites	7.5 oz	260	12

FOOD	PORTION	CALORIES	FAT
Mini Cannelloni	7.5 oz	230	7
Mini Beef Ravioli	7.5 oz	210	5
Mini Chicken Ravioli	7.5 oz	220	8
Pac Man in Chicken Sauce	7.5 oz	170	7
Pac Man in Tomato Sauce	7.5 oz	150	1
Pac Man w/ Meatballs	7.5 oz	230	9
Roller Coasters	7.5 oz	230	9
Smurf Beef in Spaghetti Sauce w/ Cheese Flavor	7.5 oz	150	1
Smurf Beef Ravioli & Pasta in Meat Sauce	7.5 oz	220	5
Smurf Pasta w/ Meatballs	7.5 oz	230	9
Spaghetti & Meat Balls	7 oz	210	8
Spaghetti & Meatballs	8.5 oz	260	11
Spaghetti & Meatballs w/ Tomato Sauce	7.5 oz	230	8
Spaghetti 'N Beef in Tomato Sauce	7 oz	220	8
Spaghetti 'N Beef in Tomato Sauce	7.5 oz	240	9
Tic Tac Toes in Spaghetti Sauce w/ Cheese Flavor	7.5 oz	160	1
Tic Tac Toes w/ Mini Meatballs	7.5 oz	240	9
Zooroni w/ Meatballs in Sauce	7.5 oz	240	8
Franco-American			
Beef RavioliO's in Meat Sauce	½ can (7.5 oz)	250	8
CircusO's Pasta in Tomato & Cheese Sauce	½ can (7.38 oz)	170	2
CircusO's Pasta w/ Meatballs in Tomato Sauce	½ can (7.38 oz)	210	8
Macaroni & Cheese	½ can (7.38 oz)	170	6
Spaghetti in Tomato Sauce w/ Cheese	½ can (7.38 oz)	180	2
Spaghetti w/ Meatballs in Tomato Sauce	½ can (7.38 oz)	220	8

FOOD	PORTION	CALORIES	FAT
Franco-American *(cont.)*			
SpaghettiO's in Tomato & Cheese Sauce	½ can (7.38 oz)	170	2
SpaghettiO's w/ Meatballs	½ can (7.38 oz)	220	9
SpaghettiO's w/ Sliced Franks	½ can (7.38 oz)	220	9
SportyO's in Tomato & Cheese Sauce	½ can (7.5 oz)	170	2
SportyO's Pasta w/ Meatballs in Tomato Sauce	½ can (7.38 oz)	210	8
TeddyO's in Tomato & Cheese Sauce	½ can (7.5 oz)	170	2
TeddyO's Pasta w/ Meatballs	½ can (7.38 oz)	210	8
Healthy Choice Lasagne w/ Meat Sauce	½ can (7.5 oz)	220	5
Healthy Choice Spaghetti Rings	½ can (7.5 oz)	140	0
Healthy Choice Spaghetti w/ Meat Sauce	½ can (7.5 oz)	150	3
Lido Club Beef Ravioli	7.5 oz	190	4
Lido Club Spaghetti Rings & Little Meat Balls	7.5 oz	220	10
Van Camp's Spaghetti Weenee	1 cup	243	7
DRY MIX			
Chef Boyardee Lasagna Dinner	1 serving (5.97 oz)	280	8
Chef Boyardee Spaghetti Dinner w/ Condensed Meat Sauce	1 serving (3.25 oz)	250	6
Chef Boyardee Spaghetti Dinner w/ Meat Sauce	1 serving (4.88 oz)	240	3
Golden Grain Macaroni & Cheese	½ cup	310	15
Kraft Dinomac Macaroni & Cheese Dinner	¾ cup	310	14
Kraft Egg Noodle & Cheese Dinner	¾ cup	340	17
Kraft Macaroni & Cheese Deluxe Dinner	¾ cup	260	8

FOOD	PORTION	CALORIES	FAT
Kraft Macaroni & Cheese Dinner	¾ cup	290	13
Kraft Macaroni & Cheese Dinner Family Size	¾ cup	290	13
Kraft Mild American Style Spaghetti Dinner	1 cup	300	7
Kraft Pasta & Cheese Fettuccini Alfredo	½ cup	180	9
Kraft Pasta & Cheese 3-Cheese w/ Vegetables	½ cup	180	8
Kraft Pasta & Cheese Cheddar Broccoli	½ cup	180	8
Kraft Pasta & Cheese Chicken w/Herbs	½ cup	170	7
Kraft Pasta & Cheese Parmesan	½ cup	180	8
Kraft Pasta & Cheese Sour Cream w/ Chives	½ cup	180	8
Kraft Spaghetti w/ Meat Sauce Dinner	1 cup	360	14
Kraft Spirals Macaroni & Cheese Dinner	¾ cup	340	18
Kraft Tangy Italian Style Spaghetti Dinner	1 cup	310	8
Kraft Teddy Bears Macaroni & Cheese Dinner	¾ cup	310	14
Kraft Wild Wheels Macaroni & Cheese Dinner	¾ cup	310	14
Lipton Pasta & Sauce			
Cheddar Broccoli w/ Fusilli	½ cup	137	2
Creamy Garlic	½ cup	144	3
Creamy Mushroom	½ cup	143	3
Herb Tomato	½ cup	130	tr
Italiano	½ cup	135	2
Mushroom & Chicken Flavored	½ cup	134	tr
Oriental w/ Fusilli	½ cup	130	tr
Primavera	½ cup	143	2

FOOD	PORTION	CALORIES	FAT
Ultra Slim-Fast Macaroni & Cheese	2.3 oz	230	3
Velveeta Bits of Bacon Shells & Cheese Dinner	½ cup	240	10
Velveeta Shells & Cheese Dinner	¾ cup	210	8
Velveeta Touch of Mexico Shells & Cheese Dinner	½ cup	210	8
FROZEN			
Banquet			
Family Entree Chicken & Vegetable Primavera	7 oz	140	3
Lasagne w/ Meat Sauce	7 oz	270	10
Macaroni & Cheese	9 oz	240	8
Macaroni & Cheese	7 oz	260	11
Mostaccioli w/ Meat Sauce	7 oz	170	3
Banquet Cookin' Bag Chicken & Vegetables Primavera	4 oz	100	2
Banquet Entree Spaghetti w/ Meat Sauce	8.5 oz	220	8
Birds Eye Pasta Primavera Style International Recipe	½ cup	121	5
Budget Gourmet			
Beef Stroganoff	1 pkg	290	12
Cheese Tortellini	1 pkg	210	8
Cheese Lasagna w/ Vegetables	1 pkg	290	9
Cheese Manicotti	1 pkg	430	25
Cheese Raviolo	1 pkg	290	10
Italian Sausage Lasagna	1 pkg	430	23
Lasagne w/ Meat Sauce	1 pkg	300	13
Linguini w/ Scallops & Clams	1 pkg	290	11
Linguini w/ Shrimp	10 oz	330	15
Linguini w/ Shrimp & Clams	1 pkg	270	10
Macaroni & Cheese	1 pkg	240	23

FOOD	PORTION	CALORIES	FAT
Pasta Alfredo w/ Broccoli	1 pkg	230	11
Shrimp w/ Fettuccini	1 pkg	370	22
Three Cheese Lasagne	1 pkg	390	18
Ziti in Marinara Sauce	1 pkg	200	9
Dining Light Cheese Cannelloni	9 oz	310	9
Dining Light Cheese Lasagna	9 oz	260	6
Dining Light Fettuccini	9 oz	290	12
Dining Light Lasagne	9 oz	240	5
Dining Light Spaghetti	9 oz	220	8
Green Giant Garden Gourmet			
Creamy Mushroom	1 pkg	220	11
Pasta Dijon	1 pkg	260	17
Pasta Florentine	1 pkg	230	9
Rotini Cheddar	1 pkg	230	10
Green Giant One Serve			
Cheese Tortellini	1 pkg	260	9
Macaroni & Cheese	1 pkg	230	9
Pasta Marinara	1 pkg	180	5
Pasta Parmesan w/ Green Peas	1 pkg	170	5
Green Giant Pasta Accents			
Creamy Cheddar	½ cup	100	5
Garden Herb	½ cup	80	3
Garlic Seasoning	½ cup	110	5
Pasta Primavera	½ cup	110	5
Healthy Choice			
Baked Cheese Ravioli	9 oz	240	2
Cheese Manicotti	9.25 oz	230	4
Chicken Fettuccini	8.5 oz	240	4
Fettuccini Alfredo	8 oz	240	7
Fettuccini w/ Turkey & Vegetables	12.5 oz	350	6
Lasagna w/ Meat Sauce	10 oz	260	5

FOOD	PORTION	CALORIES	FAT
Healthy Choice *(cont.)*			
Linguini w/ Shrimp	9.5 oz	230	2
Macaroni & Cheese	9 oz	280	6
Pasta Primavera	11 oz	280	3
Pasta w/ Shrimp	12.5 oz	270	4
Rigatoni in Meat Sauce	9.5 oz	240	4
Rigatoni w/ Chicken	12.5 oz	360	4
Spaghetti w/ Meat Sauce	10 oz	280	6
Stuffed Pasta Shells in Tomato Sauce	12 oz	330	3
Zesty Tomato Sauce over Ziti Pasta	12 oz	350	5
Zucchini Lasagna	11.5 oz	240	3
Kid Cuisine			
Macaroni & Cheese w/ Mini Franks	9 oz	360	15
Mega Meal Macaroni & Cheese	12.45 oz	470	13
Mini Cheese Ravioli	8.75 oz	290	8
Spaghetti w/ Meat Sauce	9.25 oz	310	8
Le Menu Manicotti w/ Three Cheeses	11.75 oz	390	15
Le Menu LightStyle			
3-Cheese Stuffed Shells	10 oz	280	8
Cheese Tortellini	10 oz	230	6
Garden Vegetables Lasagna	10.5 oz	260	8
Lasagna w/ Meat Sauce	10 oz	290	8
Meat Sauce & Cheese Tortellini	8 oz	250	8
Spaghetti w/ Beef Sauce & Mushrooms	9 oz	280	6
Lean Cuisine			
Baked Rigatoni w/ Meat Sauce & Cheese	9.75 oz	260	10
Beef Cannelloni w/ Mornay Sauce	9.63 oz	210	4

FOOD	PORTION	CALORIES	FAT
Cheese Cannelloni w/ Tomato Sauce	9.13 oz	270	8
Cheese Ravioli	8.5 oz	240	8
Chicken Cacciatore w/ Vermicelli	10.88 oz	280	7
Chicken Fettuccini	9 oz	280	8
Lasagne w/ Meat Sauce	10.25 oz	260	5
Linguini w/ Clam Sauce	9.63 oz	280	8
Macaroni & Beef in Tomato Sauce	10 oz	240	6
Macaroni & Cheese	9 oz	290	9
Rigatoni Bake w/ Meat Sauce & Cheese	9.75 oz	250	8
Spaghetti & Meatballs	9.5 oz	280	7
Spaghetti w/ Meat Sauce	11.5 oz	290	6
Tuna Lasagna w/ Spinach Noodles & Vegetables	9.75 oz	240	7
Zucchini Lasagna	11 oz	260	5
Morton Macaroni & Cheese	6.5 oz	290	14
Morton Spaghetti & Meat Sauce	8.5 oz	170	2
Mrs. Paul's Seafood Lasagna Light Seafood Entree	9.5 oz	290	8
Mrs. Paul's Seafood Rotini	9 oz	240	6
Mrs. Paul's Seafood Rotini Light Seafood Entree	9 oz	240	6
Swanson Lasagne w/ Meat Sauce Homestyle	10.5 oz	400	15
Swanson Macaroni & Cheese	7 oz	200	8
Swanson Macaroni & Cheese Homestyle	10 oz	390	19
Swanson Spaghetti w/ Italian Style Meatballs Homestyle	13 oz	490	18
Ultra Slim-Fast Pasta Primavera	12 oz	340	9
Ultra Slim-Fast Spaghetti w/ Beef & Mushroom Sauce	12 oz	370	10

FOOD	PORTION	CALORIES	FAT
Van De Kamp's Italian Classics Beef & Mushroom Lasagna	11 oz	430	25
Van De Kamp's Italian Classics Sausage Lasagna	11 oz	440	25
Weight Watchers			
Angel Hair Pasta	10 oz	200	4
Baked Cheese Ravioli	9 oz	240	6
Cheese Manicotti	9.25 oz	260	8
Cheese Tortellini	9 oz	310	6
Chicken Fettuccini	8.25 oz	280	9
Fettuccini Alfredo	8 oz	230	7
Garden Lasagne	11 oz	260	7
Italian Cheese Lasagne	11 oz	290	6
Lasagne	10.25 oz	240	6
Spaghetti w/ Meat Sauce	10 oz	240	7
HOME RECIPE			
macaroni & cheese	1 cup	430	22
spaghetti w/ meatballs & tomato sauce	1 cup	330	12
SHELF STABLE			
Healthy Choice Lasagne w/ Meat Sauce	7.5 oz cup	220	5
Healthy Choice Spaghetti Rings	7.5 oz cup	140	0
Healthy Choice Spaghetti w/ Meat Sauce	7.5 oz cup	150	3
TAKE-OUT			
lasagna	1 piece (2.5″ × 2.5″)	374	21
lasagna	8 oz	347	20
macaroni & cheese	1 cup	230	10
manicotti	¾ cup (6.4 oz)	273	12
rigatoni w/ sausage sauce	¾ cup	260	12

FOOD	PORTION	CALORIES	FAT
spaghetti w/ meatballs & cheese	1 cup	407	19

PASTA SALAD

FROZEN

Hanover Italian	½ cup	60	0
Hanover Milano	½ cup	60	0
Hanover Oriental	½ cup	80	0
Hanover Primavera	½ cup	50	0

MIX

Kraft Garden Primavera Pasta Salad & Dressing	½ cup	170	7
Kraft Homestyle Pasta Salad & Dressing	½ cup	240	16
Kraft Light Italian Pasta Salad & Dressing	½ cup	130	3
Kraft Light Rancher's Choice Pasta Salad & Dressing	½ cup	170	7
Kraft Pasta Salad & Dressing, Broccoli & Vegetables	½ cup	210	16
Lipton Creamy Buttermilk	½ cup	117	tr
Lipton Creamy Italian	½ cup	122	1
Lipton Garden Macaroni	½ cup	119	tr
Lipton Lemon Dill	½ cup	115	tr
Lipton Robust Italian	½ cup	128	1
Lipton Sour Cream & Dill	½ cup	120	1

TAKE-OUT

elbow macaroni salad	3.5 oz	160	5
italian style pasta salad	3.5 oz	140	7
mustard macaroni salad	3.5 oz	190	10
pasta salad w/ vegetables	3.5 oz	140	4

FOOD	PORTION	CALORIES	FAT

PÂTÉ

CANNED

FOOD	PORTION	CALORIES	FAT
chicken liver	1 tbsp	109	2
chicken liver	1 oz	238	4
goose liver, smoked	1 tbsp	60	6
goose liver, smoked	1 oz	131	12
liver	1 tbsp	41	4
liver	1 oz	90	8

PEACH

FOOD	PORTION	CALORIES	FAT
Clingstone Halves (S&W)	½ cup	100	0
Clingstone Halves Diet (S&W)	½ cup	30	0
Clingstone Halves Unsweetened (S&W)	½ cup	30	0
Clingstone Sliced Diet (S&W)	½ cup	30	0
Clingstone Sliced Unsweetened (S&W)	½ cup	30	0
Freestone Halves Diet (S&W)	½ cup	30	0
Freestone Halves in Heavy Syrup (S&W)	½ cup	100	0
Freestone Slices Diet (S&W)	½ cup	30	0
Freestone Slices in Heavy Syrup (S&W)	½ cup	100	0
Halves (Hunt's)	4 oz	90	tr
Sliced Yellow Cling Natural Style (S&W)	½ cup	90	0
Slices (Hunt's)	4 oz	90	tr
Yellow Cling Natural Lite (S&W)	½ cup	50	0
Yellow Cling Sliced Premium in Heavy Syrup	½ cup	100	0
Yellow Cling Whole Spiced in Heavy Syrup (S&W)	½ cup	90	0

FOOD	PORTION	CALORIES	FAT
halves in heavy syrup	1 half	60	tr
halves in light syrup	1 half	44	tr
halves juice pack	1 half	34	tr
halves water pack	1 half	18	tr
spiced in heavy syrup	1 fruit	66	tr
spiced in heavy syrup	1 cup	180	tr
DRIED			
Peaches (Mariani)	¼ cup	140	0
halves	10	311	1
halves	1 cup	383	1
halves, cooked w/ sugar	½ cup	139	tr
halves, cooked w/o sugar	½ cup	99	tr
FRESH			
Dole	2	70	0
peach	1	37	tr
sliced	1 cup	73	tr
FROZEN			
slices, sweetened	1 cup	235	tr
JUICE			
Dole Pure & Light	6 oz	100	tr
Goya Nectar	6 oz	110	0
Kern's Nectar	6 oz	110	0
Libby's Nectar	6 oz	100	0
Libby's Ripe Peach Nectar	8 oz	130	0
Smucker's Peach Juice	8 oz	120	0
nectar	1 cup	134	tr

PEANUT BUTTER

Arrowhead Creamy	2 tbsp	190	16
Arrowhead Crunchy	2 tbsp	190	16

FOOD	PORTION	CALORIES	FAT
BAMA Creamy	2 tbsp	200	17
BAMA Crunchy	2 tbsp	200	17
BAMA Jelly & Peanut Butter	2 tbsp	150	7
Erewhon Chunky, Salted	2 tbsp	190	14
Erewhon Chunky, Unsalted	2 tbsp	190	14
Erewhon Creamy, Salted	2 tbsp	190	14
Erewhon Creamy, Unsalted	2 tbsp	190	14
Estee Chunky	1 tbsp	100	8
Estee Creamy	1 tbsp	100	8
Health Valley Chunky, No Salt	2 tbsp	170	14
Health Valley Creamy, No Salt	2 tbsp	170	14
Home Brand Natural, Lightly Salted	2 tbsp	210	17
Home Brand Natural, Unsalted	2 tbsp	210	17
Home Brand No Sugar Added	2 tbsp	180	16
Home Brand Real Peanut Butter	2 tbsp	210	17
Jif Creamy	2 tbsp	190	16
Jif Crunchy	2 tbsp	190	16
Peter Pan Creamy	2 tbsp	190	16
Peter Pan Creamy, Salt Free	2 tbsp	190	17
Peter Pan Crunchy	2 tbsp	190	16
Peter Pan Crunchy, Salt Free	2 tbsp	190	17
Reese's Peanut Butter Flavored Chips	¼ cup	230	13
Skippy Creamy	2 tbsp	190	17
Skippy Creamy	1 cup	1540	135
Skippy Creamy, w/ 2 slices white bread	1 sandwich	340	19
Skippy Super Chunk	2 tbsp	190	17
Skippy Super Chunk	1 cup	1540	138
Skippy Super Chunk, w/ 2 slices white bread	1 sandwich	340	19

FOOD	PORTION	CALORIES	FAT
Smucker's Goober Grape	2 tbsp	180	10
Smucker's Honey Sweetened	2 tbsp	200	16
Smucker's Natural	2 tbsp	200	16
Smucker's Natural, No-Salt Added	2 tbsp	200	16
Teddie Natural Peanut Butter w/ No Salt Added	2 tbsp	200	17
chunky	2 tbsp	188	16
chunky	1 cup	1520	129
chunky w/o salt	2 tbsp	188	16
chunky w/o salt	1 cup	1520	129
smooth	2 tbsp	188	16
smooth	1 cup	1517	128
smooth w/o salt	2 tbsp	188	16
smooth w/o salt	1 cup	1517	129

PEANUTS

FOOD	PORTION	CALORIES	FAT
Cocktail Lightly Salted (Planters)	1 oz	170	14
Cocktail Unsalted (Planters)	1 oz	170	14
Dry Roasted (Guy's)	1 oz	170	14
Dry Roasted (Lance)	1.13 oz	190	15
Dry Roasted Lightly Salted (Planters)	1 oz	160	15
Dry Roasted, Unsalted (Planters)	1 oz	170	15
Fresh Roast Lightly Salted (Planters)	1 oz	160	14
Fresh Roast Salted (Planters)	1 oz	170	14
Honey Roasted (Little Debbie)	1 pkg (1.13 oz)	190	15
Honey Roasted (Planters)	1 oz	170	13
Honey Roasted (Weight Watchers)	.7 oz	100	6
Honey Roasted Dry Roasted (Planters)	1 oz	160	13
Honey Toasted P'nuts (Lance)	1.25 oz	210	16

FOOD	PORTION	CALORIES	FAT
Party Peanuts (Fisher)	1 oz	160	14
Peanuts (Beer Nuts)	1 oz	180	14
Peanuts (Planters)	½-oz bag	80	7
Redskin Salted (Lance)	1.13 oz	190	15
Roasted w/ Shell (Lance)	1.75 oz	190	15
Salted (Lance)	1.13 oz	190	15
Salted (Little Debbie)	1 pkg (1.25 oz)	220	18
Spanish (Planters)	1 oz	170	15
Spanish Raw (Planters)	1 oz	160	14
Spanish Salted (Guy's)	1 oz	170	14
cooked	½ cup	102	7
dry roasted	1 oz	164	14
dry roasted	1 cup	855	73
oil roasted	1 oz	163	14
oil roasted	1 cup	837	71
oil roasted, w/o salt	1 oz	163	14
oil roasted, w/o salt	1 cup	837	71
spanish, oil roasted	1 oz	162	14
spanish, oil roasted w/o salt	1 oz	162	14
unroasted	1 oz	159	14
valencia, oil roasted	1 oz	165	14
valencia, oil roasted	1 cup	848	74
valencia, oil roasted, w/o salt	1 oz	165	14
valencia, oil roasted, w/o salt	1 cup	848	74
virginia, oil roasted	1 oz	161	14
virginia, oil roasted	1 cup	826	70

FOOD	PORTION	CALORIES	FAT

PEAR

CANNED

FOOD	PORTION	CALORIES	FAT
Bartlett Halves in Heavy Syrup (S&W)	½ cup	100	0
Bartlett Halves Peeled Unsweetened (S&W)	½ cup	35	0
Halves (Hunt's)	4 oz	90	tr
Halves Peeled Diet (S&W)	½ cup	35	0
Quartered Peeled Diet (S&W)	½ cup	35	0
Sliced Natural Light Bartlett (S&W)	½ cup	60	0
Sliced Natural Style (S&W)	½ cup	80	0
halves in heavy syrup	1 half	68	tr
halves in heavy syrup	1 cup	188	tr
halves in light syrup	1 half	45	tr
halves juice pack	1 cup	123	tr
halves water pack	1 half	22	tr

DRIED

FOOD	PORTION	CALORIES	FAT
Pears (Mariani)	¼ cup	150	0
halves	10	459	1
halves	1 cup	472	1
halves, cooked w/ sugar	½ cup	196	tr
halves, cooked w/o sugar	½ cup	163	tr

FRESH

FOOD	PORTION	CALORIES	FAT
Dole	1	100	1
asian	1 (4.3 oz)	51	tr
pear	1	98	1
sliced w/ skin	1 cup	97	1

JUICE

FOOD	PORTION	CALORIES	FAT
Goya Nectar	6 oz	120	0
Kern's Nectar	6 oz	110	0

FOOD	PORTION	CALORIES	FAT
Libby's Nectar	6 oz	110	0
nectar	1 cup	149	tr

PEAS

CANNED

FOOD	PORTION	CALORIES	FAT
Crowder Peas Seasoned w/ Pork (Luck's)	7.5 oz	200	7
Early June or Sweet (Owatonna)	½ cup	70	0
Field Peas (Trappey's)	½ cup	90	1
Field Peas w/ Snaps (Trappey's)	½ cup	90	1
Field Peas w/ Snaps Seasoned w/ Pork (Luck's)	7.5 oz	200	7
Libby	½ cup	60	0
Natural Pack (Libby)	½ cup	60	1
Natural Pack (Seneca)	½ cup	60	0
Petit Pois (S&W)	½ cup	70	0
Seneca	½ cup	60	0
Small Pea Baked Beans (B&M)	⅞ cup	300	7
Sweet (Green Giant)	½ cup	50	0
Sweet (S&W)	½ cup	70	0
Sweet Water Pack (S&W)	½ cup	40	0
Veri-Green Sweet (S&W)	½ cup	70	0
green	½ cup	59	tr
green low sodium	½ cup	59	tr

DRIED

FOOD	PORTION	CALORIES	FAT
Arrowhead Split Peas, Green	2 oz	200	1
Hurst Brand Split Peas	1 cup	277	tr
Hurst Brand Whole Peas	1 cup	272	1
split, cooked	1 cup	231	1
split, raw	1 cup	671	2

FOOD	PORTION	CALORIES	FAT
FRESH			
Dole Sugar Peas	½ cup	30	tr
edible-pod, cooked	½ cup	34	tr
edible-pod, raw	½ cup	30	tr
green, cooked	½ cup	67	tr
green, raw	½ cup	58	tr
FROZEN			
Chinese Pea Pods (Chun King)	1.5 oz	20	0
Green (Birds Eye)	½ cup	77	tr
Harvest Fresh Early June (Green Giant)	½ cup	60	1
Harvest Fresh Sugar Snap (Green Giant)	½ cup	30	0
Harvest Fresh Sweet (Green Giant)	½ cup	50	0
In Butter Sauce (Green Giant)	½ cup	80	2
Le Suer Early (Green Giant Select)	½ cup	60	0
Le Suer Early in Butter Sauce (Green Giant Select)	½ cup	80	2
One Serve in Butter Sauce (Green Giant)	1 pkg	90	2
Peas w/ Cream Sauce (Birds Eye)	½ cup	117	6
Petite Peas (Hanover)	½ cup	70	0
Snow Pea Pods (La Choy)	½ pkg (3 oz)	35	tr
Snow Peas (Hanover)	½ cup	35	0
Sugar Snap Sweet Peas (Green Giant Select)	½ cup	30	0
Sweet Peas (Green Giant)	½ cup	50	0
Sweet Peas (Hanover)	½ cup	70	0
Tiny Tender (Birds Eye)	½ cup	62	tr
edible-pod, cooked	1 pkg (10 oz)	132	1
edible-pod, cooked	½ cup	42	tr
green, cooked	½ cup	63	tr

FOOD	PORTION	CALORIES	FAT
SHELF STABLE			
Mini Sweet (Green Giant)	½ cup	60	tr
SPROUTS			
raw	½ cup	77	tr
TAKE-OUT			
pea & potato curry	1 serving (7 oz)	284	22
pea curry	1 serving (4.4 oz)	438	42

PECANS

FOOD	PORTION	CALORIES	FAT
Halves (Planters)	1 oz	190	20
Pieces (Planters)	1 oz	190	20
dried	1 oz	190	19
dry roasted	1 oz	187	18
dry roasted, salted	1 oz	187	18
halves, dried	1 cup	721	73
oil roasted	1 oz	195	20
oil roasted, salted	1 oz	195	20

PECTIN
(see also FIBER)

FOOD	PORTION	CALORIES	FAT
Certo	1 tbsp	2	0
Slim Set	1 pkg	208	0
Slim Set	1 tbsp	3	0
Sure-Jell	¼ pkg	38	0
Sure-Jell Light	¼ pkg	33	0

PEPPER

FOOD	PORTION	CALORIES	FAT
Spice Lemon Pepper (Nile Spice)	⅛ tsp	0	0
black	1 tsp	5	tr
cayenne	1 tsp	6	tr
red	1 tsp	6	tr

FOOD	PORTION	CALORIES	FAT
white	1 tsp	7	tr

PEPPERS

CANNED
Hot Banana Pepper Rings (Vlasic)	1 oz	4	0
Hot Cherry (Vlasic)	1 oz	10	0
Jalapeno Mexican Hot (Vlasic)	1 oz	8	0
Jalapeno Whole (Trappey's)	2 med	8	0
Mexican Tiny Hot (Vlasic)	1 oz	6	0
Mild Cherry (Vlasic)	1 oz	8	0
Mild Greek Pepperoncini Salad Peppers (Vlasic)	1 oz	4	0
chili, red hot	1 (2.6 oz)	18	tr
chili, red hot, chopped	½ cup	17	tr
green chili, hot	1 (2.6 oz)	18	tr
green chili, hot, chopped	½ cup	17	tr
green halves	½ cup	13	tr
jalapeno, chopped	½ cup	17	tr
red halves	½ cup	13	tr

DRIED
green	1 tbsp	1	tr
red	1 tbsp	1	tr

FRESH
Dole Bell	1 med	25	1
chili, red, raw, chopped	½ cup	30	tr
chili, red hot, raw	1 (1.6 oz)	18	tr
green chili, hot, raw	1	18	tr
green chili, hot, raw, chopped	½ cup	30	tr
green, raw, chopped	½ cup	13	tr
green, chopped, cooked	½ cup	19	tr

FOOD	PORTION	CALORIES	FAT
green, cooked	1 (2.6 oz)	20	tr
green, raw	1 (2.6 oz)	20	tr
red, chopped, cooked	½ cup	19	tr
red, cooked	1 (2.6 oz)	20	tr
red, raw	1 (2.6 oz)	20	tr
red, raw, chopped	½ cup	13	tr
yellow, raw	1 (6.5 oz)	50	tr
yellow, raw	10 strips	14	tr
FROZEN			
Green, Diced (Southland)	2 oz	10	0
Sweet Red & Green, Cut (Southland)	2 oz	15	0
green, chopped, not prep	1 oz	6	tr
red, chopped, not prep	1 oz	6	tr

PERCH

FOOD	PORTION	CALORIES	FAT
FRESH			
cooked	1 fillet (1.6 oz)	54	1
cooked	3 oz	99	1
ocean perch, atlantic, cooked	1 fillet (1.8 oz)	60	1
ocean perch, atlantic, cooked	3 oz	103	2
red, raw	3½ oz	114	4
FROZEN			
Fishmarket Fresh Ocean Perch (Gorton's)	5 oz	140	3
Ocean Perch Batter-Dipped (Van De Kamp's)	2 pieces	270	15
Ocean Perch Breaded (Van De Kamp's)	1 piece	170	12
Ocean Perch Lightly Breaded (Van De Kamp's)	5 oz	300	20
Ocean Perch Microwave Lightly Breaded (Van De Kamp's)	5 oz	300	20

FOOD	PORTION	CALORIES	FAT
Perch, Today's Catch (Van De Kamp's)	5 oz	160	2

PERSIMMONS

dried, japanese	1	93	tr
fresh	1	32	tr
fresh, japanese	1	118	tr

PHEASANT

FRESH

breast w/o skin, raw	½ breast (6.4 oz)	243	6
leg w/o skin, raw	1 (3.6 oz)	143	5
w/ skin, raw	½ pheasant (14 oz)	723	37
w/o skin, raw	½ pheasant (12.4 oz)	470	13

PHYLLO

Ekizian Phyllo Dough	½ lb	865	17

PICKLES

Bread & Butter Chips (Vlasic)	1 oz	30	0
Bread & Butter Chunks (Vlasic)	1 oz	25	0
Bread 'N Butter Slices (Claussen)	1	7	tr
Bread & Butter Stixs (Vlasic)	1 oz	18	0
Deli Bread & Butter (Vlasic)	1 oz	25	0
Deli Dill Halves (Vlasic)	1 oz	4	0
Dill Spears (Claussen)	1	4	tr
Half-the-Salt Hamburger Dill Chips (Vlasic)	1 oz	2	0
Half-the-Salt Kosher Crunchy Dills (Vlasic)	1 oz	4	0

FOOD	PORTION	CALORIES	FAT
Half-the-Salt Kosher Dill Spears (Vlasic)	1 oz	4	0
Half-the-Salt Sweet Butter Chips (Vlasic)	1 oz	30	0
Hot & Spicy Garden Mix (Vlasic)	1 oz	4	0
Kosher Baby Dills (Vlasic)	1 oz	4	0
Kosher Crunchy Dills (Vlasic)	1 oz	4	0
Kosher Dill Gherkins (Vlasic)	1 oz	4	0
Kosher Dill Spears (Vlasic)	1 oz	4	0
Kosher Halves (Claussen)	1 half	9	tr
Kosher Slices (Claussen)	1	1	tr
Kosher Snack Chunks (Vlasic)	1 oz	4	0
Kosher Whole (Claussen)	1	9	tr
No Garlic Dill Spears (Vlasic)	1 oz	4	0
No Garlic Dills (Claussen)	1	17	tr
Original Dills (Vlasic)	1 oz	2	0
Polish Snack Chunk Dills (Vlasic)	1 oz	4	0
Relish (Claussen)	1 tbsp	14	tr
Zesty Crunch Dills (Vlasic)	1 oz	4	0
Zesty Dill Snack Chunks (Vlasic)	1 oz	4	0
Zesty Dill Spears (Vlasic)	1 oz	4	0
dill	1 (2.3 oz)	12	tr
dill, low sodium	1 (2.3 oz)	12	tr
dill, low sodium, sliced	1 slice	1	tr
dill, sliced	1 slice	1	tr
gherkins	3.5 oz	21	tr
kosher dill	1 (2.3 oz)	12	tr
piccalilli	1.4 oz	13	tr
polish dill	1 (2.3 oz)	12	tr
quick sour	1 (1.2 oz)	4	tr

FOOD	PORTION	CALORIES	FAT
quick sour, low sodium	1 (1.2 oz)	4	tr
quick sour, sliced	1 slice	1	tr
sweet	1 (1.2 oz)	41	tr
sweet, low sodium	1 (1.2 oz)	41	tr
sweet, sliced	1 slice	7	tr
sweet gherkin	1 sm (½ oz)	20	tr

PIE

(*see also* PIE CRUST)

FOOD	PORTION	CALORIES	FAT
CANNED FILLING			
Mincemeat Condensed (None Such)	¼ pkg	220	2
Mincemeat Old Fashioned (S&W)	½ cup	206	2
Mincemeat Ready-to-Use (None Such)	⅓ cup	200	1
Mincemeat Ready-to-Use w/ Brandy & Rum (None Such)	⅓ cup	220	2
Pumpkin (Libby's)	1 cup	210	0
pumpkin pie mix	1 cup	282	tr
FROZEN			
Apple (Banquet)	1 slice (3.3 oz)	250	11
Apple (Mrs. Smith's)	⅛ of 9⅝" pie	390	17
Apple (Weight Watchers)	1 slice (3.5 oz)	165	4
Apple Homestyle (Sara Lee)	1 slice (4 oz)	280	12
Apple Homestyle High (Sara Lee)	1 slice (4.9 oz)	400	23
Apple Natural Juice (Mrs. Smith's)	⅐ of 9" pie	420	22
Apple Streusel Natural Juice (Mrs. Smith's)	⅐ of 9" pie	420	16
Banana (Banquet)	1 slice (2.3 oz)	180	10
Blackberry (Banquet)	1 slice (3.3 oz)	270	11
Blueberry (Banquet)	1 slice (3.3 oz)	270	11
Blueberry (Mrs. Smith's)	⅛ of 9⅝" pie	380	17

FOOD	PORTION	CALORIES	FAT
Blueberry Homestyle (Sara Lee)	1 slice (4 oz)	300	12
Cherry (Banquet)	1 slice (3.3 oz)	250	11
Cherry (Mrs. Smith's)	⅛ of 9⅝″ pie	400	16
Cherry Homestyle (Sara Lee)	1 slice (4 oz)	270	13
Cherry Natural Juice (Mrs. Smith's)	⅐ of 9″ pie	410	18
Chocolate (Banquet)	1 slice (2.3 oz)	190	10
Chocolate Mocha (Weight Watchers)	1 (2.75 oz)	180	4
Coconut (Banquet)	1 slice (2.3 oz)	190	11
Coconut Custard (Mrs. Smith's)	⅛ of 9⅝″ pie	330	15
Dutch Apple Homestyle (Sara Lee)	1 slice (4 oz)	300	12
Hyannis Boston Cream Pie (Pepperidge Farm)	1 slice	230	10
Lemon (Banquet)	1 slice (2.3 oz)	170	9
Mince Homestyle (Sara Lee)	1 slice (4 oz)	300	13
Mincemeat (Banquet)	1 slice (3.3 oz)	260	11
Mississippi Mud (Pepperidge Farm)	1 slice	310	23
Peach (Banquet)	1 slice (3.3 oz)	245	11
Peach (Mrs. Smith's)	⅛ of 9⅝″ pie	365	16
Peach Homestyle (Sara Lee)	1 slice (3.4 oz)	280	12
Pecan Homestyle (Sara Lee)	1 slice (3.4 oz)	400	18
Pecan Thaw 'N' Serve (Mrs. Smith's)	⅛ of 9⅝″ pie	510	23
Pumpkin (Banquet)	1 slice (3.3 oz)	200	8
Pumpkin Homestyle (Sara Lee)	1 slice (4 oz)	240	10
Pumpkin Custard (Mrs. Smith's)	⅛ of 9⅝″ pie	310	11
Raspberry Homestyle (Sara Lee)	1 slice (4 oz)	280	13
Strawberry (Banquet)	1 slice (2.3 oz)	170	9
HOME RECIPE			
pecan	⅙ of 9″ pie	575	19
pumpkin, as prep w/ Libby's Solid Pack	⅙ of 9″ pie	330	17

FOOD	PORTION	CALORIES	FAT
MIX			
Banana Cream (Jell-O)	⅙ of 8" pie	107	3
Banana Cream No Bake Dessert (Jell-O)	⅛ pie	233	12
Cheese Cake Lite No-Bake (Royal)	⅛ pie	130	3
Cheese Cake Real No-Bake (Royal)	⅛ pie	160	3
Chocolate Cream Pie No Bake Dessert (Jell-O)	⅛ pie	260	17
Chocolate Mousse No-Bake (Royal)	⅛ pie	130	4
Chocolate Mousse No Bake Dessert (Jell-O)	⅛ pie	262	15
Coconut Cream (Jell-O)	⅙ of 8" pie	115	5
Key Lime Filling (Royal)	mix for 1 serving	50	0
Lemon (Jell-O)	⅙ of 8" pie	180	2
Lemon Filling (Royal)	mix for 1 serving	50	0
Lemon Meringue No-Bake (Royal)	⅛ pie	210	5
READY-TO-USE			
apple	⅙ of 9" pie	405	18
blueberry	⅙ of 9" pie	380	17
cherry	⅙ of 9" pie	410	18
creme	⅙ of 9" pie	455	23
custard	⅙ of 9" pie	330	17
lemon meringue	⅙ of 9" pie	355	14
peach	⅙ of 9" pie	405	17
pumpkin	⅙ of 9" pie	320	17
SNACK			
Apple (Little Debbie)	1 pkg (3 oz)	310	9
Apple (Tastykake)	1	345	12
Blueberry (Tastykake)	1	359	12
Cherry (Tastykake)	1	368	13

FOOD	PORTION	CALORIES	FAT
Chocolate Pudding (Tastykake)	1	443	16
Coconut Creme (Tastykake)	1	432	22
Dutch Apple (Little Debbie)	1 pkg (2.17 oz)	270	12
French Apple (Tastykake)	1	399	13
Lemon (Tastykake)	1	361	13
Marshmallow Banana (Little Debbie)	1 pkg (1.38 oz)	170	6
Marshmallow Chocolate (Little Debbie)	1 pkg (1.38 oz)	170	6
Oatmeal Creme (Little Debbie)	1 pkg (1.33 oz)	170	8
Peach (Tastykake)	1	343	12
Pecan (Little Debbie)	1 pkg (1.83 oz)	200	7
Pineapple (Tastykake)	1	362	12
Pumpkin (Tastykake)	1	356	14
Raisin Creme (Little Debbie)	1 pkg (1.17 oz)	170	9
Strawberry (Tastykake)	1	373	12
Tasty Klair (Tastykake)	1	436	19
Vanilla Pudding (Tastykake)	1	437	19
apple	1 (3 oz)	266	14
cherry	1 (3 oz)	266	14
lemon	1 (3 oz)	266	14

PIE CRUST

FOOD	PORTION	CALORIES	FAT
FROZEN			
Patty Shells (Pepperidge Farm)	1	210	15
Pie Shell (Mrs. Smith's)	⅛ of 9⅝" pie	130	8
Puff Pastry Sheets (Pepperidge Farm)	¼ sheet	260	17
HOME RECIPE			
9-inch crust	1	900	60
MIX			
Flako	⅙ of 9" pie	250	15

FOOD	PORTION	CALORIES	FAT
Pillsbury Mix	⅛ of 2-crust pie	270	17
Pillsbury Stick	⅛ of 2-crust pie	270	17
as prep	2 crusts	1485	93
READY-TO-USE Ready Crust Chocolate	1	110	5
Ready Crust Chocolate	⅛ of 9″ pie	100	5
Ready Crust Graham	1	110	5
Ready Crust Graham	⅛ of 9″ pie	100	5
REFRIGERATED Pillsbury All Ready	⅛ of 2-crust pie	240	15

PIEROGI

FROZEN Potato Cheese (Mrs. T's)	1	70	1
Potato Onion (Mrs. T's)	1	50	tr
Sauerkraut (Mrs. T's)	1	60	0
TAKE-OUT pierogi	¾ cup (4.4 oz)	307	19

PIGEON PEAS

DRIED cooked	½ cup	86	1
cooked	1 cup	204	1
raw	1 cup	704	3

PIGNOLIA
(*see* PINE NUTS)

PIG'S EARS AND FEET

ears, frzn, simmered	1 ear (3.7 oz)	183	12
feet, pickled	1 oz	58	5

FOOD	PORTION	CALORIES	FAT
feet, pickled	1 lb	923	73
feet, simmered	2.5 oz	138	9

PIKE

FRESH
northern, cooked	3 oz	96	1
northern, cooked	½ fillet (5.4 oz)	176	1
roe, raw	3.5 oz	130	2
walleye, baked	3 oz	101	1
walleye, fillet, baked	4.4 oz	147	2

PILLNUTS

pillnuts, canarytree, dried	1 oz	204	23

PIMIENTOS

Dromedary	1 oz	10	0
canned	1 tbsp	3	tr
canned	1 slice	0	0

PINE NUTS

pignolia, dried	1 tbsp	51	5
pignolia, dried	1 oz	146	14
pinyon, dried	1 oz	161	17

PINEAPPLE

CANNED
All Cuts Juice Pack (Dole)	½ cup	70	tr
All Cuts Syrup Pack (Dole)	½ cup	90	tr
Chunk (Empress)	4 oz	70	0
Crushed (Empress)	4 oz	70	0

FOOD	PORTION	CALORIES	FAT
Hawaiian Slice in Heavy Syrup (S&W)	½ cup	90	0
Hawaiian Slice Juice Pack (S&W)	½ cup	70	0
Sliced (Empress)	4 oz	70	0
Sliced Unsweetened	½ cup	60	0
chunks in heavy syrup	1 cup	199	tr
chunks juice pack	1 cup	150	tr
crushed in heavy syrup	1 cup	199	tr
slices in heavy syrup	1 slice	45	tr
slices in light syrup	1 slice	30	tr
slices juice pack	1 slice	35	tr
slices water pack	1 slice	19	tr
tidbits in heavy syrup	1 cup	199	tr
tidbits in juice	1 cup	150	tr
tidbits in water	1 cup	79	tr
FRESH			
Chiquita	1 cup	90	1
Dole	2 slices	90	1
diced	1 cup	77	tr
slice	1 slice	42	tr
FROZEN			
chunks sweetened	½ cup	104	tr
JUICE			
Dole	6 oz	100	tr
Dole New Breakfast Juice	6 oz	100	tr
Libby's Nectar	6 oz	110	0
Mott's	9.5 oz	169	0
S&W Unsweetened	6 oz	100	0
Tree Top	6 oz	100	0
canned	1 cup	139	tr

FOOD	PORTION	CALORIES	FAT
frzn, as prep	1 cup	129	tr
frzn, not prep	6 oz	387	tr

PINK BEANS

CANNED Spanish Style (Goya)	7.5 oz	140	tr
DRIED cooked	1 cup	252	1
raw	1 cup	721	2

PINTO BEANS

CANNED Gebhardt	4 oz	100	tr
Goya Spanish	7.5 oz	140	1
Green Giant	½ cup	90	1
Green Giant Picante	½ cup	100	1
Luck's Seasoned w/ Pork	7.25 oz	220	6
Luck's Seasoned w/ Pork & Onions	7.5 oz	220	6
Ranch Style Premium	7.5 oz	160	1
Ranch Style w/ Jalapeno	7.5 oz	180	2
Trappey's	½ cup	90	1
Trappey's Hearty Texas	½ cup	110	2
Trappey's Jalapinto	½ cup	90	1
pinto	1 cup	186	1
DRIED Arrowhead Red	2 oz	200	1
Hurst Brand	1 cup	265	tr
cooked	1 cup	235	1
raw	1 cup	656	2

FOOD	PORTION	CALORIES	FAT
FROZEN			
cooked	3 oz	152	tr
SPROUTS			
cooked	3.5 oz	22	tr
raw	3.5 oz	62	1

PINYON
(*see* PINE NUTS)

PISTACHIOS

California Natural (Dole)	1 oz	90	7
Dry Roasted (Planters)	1 oz	170	15
Lance	1.13 oz	180	14
Red Salted (Planters)	1 oz	170	14
Shelled & Roasted (Dole)	1 oz	163	14
dried	1 oz	164	14
dried	1 cup	739	62
dry roasted	1 oz	172	15
dry roasted salted	1 oz	172	15
dry roasted salted	1 cup	776	68

PITANGA

fresh	1	2	tr
fresh	1 cup	57	1

PIZZA

FROZEN			
Celeste			
Canadian Style Bacon	1 (9.25 oz)	550	26
Cheese	1 (6.5 oz)	500	24
Deluxe	1 (8.25 oz)	600	32

FOOD	PORTION	CALORIES	FAT
Celeste *(cont.)*			
Pepperoni	1 (6.75 oz)	540	29
Sausage	1 (7.5 oz)	580	32
Sausage & Mushroom	1 (9.25 oz)	600	32
Supreme	1 (9 oz)	690	39
Fox Deluxe			
Golden Topping	½ pizza	240	11
Hamburger	½ pizza	260	12
Pepperoni	½ pizza	250	13
Sausage	½ pizza	260	13
Sausage & Pepperoni	½ pizza	260	13
Healthy Choice			
French Bread Cheese	1 (5.3 oz)	270	2
French Bread Deluxe	1 (6.25 oz)	330	8
French Bread Italian Turkey Sausage	1 (6.45 oz)	320	7
French Bread Pepperoni	1 (6.25 oz)	320	8
Jeno's			
4-Pack Cheese	1 pizza	160	8
4-Pack Combination	1 pizza	180	9
4-Pack Hamburger	1 pizza	180	9
4-Pack Pepperoni	1 pizza	170	9
4-Pack Sausage	1 pizza	180	9
Crisp 'N Tasty Sausage & Pepperoni	½ pizza	300	16
Crisp 'N Tasty Canadian Bacon	½ pizza	250	11
Crisp 'N Tasty Cheese	½ pizza	270	14
Crisp 'N Tasty Hamburger	½ pizza	290	15
Crisp 'N Tasty Pepperoni	½ pizza	280	15
Crisp 'N Tasty Sausage	½ pizza	300	16
Microwave Pizza Rolls Pepperoni & Cheese	6	240	13

FOOD	PORTION	CALORIES	FAT
Microwave Pizza Rolls Sausage & Cheese	6	250	13
Pizza Rolls Cheese	6	240	12
Pizza Rolls Hamburger	6	240	13
Pizza Rolls Pepperoni & Cheese	6	230	13
Pizza Rolls Sausage & Pepperoni	6	230	13
Kid Cuisine			
Cheese	1 (6.85 oz)	380	12
Hamburger	6.85 oz	330	10
Mega Meal Cheese	1 (9.7 oz)	430	7
MicroMagic			
Deep Dish Combination	1 (6.5 oz)	605	34
Deep Dish Pepperoni	1 (6.5 oz)	615	32
Deep Dish Sausage	1 (6.5 oz)	590	31
Mr. P's			
Combination	½ pizza	260	13
Golden Topping	½ pizza	240	11
Hamburger	½ pizza	260	12
Pepperoni	½ pizza	250	13
Sausage	½ pizza	260	13
Pappalo's			
Combination Pan	⅙ pizza	340	15
French Bread Cheese	1 pizza	360	15
French Bread Combination	1 pizza	430	21
French Bread Pepperoni	1 pizza	410	20
French Bread Sausage	1 pizza	410	18
Hamburger Pan	⅙ pizza	310	12
Pepperoni Pan	⅙ pizza	330	14
Sausage Pan	⅙ pizza	360	18
Thin Crust Combination	⅙ pizza	260	10
Thin Crust Hamburger	⅙ pizza	240	8
Thin Crust Pepperoni	⅙ pizza	270	11
Thin Crust Sausage	⅙ pizza	250	9

FOOD	PORTION	CALORIES	FAT
Pepperidge Farm			
Croissant Pastry Cheese	1	430	23
Croissant Pastry Deluxe	1	440	23
Croissant Pastry Pepperoni	1	420	22
Pillsbury Microwave			
Cheese	½ pizza	240	10
Combination	½ pizza	310	15
French Bread	1 pizza	370	15
French Bread Pepperoni	1 pizza	430	19
French Bread Sausage	1 pizza	410	16
French Bread Sausage & Pepperoni	1 pizza	450	21
Pepperoni	½ pizza	300	15
Sausage	½ pizza	280	13
Totino's			
Bacon Party	½ pizza	370	20
Canadian Bacon Party	½ pizza	310	14
Cheese Party	½ pizza	340	17
Cheese Slices	1	170	7
Combination Party	½ pizza	380	21
Combination Slices	1	200	10
Hamburger Party	½ pizza	370	19
Mexican Style Party	½ pizza	380	21
Microwave Cheese	1 pizza	250	8
Microwave Pepperoni	1 pizza	280	12
Microwave Sausage	1 pizza	320	16
Microwave Sausage Pepperoni Combination	1 pizza	310	15
My Classic Deluxe Cheese	⅙ pizza	210	9
My Classic Deluxe Combination	⅙ pizza	270	14
My Classic Deluxe Pepperoni	⅙ pizza	260	13

FOOD	PORTION	CALORIES	FAT
Pepperoni Pan	⅙ pizza	330	14
Pepperoni Party	½ pizza	370	20
Pepperoni Slices	1	190	9
Sausage & Pepperoni Combination Pan	⅙ pizza	340	15
Sausage Pan	⅙ pizza	320	13
Sausage Party	½ pizza	390	21
Sausage Slices	1	200	10
Three Cheese Pan	⅙ pizza	290	10
Vegetable Party	½ pizza	300	13
Weight Watchers			
Cheese	1 (6.03 oz)	300	7
Deluxe Combination	1 (7.32 oz)	320	9
Deluxe French Bread	1 (5.94 oz)	260	7
Pepperoni	1 (6.08 oz)	320	8
Sausage	1 (6.43 oz)	340	10
MIX			
Chef Boyardee 2 Complete Cheese	1 serving (3.16 oz)	210	5
Chef Boyardee 2 Complete Pepperoni	1 serving (3.75 oz)	210	7
Chef Boyardee Complete Cheese	1 serving (3.84 oz)	230	6
Chef Boyardee Complete Pepperoni	1 serving (4.16 oz)	250	9
Chef Boyardee Complete Sausage	1 serving (4.22 oz)	270	10
Chef Boyardee Plain	1 serving (3.5 oz)	180	3
Chef Boyardee Quick & Easy Crust Mix	1 serving (1.5 oz)	150	2

FOOD	PORTION	CALORIES	FAT
SAUCE			
Chef Boyardee Pizza Sauce w/ Cheese	3.88 oz	90	6
Contadina Original Quick & Easy	¼ cup	30	1
Contadina Pizza Sauce w/ Italian Cheese	¼ cup	30	1
Contadina Pizza Sauce w/ Pepperoni	¼ cup	40	2
Ragu Pizza Quick Sauce Traditional	1.7 oz	35	2
Ragu Pizza Quick Sauce w/ Cheese	1.7 oz	35	2
Ragu Pizza Quick Sauce w/ Garlic & Basil	1.7 oz	35	2
Ragu Pizza Quick Sauce w/ Mushrooms	1.7 oz	35	2
Ragu Pizza Quick Sauce w/ Pepperoni	1.7 oz	35	2
Ragu Pizza Quick Sauce w/ Sausage	3 tbsp	35	2
TAKE-OUT			
cheese	⅛ of 12" pie	140	3
cheese	12" pie	1121	26
cheese, meat & vgetables	⅛ of 12" pie	184	5
cheese, meat & vegetables	12" pie	1472	43
pepperoni	⅛ of 12" pie	181	7
pepperoni	12" pie	1445	56

PLANTAINS

FOOD	PORTION	CALORIES	FAT
All Natural Plantain Chips (Top Banana)	1 oz	150	8
FRESH			
sliced, cooked	½ cup	89	tr
uncooked	1	218	1
TAKE-OUT			
ripe, fried	2.8 oz	214	7

FOOD	PORTION	CALORIES	FAT

PLUMS

CANNED

FOOD	PORTION	CALORIES	FAT
Halves Purple Fancy Unpeeled in Extra Heavy Syrup (S&W)	½ cup	135	0
Halves Unpeeled Diet (S&W)	½ cup	52	0
Whole Purple Fancy Unpeeled In Extra Heavy Syrup (S&W)	½ cup	135	0
Whole Unpeeled Diet (S&W)	½ cup	52	0
purple in heavy syrup	3	119	tr
purple in heavy syrup	1 cup	320	tr
purple in light syrup	3	83	tr
purple in light syrup	1 cup	158	tr
purple juice pack	3	55	tr
purple juice pack	1 cup	146	tr
purple water pack	3	39	tr
purple water pack	1 cup	102	tr

FRESH

FOOD	PORTION	CALORIES	FAT
Dole	2	70	1
plum	1	36	tr
sliced	1 cup	91	1

JUICE

FOOD	PORTION	CALORIES	FAT
Kern's Nectar	6 oz	110	0

POI

FOOD	PORTION	CALORIES	FAT
POI	½ cup	134	tr

POKEBERRY SHOOTS

FRESH

FOOD	PORTION	CALORIES	FAT
cooked	½ cup	16	tr
raw	½ cup	18	tr

FOOD	PORTION	CALORIES	FAT

POLLACK

atlantic, baked	3 oz	100	1
atlantic fillet, baked	5.3 oz	178	2
FROZEN			
Light Fillets (Mrs. Paul's)	1 fillet (4.5 oz)	240	11

POMEGRANATES

pomegranates	1	104	tr

POMPANO

florida, cooked	3 oz	179	10

POPCORN
(see also CHIPS, PRETZELS, SNACKS)

Bachman	1 oz	160	11
Cracker Jack	1 oz	120	3
Jiffy Pop Microwave Butter	4 cups	140	7
Jiffy Pop Microwave Regular	4 cups	140	7
Jiffy Pop Pan Butter	4 cups	130	6
Jiffy Pop Pan Regular	4 cups	130	6
Lance Cheese	1 pkg (⅞ oz)	130	8
Lance Cheese	1 oz	150	9
Lance Plain	1 pkg (1 oz)	140	8
Newman's Own			
Microwave Butter	3 cups	140	7
Microwave Light Butter	3 cups	90	3
Microwave Light Natural	3 cups	90	3
Microwave Natural	3 cups	140	7
Microwave Natural No Salt	3 cups	140	7
Orville Redenbacher			
Gourmet Hot Air	3 cups	40	tr

FOOD	PORTION	CALORIES	FAT
Gourmet Original	3 cups	80	4
Gourmet White	3 cups	80	4
Microwave Gourmet	3 cups	100	6
Microwave Gourmet Butter	3 cups	100	6
Microwave Gourmet Butter Toffee	2 ½ cups	210	12
Microwave Gourmet Caramel	2 ½ cups	240	14
Microwave Gourmet Cheddar Cheese	3 cups	130	8
Microwave Gourmet Frozen	3 cups	100	6
Microwave Gourmet Frozen Butter	3 cups	100	6
Microwave Gourmet Light	3 cups	70	3
Microwave Gourmet Light Butter	3 cups	70	3
Microwave Gourmet Salt Free	3 cups	100	6
Microwave Gourmet Salt Free Butter	3 cups	100	6
Microwave Gourmet Sour Cream 'N Onion	3 cups	160	12
Pillsbury Microwave Butter	3 cups	210	13
Pillsbury Microwave Original	3 cups	210	13
Pillsbury Microwave Salt Free	3 cups	170	7
Ultra Slim-Fast Lite N' Tasty	½ oz	60	2
Weight Watchers Microwave	1 oz	100	1
Weight Watchers Ready-to-Eat Butter	.7 oz	90	3
Weight Watchers Ready-to-Eat White Cheddar Cheese	.7 oz	90	4
Wise Tender Eating	½ oz	70	6
Wise w/ Real Premium White Cheddar Cheese	½ oz	70	5
air-popped	1 cup	30	tr
popped w/ vegetable oil	1 cup	55	3
sugar syrup coated	1 cup	135	1

FOOD	PORTION	CALORIES	FAT

POPPY SEEDS

poppy seeds	1 tsp	15	1

PORK

(*see also* BACON, CANADIAN BACON, HAM, HOT DOG, LUNCHEON MEATS/
COLD CUTS, SAUSAGE)

The values for cooked pork may differ slightly from values for raw pork.
When meat is cooked some moisture and fat are lost, changing the nutritive
value slightly. As a rule of thumb, it can be assumed that a 4-oz. raw
portion will equal a 3-oz. cooked portion of meat.

FOOD	PORTION	CALORIES	FAT
FRESH			
blade chop, roasted	1 (3.1 oz)	321	27
center loin			
lean & fat, braised	3 oz	301	22
lean & fat, pan-fried	3 oz	318	26
lean only, broiled	3 oz	196	9
lean only, pan-fried	3 oz	226	14
lean only, roasted	3 oz	204	11
center loin chop			
lean & fat, braised	1 (2.6 oz)	266	19
lean & fat, broiled	1 (3.1 oz)	275	19
lean & fat, pan-fried	1 (3.1 oz)	333	27
lean & fat, roasted	1 (3.1 oz)	268	19
lean only, braised	1 (2.1 oz)	166	8
lean only, broiled	1 (2.5 oz)	166	8
lean only, pan-fried	1 (2.4 oz)	178	11
lean only, roasted	1 (2.4 oz)	180	10
ham, fresh			
shank half, lean & fat, roasted	3 oz	258	19
shank half, lean only, roasted	3 oz	183	9
whole, lean & fat, roasted	3 oz	250	18
whole, lean only, roasted	3 oz	187	9

FOOD	PORTION	CALORIES	FAT
half, lean & fat, roasted	3 oz	233	23
half, lean only, roasted	3 oz	187	9
leg, loin & shoulder, lean only, roasted	3 oz	198	11
loin			
lean & fat, braised	3 oz	312	24
lean & fat, broiled	3 oz	294	23
lean only, braised	3 oz	232	12
lean only, broiled	3 oz	218	13
lean only, roasted	3 oz	204	12
loin blade			
lean & fat, braised	3 oz	348	29
lean & fat, broiled	3 oz	334	29
lean & fat, pan-fried	3 oz	352	31
lean & fat, roasted	3 oz	310	26
lean only, broiled	3 oz	255	18
lean only, pan-fried	3 oz	240	17
lean only, roasted	3 oz	238	16
loin blade chop			
lean & fat, braised	1 (3.1 oz)	321	27
lean & fat, braised	1 (2.4 oz)	275	23
lean & fat, pan-fried	1 (3.1 oz)	368	33
lean only, braised	1 (1.8 oz)	156	10
lean only, broiled	1 (2.1 oz)	177	13
lean only, pan-fried	1 (2.2 oz)	175	12
lean only, roasted	1 (2.5 oz)	198	14
loin chop			
lean & fat, braised	1 (2.3 oz)	267	20
lean & fat, braised	1 (2.5 oz)	261	20
lean & fat, broiled	1 (2.7 oz)	295	23
lean & fat, pan-fried	1 (2.9 oz)	337	29

FOOD	PORTION	CALORIES	FAT
loin chop *(cont.)*			
lean & fat, roasted	1 (2.8 oz)	274	21
lean & fat, roasted	1 (2.9 oz)	262	20
lean only, braised	1 (1.8 oz)	147	8
lean only, broiled	1 (2.1 oz)	165	10
lean only, pan-fried	1 (2 oz)	157	9
lean only, roasted	1 chop (2.3 oz)	167	9
lungs, braised	3 oz	84	3
pancreas, braised	3 oz	186	9
rib chop			
lean & fat, braised	1 (2.2 oz)	246	18
lean & fat, broiled	1 (2.6 oz)	264	20
lean & fat, pan-fried	1 (2.9 oz)	343	29
lean & fat, roasted	1 (2.6 oz)	252	19
lean only, braised	1 (1.8 oz)	147	8
lean only, broiled	1 (2.1 oz)	162	9
lean only, pan-fried	1 (2 oz)	160	9
lean only, roasted	1 (2.2 oz)	162	9
shoulder blade boston steak			
lean & fat, braised	1 (5.6 oz)	594	46
lean & fat, broiled	1 (6.5 oz)	647	53
lean & fat, roasted	1 (6.5 oz)	594	47
lean only, braised	1 (4.6 oz)	382	23
lean only, broiled	1 (5.3 oz)	413	28
lean only, roasted	1 (5.5 oz)	404	27
shoulder, arm picnic			
cured, lean & fat, roasted	3 oz	238	18
cured, lean only, roasted	3 oz	145	6
lean & fat, braised	3 oz	293	22
lean & fat, roasted	3 oz	281	22
lean only, braised	3 oz	211	10

FOOD	PORTION	CALORIES	FAT
lean only, roasted	3 oz	194	11
shoulder, blade roll, cured, lean & fat	3 oz	304	25
shoulder, boston blade			
lean & fat, braised	3 oz	316	24
lean & fat, broiled	3 oz	297	24
lean & fat, roasted	3 oz	273	21
lean only, braised	3 oz	250	15
lean only, broiled	3 oz	233	16
lean only, roasted	3 oz	218	14
shoulder, whole, roasted	3 oz	277	22
shoulder, whole, lean only, roasted	3 oz	207	13
sirloin chop			
lean & fat, braised	1 (2.4 oz)	250	18
lean & fat, broiled	1 (2.8 oz)	278	21
lean & fat, roasted	1 (2.8 oz)	244	17
lean only, braised	1 (1.9 oz)	149	7
lean only, broiled	1 (2.3 oz)	165	9
lean only, roasted	1 (2.5 oz)	175	10
spareribs, braised	3 oz	338	26
spleen, braised	3 oz	127	3
tail, simmered	3 oz	336	30
tenderloin, lean only, roasted	3 oz	141	4

POSOLE
(*see* HOMINY)

POT PIE

FROZEN			
Beef (Morton)	7 oz	430	31
Beef (Swanson)	7 oz	370	19
Beef Hungry Man (Swanson)	16 oz	610	31

FOOD	PORTION	CALORIES	FAT
Chicken (Swanson)	7 oz	380	22
Chicken Hungry Man (Swanson)	16 oz	630	35
Turkey (Swanson)	7 oz	380	21
Turkey Hungry Man (Swanson)	16 oz	650	36
Vegetable Pie w/ Beef (Banquet)	7 oz	510	33
Vegetable Pie w/ Beef (Morton)	7 oz	430	31
Vegetable Pie w/ Chicken (Banquet)	7 oz	550	36
Vegetable Pie w/ Chicken (Morton)	7 oz	420	28
Vegetable Pie w/ Turkey (Banquet)	7 oz	510	31
Vegetable Pie w/ Turkey (Morton)	7 oz	420	28
HOME RECIPE			
beef, baked	⅓ of 9" pie (7.4 oz)	515	30
chicken	⅓ of 9" pie (8.1 oz)	545	31

POTATO
(see also CHIPS)

CANNED			
Libby	½ cup	45	0
Seneca	½ cup	45	0
New Potatoes Extra Small (S&W)	½ cup	45	0
Whole New (Hunt's)	4 oz	70	tr
potatoes	½ cup	54	tr
FRESH			
Yukon Gold	1 (5.3 oz)	110	0
baked, skin only	1 skin (2 oz)	115	tr
baked w/ skin	1 (6.5 oz)	220	tr
baked w/o skin	1 (5 oz)	145	tr
baked w/o skin	½ cup	57	tr
boiled	½ cup	68	tr

FOOD	PORTION	CALORIES	FAT
microwaved	1 (7 oz)	212	tr
microwaved w/o skin	½ cup	78	tr
raw w/o skin	1 (3.9 oz)	88	tr
FROZEN			
Baked Potato Broccoli & Cheddar (Lean Cuisine)	10⅜ oz	290	9
Baked Potato Broccoli & Cheese (Weight Watchers)	1	270	6
Baked Potato Broccoli & Ham (Weight Watchers)	11.5 oz	280	17
Baked Potato Chicken Divan (Weight Watchers)	1	280	7
Baked Potato Homestyle Turkey (Weight Watchers)	1	250	7
Baked Potato w/ Broccoli & Cheese Sauce (Healthy Choice)	10 oz	240	5
Cheddar Browns (Ore Ida)	3 oz	90	2
Cheddared Potatoes (Budget Gourmet)	1 pkg	260	16
Cheddared Potatoes w/ Broccoli (Budget Gourmet)	1 pkg	150	8
Cottage Fries (Ore Ida)	3 oz	130	4
Crispers! (Ore Ida)	3 oz	220	13
Crispy Crowns! (Ore Ida)	3 oz	190	11
Crispy Crunchers (Ore Ida)	3 oz	180	9
Deep Fries Crinkle Cuts (Ore Ida)	3 oz	160	7
Deep Fries French Fries (Ore Ida)	3 oz	170	7
Dinner Fries Country Style (Ore Ida)	3 oz	110	2
French Fries (MicroMagic)	1 pkg (3 oz)	290	13
Golden Crinkles (Ore Ida)	3 oz	120	3
Golden Fries (Ore Ida)	3 oz	120	3
Golden Patties (Ore Ida)	1 (2.5 oz)	130	7

FOOD	PORTION	CALORIES	FAT
Golden Twirls (Ore Ida)	3 oz	160	7
Hash Browns Shredded (Ore Ida)	3 oz	70	tr
Hash Browns Southern Style (Ore Ida)	3 oz	70	tr
Lite Crinkle Cuts (Ore Ida)	3 oz	90	2
Microwave Crinkle Cuts (Ore Ida)	3.5 oz	190	8
Microwave Hash Browns (Ore Ida)	2 oz	110	6
Microwave Tater Tots (Ore Ida)	4 oz	210	9
Nacho Potatoes (Budget Gourmet)	1 pkg	200	12
O'Brien Potatoes (Ore Ida)	3 oz	60	tr
One Serve Potatoes & Broccoli in Cheese Sauce (Green Giant)	1 pkg	130	5
One Serve Potatoes Au Gratin (Green Giant)	1 pkg	200	10
Pixie Crinkles (Ore Ida)	3 oz	140	5
Shoestrings (Ore Ida)	3 oz	150	6
Skinny Fries (MicroMagic)	1 pkg (3 oz)	350	15
Stuffed Potatoes w/ Cheddar Cheese (Oh Boy!)	1 (6 oz)	150	4
Stuffed Potatoes w/ Real Bacon (Oh Boy!)	1 (6 oz)	120	3
Stuffed Potatoes w/ Sour Cream & Chives (Oh Boy!)	1 (6 oz)	110	2
Tater Tots (Ore Ida)	3 oz	160	8
Tater Tots w/ Bacon (Ore Ida)	3 oz	150	7
Tater Tots w/ Onion (Ore Ida)	3 oz	150	7
Three Cheese Potatoes (Budget Gourmet)	1 pkg	230	11
Toaster Hash Browns (Ore Ida)	1 (1.75 oz)	100	5
Topped Broccoli & Cheese (Ore Ida)	1 (5.63 oz)	160	4
Topped Vegetable Primavera (Ore Ida)	1 (6.13 oz)	160	5

FOOD	PORTION	CALORIES	FAT
Twice Baked Butter Flavor (Ore Ida)	1 (5 oz)	200	8
Twice Baked Cheddar Cheese (Ore Ida)	1 (5 oz)	210	9
Twice Baked Sour Cream & Chives (Ore Ida)	1 (5 oz)	190	8
Wedges Home Style (Ore Ida)	3 oz	110	2
Zesties! (Ore Ida)	3 oz	160	8
french fries	10	111	4
french fries, thick cut	10	109	4
hash browns	½ cup	170	9
potato puffs	1 puff	16	1
potato puffs	½ cup	138	7
HOME RECIPE			
au gratin	½ cup	160	9
hash browns	½ cup	163	11
mashed	½ cup	111	4
o'brien	1 cup	157	3
potato dumpling	3.5 oz	334	1
potato pancakes	1 (2.7 oz)	495	13
scalloped	½ cup	105	5
MIX			
Cheddar & Bacon Casserole (French's)	½ cup	130	5
Creamy Italian Scalloped (French's)	½ cup	120	3
Creamy Stroganoff (French's)	½ cup	130	4
Crispy Top Scalloped w/ Savory Onion (French's)	½ cup	140	5
Mashed Potato Flakes (Hungry Jack)	½ cup	40	7
Mashed, not prep (Country Store)	⅓ cup	70	0
Potato Salad Classic Idaho (Lipton)	½ cup	94	tr
Potato Salad German (Lipton)	½ cup	99	tr

FOOD	PORTION	CALORIES	FAT
Potatoes & Cheese (Kraft)			
2-Cheese	½ cup	130	4
Au Gratin	½ cup	130	5
Broccoli Au Gratin	½ cup	120	5
Scalloped	½ cup	140	5
Scalloped w/ Ham	½ cup	150	5
Sour Cream w/ Chives	½ cup	150	5
Potatoes & Sauce (Lipton)			
Au Gratin	½ cup	108	tr
Beef & Mushroom	½ cup	95	tr
Cheddar Bacon	½ cup	106	1
Cheddar Broccoli	½ cup	104	1
Chicken Flavored Mushroom	½ cup	90	tr
Italiano	½ cup	107	2
Nacho	½ cup	103	1
Scalloped	½ cup	102	2
Sour Cream & Chives	½ cup	113	2
Real Cheese Scalloped Potatoes (French's)	½ cup	140	5
Real Sour Cream & Chives Potatoes (French's)	½ cup	150	7
Spuds Mashed (French's)	½ cup	140	7
Tangy Au Gratin (French's)	½ cup	130	5
au gratin	4½ oz	127	6
instant mashed flakes, as prep w/ whole milk & butter	½ cup	118	6
instant mashed flakes, not prep	½ cup	78	tr
instant mashed granules, as prep w/ whole milk & butter	½ cup	114	5
instant mashed granules, not prep	½ cup	372	1
scalloped	4 ½ oz	127	6

FOOD	PORTION	CALORIES	FAT
SHELF STABLE			
Augratin (Pantry Express)	½ cup	120	5
TAKE-OUT			
au gratin w/ cheese	½ cup	178	10
baked, topped w/ cheese sauce	1	475	29
baked, topped w/ cheese sauce & bacon	1	451	26
baked, topped w/ cheese sauce & broccoli	1	402	14
baked, topped w/ cheese sauce & chili	1	481	22
baked, topped w/ sour cream & chives	1	394	22
curry	1 serving (6 oz)	292	16
french fried in vegetable oil	1 reg	235	12
french fried in vegetable oil	1 lg	355	19
french fried in beef tallow	1 reg	237	12
french fried in beef tallow	1 lg	358	19
hash browns	½ cup	151	9
mashed w/ whole milk & margarine	⅓ cup	66	tr
mustard potato salad	3.5 oz	120	6
potato salad	⅓ cup	108	6
potato salad	½ cup	179	10
potato salad w/ vegetables	3.5 oz	120	3
scalloped	½ cup	127	5

POTATO STARCH

Manischewitz	1 cup	570	0
potato starch	3.5 oz	335	tr

FOOD	PORTION	CALORIES	FAT

POUT

FRESH

FOOD	PORTION	CALORIES	FAT
ocean, baked	3 oz	86	1
ocean fillet, baked	4.8 oz	139	2

PRESERVE
(*see* JAM/JELLY/PRESERVES)

PRETZELS
(*see also* CHIPS, POPCORN, SNACKS)

FOOD	PORTION	CALORIES	FAT
Bachman Rods	1 (1 oz)	110	2
Estee Unsalted	7	50	tr
J&J Soft	1 (2.25 oz)	170	0
J&J Soft Bites	5	110	0
Lance	1 oz	100	1
Lance Twist	1.5 oz	150	1
Mister Salty Fat Free Sticks	1 oz	100	0
Mister Salty Fat Free Twists	1 oz	100	0
Mister Salty Twists	1 oz	110	2
Mister Salty Very Thin Sticks	1 oz	110	1
Mr. Phipps Chips	8	60	1
Mr. Phipps Chips Lightly Salted	8	60	1
Mr. Phipps Chips Sesame	8	60	2
Quinlan Artificial Butter Tiny Thins	1 oz	108	1
Quinlan Beers	1 oz	110	1
Quinlan Cheese Tiny Thins	1 oz	109	2
Quinlan Logs	1 oz	103	tr
Quinlan Party Thins	1 oz	109	tr
Quinlan Philly Style	1 oz	107	tr
Quinlan Rods	1 oz	100	tr

FOOD	PORTION	CALORIES	FAT
Quinlan Sour Cheese Tiny Thins	1 oz	100	0
Quinlan Sourdough Thins, Hard	1 oz	100	0
Quinlan Sticks	1 oz	105	tr
Quinlan Thins	1 oz	104	tr
Quinlan Tiny Thins	1 oz	109	2
Quinlan Tiny Thins No-Salt	1 oz	115	2
Quinlan Ultra Thins	1 oz	106	tr
Seyfert's Butter Rods	1 oz	110	1
Ultra Slim-Fast Lite N' Tasty	1 oz	100	tr
Wege Sourdough	1 oz	102	tr
Wege Unsalted	1 oz	102	tr
Wege Whole Wheat	1 oz	109	1
sticks	10	10	tr
twists	1 (½ oz)	65	1
twists, thin	10 (2 oz)	240	2

PRICKLY PEAR

fresh	1	42	1

PRUNES

CANNED

in heavy syrup	5	90	tr
in heavy syrup	1 cup	245	tr

DRIED

Mariani Pitted	¼ cup	140	1
Mariani Whole	¼ cup	140	1
cooked w/ sugar	½ cup	147	tr
cooked w/o sugar	½ cup	113	tr
dried	10	201	tr
dried	1 cup	385	1

FOOD	PORTION	CALORIES	FAT
JUICE			
Mott's	6 oz	130	0
Mott's Country Style	6 oz	130	0
S&W Unsweetened	6 oz	120	0
canned	1 cup	181	tr

PUDDING
(*see also* CUSTARD, PUDDING POPS)

FOOD	PORTION	CALORIES	FAT
HOME RECIPE			
bread w/ raisins	½ cup	180	5
corn	½ cup	97	1
corn	⅔ cup	181	9
yorkshire, as prep w/ skim milk	3.5 oz	93	4
yorkshire, as prep w/ whole milk	3.5 oz	104	5
MIX WITH 2% MILK			
Butterscotch Instant Sugar Free (Jell-O)	½ cup	88	2
Chocolate Fudge Instant Sugar Free (Jell-O)	½ cup	100	3
Chocolate Instant Sugar Free (Jell-O)	½ cup	96	3
Chocolate Sugar Free (Jell-O)	½ cup	91	3
Pistachio Instant Sugar Free (Jell-O)	½ cup	94	3
Vanilla Instant Sugar Free (Jell-O)	½ cup	90	2
Vanilla Sugar Free (Jell-O)	½ cup	82	2
MIX WITH SKIM MILK			
Butterscotch w/ Nutrasweet (D-Zerta)	½ cup	69	tr
Chocolate w/ Nutrasweet (D-Zerta)	½ cup	65	tr
Vanilla w/ Nutrasweet (D-Zerta)	½ cup	69	tr
MIX WITH WHOLE MILK			
Banana Cream Instant (Jell-O)	½ cup	168	5

FOOD	PORTION	CALORIES	FAT
Butter Pecan Instant (Jell-O)	½ cup	174	5
Butterscotch (Jell-O)	½ cup	171	4
Butterscotch Instant (Jell-O)	½ cup	168	5
Chocolate (Jell-O)	½ cup	165	5
Chocolate Fudge (Jell-O)	½ cup	164	5
Chocolate Fudge Instant (Jell-O)	½ cup	174	5
Chocolate Instant (Jell-O)	½ cup	176	5
Chocolate Tapioca Americana (Jell-O)	½ cup	173	5
Coconut Cream Instant (Jell-O)	½ cup	182	6
French Vanilla (Jell-O)	½ cup	171	4
French Vanilla Instant (Jell-O)	½ cup	168	5
Golden Egg Custard Americana (Jell-O)	½ cup	167	6
Golden Egg Custard Americana (Jell-O)	1 pkg (3.5 oz)	378	2
Lemon Instant (Jell-O)	½ cup	172	5
Milk Chocolate (Jell-O)	½ cup	168	5
Milk Chocolate Instant (Jell-O)	½ cup	178	5
Pineapple Cream Instant (Jell-O)	½ cup	168	5
Pistachio Instant (Jell-O)	½ cup	172	5
Rice Americana (Jell-O)	½ cup	177	4
Vanilla (Jell-O)	½ cup	162	4
Vanilla Instant (Jell-O)	½ cup	171	5
Vanilla Tapioca Americana (Jell-O)	½ cup	166	4
chocolate, instant	½ cup	155	4
chocolate, regular	½ cup	150	4
rice	½ cup	155	4
tapioca	½ cup	145	4
vanilla, instant	½ cup	150	4
vanilla, regular	½ cup	145	4

FOOD	PORTION	CALORIES	FAT
READY-TO-USE			
Banana (Snack Pack)	4.25 oz	145	6
Butterscotch (Snack Pack)	4.25 oz	170	6
Butterscotch (Swiss Miss)	4 oz	180	6
Butterscotch (Ultra Slim-Fast)	4 oz	100	tr
Butterscotch Sugar Free (Diamond Crystal)	½ cup	80	tr
Chocolate (Snack Pack)	4.25 oz	170	6
Chocolate (Swiss Miss)	4 oz	180	6
Chocolate (Ultra Slim-Fast)	4 oz	100	tr
Chocolate Fudge (Snack Pack)	4.25 oz	165	6
Chocolate Fudge (Swiss Miss)	4 oz	220	6
Chocolate Fudge Light (Swiss Miss)	4 oz	100	1
Chocolate Light (Snack Pack)	4.25 oz	100	2
Chocolate Light (Swiss Miss)	4 oz	100	1
Chocolate Marshmallow (Snack Pack)	4.25 oz	165	6
Chocolate Parfait (Swiss Miss)	4 oz	170	6
Chocolate Sugar Free (Diamond Crystal)	½ cup	70	tr
Chocolate Sundae (Swiss Miss)	4 oz	220	7
Lemon (Snack Pack)	4.25 oz	150	4
Tapioca (Snack Pack)	4.25 oz	150	5
Tapioca (Swiss Miss)	4 oz	160	5
Tapioca Light (Snack Pack)	4.25 oz	100	2
Vanilla (Snack Pack)	4.25 oz	170	6
Vanilla (Swiss Miss)	4 oz	190	7
Vanilla (Ultra Slim-Fast)	4 oz	100	tr
Vanilla Chocolate Parfait Light (Swiss Miss)	4 oz	100	1
Vanilla Light (Swiss Miss)	4 oz	100	1

FOOD	PORTION	CALORIES	FAT.
Vanilla Parfait (Swiss Miss)	4 oz	180	6
Vanilla Sugar Free (Diamond Crystal)	½ cup	80	tr
Vanilla Sundae (Swiss Miss)	4 oz	200	7
TAKE-OUT			
blancmange	1 serving (4.7 oz)	154	5
bread	1 serving (6.7 oz)	564	18
queen of puddings	1 serving (4.4 oz)	266	10
rice	1 serving (3 oz)	110	4
rice w/ raisins	½ cup	246	6
tapioca	½ cup	169	6

PUDDING POPS

(*see also* ICE CREAM AND FROZEN DESSERTS, PUDDING)

Jell-O			
Chocolate	1 pop	80	2
Chocolate/Caramel Swirl	1 pop	78	2
Chocolate Covered Chocolate	1 pop	130	8
Chocolate Covered Vanilla	1 pop	130	8
Chocolate Fudge	1 pop	73	2
Chocolate w/ Chocolate Chips	1 pop	82	3
Chocolate/Vanilla Swirl	1 pop	77	2
Double Chocolate Swirl	1 pop	74	2
Milk Chocolate	1 pop	75	2
Vanilla	1 pop	75	2
Vanilla w/ Chocolate Chips	1 pop	82	3

PUMMELO

fresh	1	228	tr
sections	1 cup	71	tr

FOOD	PORTION	CALORIES	FAT

PUMPKIN

CANNED

Libby's Solid Pack	1 cup	80	1
Owatonna	½ cup	40	1
pumpkin	½ cup	41	tr

FRESH

cooked, mashed	½ cup	24	tr
flowers, cooked	½ cup	10	tr
flowers, raw	1	0	0
leaves, cooked	½ cup	7	tr
leaves, raw	½ cup	4	tr
raw, cubed	½ cup	15	tr

SEEDS

dried	1 oz	154	13
roasted	1 oz	148	12
roasted	1 cup	1184	96
salted & roasted	1 oz	148	12
salted & roasted	1 cup	1184	96
whole, roasted	1 oz	127	6
whole, roasted	1 cup	285	12
whole, salted & roasted	1 oz	127	6
whole, salted & roasted	1 cup	285	12

PURSLANE

cooked	1 cup	21	tr
raw	1 cup	7	tr

QUAHOGS
(*see* CLAMS)

FOOD	PORTION	CALORIES	FAT
QUAIL			
FRESH			
breast w/o skin, raw	1 (2 oz)	69	2
w/ skin, raw	1 quail (3.8 oz)	210	13
w/o skin, raw	1 quail (3.2 oz)	123	4
QUICHE			
HOME RECIPE			
lorraine	⅛ of 8″ pie	600	48
TAKE-OUT			
cheese	1 slice (3 oz)	283	20
lorraine	1 slice (3 oz)	352	25
mushroom	1 slice (3 oz)	256	18
QUINCE			
fresh	1	53	tr
QUINOA			
Arrowhead Quinoa Seeds	2 oz	200	3
quinoa	½ cup	318	5
RABBIT			
domestic, w/o bone, roasted	3 oz	167	7
wild, w/o bone, stewed	3 oz	147	3
RACCOON			
roasted	3 oz	217	12
RADICCHIO			
raw, shredded	½ cup	5	tr

FOOD	PORTION	CALORIES	FAT

RADISH

DRIED

chinese	½ cup	157	tr
daikon	½ cup	157	tr

FRESH

Dole	7	20	0
chinese, raw	1 (12 oz)	62	tr
chinese, raw, sliced	½ cup	8	tr
chinese, sliced, cooked	½ cup	13	tr
daikon, raw	1 (12 oz)	62	tr
daikon, raw, sliced	½ cup	8	tr
daikon, sliced, cooked	½ cup	13	tr
red, raw	10	7	tr
red, sliced	½ cup	10	tr
white icicle, raw	1 (½ oz)	2	tr
white icicle, raw, sliced	½ cup	7	tr

SPROUTS

raw	½ cup	8	tr

RAISINS

Cinderella Seedless	½ cup	250	0
Dole Golden	½ cup	260	0
Dole Seedless	½ cup	260	0
Sunbelt	1 bar (1 oz)	90	tr
golden seedless	1 cup	437	1
seedless	1 tbsp	27	tr
seedless	1 cup	434	1
sultanas	1 oz	88	0

FOOD	PORTION	CALORIES	FAT

RASPBERRIES

CANNED
in heavy syrup	½ cup	117	tr

FRESH
Dole	1 cup	45	0
raspberries	1 cup	61	1
raspberries	1 pint	154	2

FROZEN
Whole in Lite Syrup (Birds Eye)	½ cup	99	tr
sweetened	1 cup	256	tr
sweetened	1 pkg (10 oz)	291	tr

JUICE
Dole Pure & Light	6 oz	90	tr
Smucker's	8 oz	120	0
Smucker's Juice Sparkler	10 oz	130	tr

RED BEANS

CANNED
Green Giant	½ cup	90	1
Van Camp's	1 cup	194	1
Small (Hunt's)	4 oz	90	tr

RELISH

Dill (Vlasic)	1 oz	2	0
Hamburger (Vlasic)	1 oz	40	0
Hot Dog (Vlasic)	1 oz	40	1
Hot Piccalilli (Vlasic)	1 oz	35	0
India (Vlasic)	1 oz	30	0
Sandwich Spred (Hellmann's)	1 tbsp	55	5
Sweet (Vlasic)	1 oz	30	0

FOOD	PORTION	CALORIES	FAT
cranberry orange	½ cup	246	tr
hamburger	1 tbsp	19	tr
hamburger	½ cup	158	1
hot dog	1 tbsp	14	tr
hot dog	½ cup	111	1
piccalilli	1.4 oz	13	tr
sweet	1 tbsp	19	tr
sweet	1 cup	159	1

RHUBARB

FOOD	PORTION	CALORIES	FAT
fresh	½ cup	13	tr
frzn	½ cup	60	tr
frzn, as prep w/ sugar	½ cup	139	tr

RICE
(*see also* BRAN; CEREAL, COOKED; FLOUR; RICE CAKES; WILD RICE)

BROWN

FOOD	PORTION	CALORIES	FAT
Arrowhead Basmati	2 oz	200	1
Arrowhead Brown Long	2 oz	200	1
Arrowhead Brown Medium	2 oz	200	1
Arrowhead Brown Short	2 oz	200	1
Arrowhead Quick Original	2 oz	200	1
Arrowhead Quick Spanish Style	2 oz	150	1
Arrowhead Quick Vegetable Herb	2 oz	150	1
Arrowhead Quick Wild Rice & Herb	2 oz	140	1
Pritikin Pilaf	½ cup	90	tr
Pritikin Spanish	½ cup	100	tr
S&W Quick Natural Long Grain	3.5 oz	110	0
S&W Quick Natural Long Grain, cooked	3.5 oz	119	0
long-grain, cooked	½ cup	109	tr

FOOD	PORTION	CALORIES	FAT
medium-grain, cooked	½ cup	109	tr
CANNED			
Ranch Style Spanish	7.5 oz	160	3
Van Camp's Spanish	1 cup	160	4
DRY MIX			
Chun King Entree Stir Fry	.25 oz	20	0
Kikkoman Fried Rice Seasoning Mix	1 oz pkg	91	tr
Knorr			
Risotto Milanese w/ Saffron	½ cup	130	3
Risotto Tomato	½ cup	110	tr
Risotto w/ Mushrooms	½ cup	110	tr
Risotto w/ Onion	½ cup	110	tr
Risotto w/ Peas & Corn	½ cup	110	1
La Choy Chinese Fried Rice	¾ cup	190	1
Lipton Rice & Sauce			
Almondine	½ cup	140	2
Beef	½ cup	124	tr
Chicken	½ cup	126	1
Florentine	½ cup	134	1
Herbs & Butter	½ cup	127	2
Long Grain & Wild Mushroom & Herb	½ cup	42	2
Long Grain & Wild Oriental	½ cup	121	tr
Medley	½ cup	124	tr
Mushroom	½ cup	123	tr
Oriental	½ cup	131	1
Spanish	½ cup	120	tr
With Peas	½ cup	128	1
With Vegetables, Broccoli & Cheddar	½ cup	128	2
Lipton Rice Asparagus w/ Hollandaise	½ cup	123	tr

FOOD	PORTION	CALORIES	FAT
Lipton Rice Salad Herbal Vinaigrette	½ cup	111	tr
Nile Spice Rozdali Spicy Currant	½ cup	161	4
Nile Spice Rozdali Vegetable Curry	½ cup	154	4
Rice-A-Roni			
Beef	½ cup	140	4
Beef & Mushroom	½ cup	150	3
Chicken	½ cup	150	3
Chicken & Broccoli	½ cup	150	3
Chicken & Mushroom	½ cup	180	7
Chicken & Vegetables	½ cup	140	3
Fried Rice	½ cup	110	5
Herb & Butter	½ cup	130	4
Long Grain & Wild, Chicken w/ Almonds	½ cup	140	4
Long Grain & Wild, Original	½ cup	130	3
Long Grain & Wild, Pilaf	½ cup	130	3
Pilaf	½ cup	150	4
Risotto	½ cup	200	6
Spanish	½ cup	150	4
Stroganoff	½ cup	200	8
Yellow Rice	½ cup	140	4
Ultra Slim-Fast Oriental Style	2.3 oz	240	1
Ultra Slim-Fast Rice & Chicken Sauce	2.3 oz	240	1
FROZEN			
Birds Eye			
International French Style	½ cup	106	tr
International Italian Style	½ cup	119	tr
International Spanish Style	½ cup	111	tr
Rice & Peas w/ Mushrooms	⅔ cup	108	tr
Budget Gourmet			
Oriental Rice w/ Vegetables	1 pkg	240	12

FOOD	PORTION	CALORIES	FAT
Rice Mexicana	1 pkg	240	9
Rice Pilaf w/ Green Beans	1 pkg	240	11
Green Giant			
Garden Gourmet Asparagus Pilaf	1 pkg	190	4
Garden Gourmet Sherry Wild Rice	1 pkg	210	4
One Serve Rice 'N Broccoli in Cheese Sauce	1 pkg	180	6
One Serve Rice, Peas & Mushrooms w/ Sauce	1 pkg	130	2
Rice Originals Italian Rice & Spinach in Cheese Sauce	½ cup	140	4
Rice Originals Pilaf	½ cup	110	1
Rice Originals Rice 'N Broccoli in Cheese Sauce	½ cup	120	4
Rice Originals Rice Medley	½ cup	100	1
Rice Originals White & Wild	½ cup	130	2
TAKE-OUT			
pilaf	½ cup	84	3
risotto	6.6 oz	426	18
spanish	¾ cup	363	27
WHITE			
General Foods Minute Rice, as prep	½ cup	164	5
Drumstick, as prep	½ cup	143	4
Long Grain & Wild, as prep	½ cup	149	5
Rib Roast, as prep	½ cup	152	4
S&W Long Grain, cooked	3.5 oz	106	0
Superfino Arborio Rice	½ cup	100	0
glutinous, cooked	½ cup	116	tr
long-grain, cooked	½ cup	131	tr
long-grain instant, cooked	½ cup	80	tr
long-grain parboiled, cooked	½ cup	100	tr
medium-grain, cooked	½ cup	132	tr

FOOD	PORTION	CALORIES	FAT
short-grain, cooked	½ cup	133	tr
starch	3.5 oz	343	0

RICE CAKES

7 Grain (Pritikin)	1	35	0
Plain (Pritikin)	1	35	0
Sesame (Pritikin)	1	35	0

ROCKFISH

FRESH

pacific, cooked	3 oz	103	2
pacific, cooked	1 fillet (5.2 oz)	180	3

ROE
(see also individual fish names)

baked	3 oz	173	7
baked	1 oz	58	2

ROLL
(see also BISCUIT, CROISSANT, ENGLISH MUFFIN, MUFFIN, SCONE)

FROZEN

All Butter Cinnamon Roll w/ Icing (Sara Lee)	1	280	11
All Butter Cinnamon Roll w/o Icing (Sara Lee)	1	230	11

HOME RECIPE

dinner	1 (1.2 oz)	120	3

MIX

Hot Roll Mix (Dromedary)	2	239	5
Hot Roll Mix (Pillsbury)	2	240	4

FOOD	PORTION	CALORIES	FAT
READY-TO-EAT			
Big Marty Poppy (Martin's)	1	170	2
Big Marty Sesame (Martin's)	1	170	2
Brown 'N Serve Club (Pepperidge Farm)	1	100	1
Brown 'N Serve French (Pepperidge Farm)	½ roll	180	2
Brown 'N Serve Hearth (Pepperidge Farm)	1	50	1
Buns (Wonder)	1	70	2
Dark Bread (Hollywood)	1	40	tr
Dinner (Pepperidge Farm)	1	60	2
Dinner (Roman Meal)	1	45	tr
Dinner Country Style Classic (Pepperidge Farm)	1	50	1
Dinner Light Pan Special Formula (Hollywood)	1	60	tr
Finger Poppy Seed (Pepperidge Farm)	1	50	2
Finger Sesame Seed (Pepperidge Farm)	1	60	2
Frankfurter (Country Kitchen)	1	120	2
Frankfurter Dijon (Pepperidge Farm)	1	160	5
Frankfurter Side Sliced (Pepperidge Farm)	1	140	3
Frankfurter Top Sliced (Pepperidge Farm)	1	140	3
Frankfurter w/ Poppy Seeds (Pepperidge Farm)	1	130	2
French Style (Pepperidge Farm)	1	100	1
Hamburger (Pepperidge Farm)	1	130	2
Hamburger (Roman Meal)	1	113	2
Hamburger (Shop 'n Save)	1	120	2

FOOD	PORTION	CALORIES	FAT
Hamburger Light (Wonder)	1	80	1
Heat & Serve Butter Crescent (Pepperidge Farm)	1	110	6
Heat & Serve Golden Twist (Pepperidge Farm)	1	110	5
Hoagie (Martin's)	1	240	3
Hoagie Sesame (Martin's)	1	240	3
Hoagie Soft (Pepperidge Farm)	1	210	5
Hotdog (Roman Meal)	1	104	2
Hotdog Light (Wonder)	1	80	1
Old Fashioned (Pepperidge Farm)	1	50	2
Parker House (Pepperidge Farm)	1	60	1
Party (Pepperidge Farm)	1	30	1
Potato Dinner (Martin's)	1	100	1
Potato Long (Martin's)	1	140	1
Potato Party (Martin's)	1	50	1
Potato Sandwich (Martin's)	1	140	1
Potato Sandwich (Pepperidge Farm)	1	160	4
Salad Roll (Matthew's)	1	110	2
Sandwich (Matthew's)	1	110	2
Sandwich Onion w/ Poppy Seeds (Pepperidge Farm)	1	150	3
Sandwich Salad (Pepperidge Farm)	1	110	4
Sandwich Whole Wheat 100% Stoneground (Martin's)	1	160	2
Sandwich w/ Sesame Seeds (Pepperidge Farm)	1	140	3
Sliced Light Special Formula (Hollywood)	1	80	tr
Soft Family (Pepperidge Farm)	1	100	2
Sourdough French (Pepperidge Farm)	1	100	1

FOOD	PORTION	CALORIES	FAT
dinner	1 (1 oz)	85	2
frankfurter	1 (8/pkg)	115	2
hamburger	1 (8/pkg)	115	2
hard	1	155	2
hot cross bun	1	202	4
submarine	1 (4.7 oz)	155	2
REFRIGERATED			
Pillsbury Best Quick Cinnamon w/ Icing	1	110	5
Pillsbury Butterflake	1	140	5
Pillsbury Crescent	1	100	6

ROSE APPLE
fresh	3.5 oz	32	tr

ROSE HIP
fresh	3.5 oz	91	0

ROSELLE
fresh	1 cup	28	tr

ROSEMARY
dried	1 tsp	4	tr

ROUGHY
orange, baked	3 oz	75	1

RUTABAGA
fresh, cooked, mashed	½ cup	41	tr
fresh, raw, cubed	½ cup	25	tr

FOOD	PORTION	CALORIES	FAT

SABLEFISH

FRESH

FOOD	PORTION	CALORIES	FAT
baked	.3 oz	213	17
fillet, baked	5.3 oz	378	30

SMOKED

FOOD	PORTION	CALORIES	FAT
sablefish	1 oz	72	6
sablefish	3 oz	218	17

SAFFLOWER
(see also OIL)

FOOD	PORTION	CALORIES	FAT
seeds, dried	1 oz	147	11

SAFFRON

FOOD	PORTION	CALORIES	FAT
saffron	1 tsp	2	tr

SAGE

FOOD	PORTION	CALORIES	FAT
ground	1 tsp	2	tr

SALAD
(see also PASTA SALAD)

TAKE-OUT

FOOD	PORTION	CALORIES	FAT
chef w/o dressing	1½ cup	386	28
tossed w/o dressing	1½ cup	32	tr
tossed w/o dressing	¾ cup	16	0
tossed w/o dressing w/ cheese & egg	1½ cup	102	6
tossed w/o dressing w/ chicken	1½ cup	105	2
tossed w/o dressing w/ pasta & seafood	1½ cup	380	21
tossed w/o dressing w/ shrimp	1½ cup	107	2
waldorf	½ cup	79	6

FOOD	PORTION	CALORIES	FAT

SALAD DRESSING

HOME RECIPE

FOOD	PORTION	CALORIES	FAT
french	1 tbsp	88	10
vinegar & oil	1 tbsp	72	8

MIX
Good Seasons

FOOD	PORTION	CALORIES	FAT
Bleu Cheese & Herbs	1 pkg	4	tr
Bleu Cheese & Herbs, as prep	1 tbsp	72	8
Buttermilk Farm, as prep	1 tbsp	58	6
Cheese Garlic, as prep	1 tbsp	72	8
Cheese Italian, as prep	1 tbsp	72	8
Classic Herb, as prep	1 tbsp	83	9
Garlic & Herbs, as prep	1 tbsp	84	9
Italian, as prep	1 tbsp	71	8
Italian Lite, as prep	1 tbsp	27	3
Italian No Oil, as prep	1 tbsp	7	tr
Lemon & Herbs, as prep	1 tbsp	83	9
Mild Italian, as prep	1 tbsp	73	8
Zesty Italian, as prep	1 tbsp	71	8
Zesty Italian Lite, as prep	1 tbsp	31	3

READY-TO-USE

FOOD	PORTION	CALORIES	FAT
Catalina	1 tbsp	15	1
Catalina French	1 tbsp	60	5
Diamond Crystal Blue Cheese	1 tbsp	20	1
Diamond Crystal Home Style	1 tbsp	20	1
Diamond Crystal Thousand Island	1 tbsp	20	1
Kraft Bacon & Tomato	1 tbsp	70	7
Kraft Bacon Creamy	1 tbsp	30	2
Kraft Blue Cheese Chunky	1 tbsp	60	6
Kraft Buttermilk Creamy	1 tbsp	80	8

FOOD	PORTION	CALORIES	FAT
Kraft Coleslaw	1 tbsp	70	6
Kraft Creamy Garlic	1 tbsp	50	5
Kraft Creamy Italian w/ Real Sour Cream	1 tbsp	50	5
Kraft Cucumber Creamy	1 tbsp	70	8
Kraft Free Catalina Nonfat	1 tbsp	16	0
Kraft Free French Nonfat	1 tbsp	26	0
Kraft Free Ranch Nonfat	1 tbsp	16	0
Kraft Free Thousand Island Nonfat	1 tbsp	20	0
Kraft French	1 tbsp	60	6
Kraft Golden Caesar	1 tbsp	70	7
Kraft House Italian	1 tbsp	60	3
Kraft Miracle French	1 tbsp	70	6
Kraft Oil & Vinegar	1 tbsp	70	7
Kraft Onion & Chives Creamy	1 tbsp	70	7
Kraft Presto Italian	1 tbsp	70	7
Kraft Red Wine Vinegar & Oil	1 tbsp	50	4
Kraft Russian Creamy	1 tbsp	60	5
Kraft Russian w/ Pure Honey	1 tbsp	60	5
Kraft Thousand Island	1 tbsp	60	5
Kraft Thousand Island & Bacon	1 tbsp	60	6
Kraft Zesty Italian	1 tbsp	50	5
Newman's Own Italian Light	1 tbsp	40	4
Newman's Own Olive Oil & Vinegar	1 tbsp	80	9
Ott's Famous Chef	1 tbsp	40	3
Ott's Italian Chef	1 tbsp	80	9
Seven Seas Buttermilk	1 tbsp	80	8
Seven Seas Buttermilk Ranch Light	1 tbsp	50	5
Seven Seas French Creamy	1 tbsp	60	6
Seven Seas French Light	1 tbsp	35	3

FOOD	PORTION	CALORIES	FAT
Seven Seas Herb & Spice	1 tbsp	60	6
Seven Seas Italian Creamy	1 tbsp	70	7
Seven Seas Thousand Island Creamy	1 tbsp	50	5
Seven Seas Thousand Island Light	1 tbsp	30	2
Seven Seas Free Ranch Nonfat	1 tbsp	16	0
Seven Seas Viva Herbs & Spices Light	1 tbsp	30	3
blue cheese	1 tbsp	77	8
french	1 tbsp	67	6
italian	1 tbsp	69	7
russian	1 tbsp	76	8
sesame seed	1 tbsp	68	7
thousand island	1 tbsp	59	6
READY-TO-USE REDUCED CALORIE			
Estee Blue Cheese	1 tbsp	8	tr
Estee Dijon Creamy	1 tbsp	8	tr
Estee French	1 tbsp	4	0
Estee Garlic Creamy	1 tbsp	2	0
Estee Italian Creamy	1 tbsp	4	0
Estee Thousand Island	1 tbsp	8	0
Herb Magic Vinaigrette	1 tbsp	6	0
Kraft Bacon & Tomato	1 tbsp	30	2
Kraft Buttermilk Creamy	1 tbsp	30	3
Kraft Chunky Blue Cheese	1 tbsp	30	2
Kraft Cucumber Creamy	1 tbsp	25	2
Kraft French	1 tbsp	20	1
Kraft Italian Creamy	1 tbsp	25	2
Kraft Russian	1 tbsp	30	1
Kraft Thousand Island	1 tbsp	20	1
Kraft Zesty Italian	1 tbsp	20	2

FOOD	PORTION	CALORIES	FAT
Magic Mountain Bleu Cheese	1 tbsp	5	tr
Magic Mountain French	1 tbsp	4	tr
Magic Mountain Herb & Spice No Oil	1 tbsp	2	tr
Magic Mountain Northern Italian	1 tbsp	2	tr
S&W Italian Creamy	1 tbsp	10	1
S&W Italian No-Oil	1 tbsp	2	0
Seven Seas Viva Free Italian Nonfat	1 tbsp	4	0
Ultra Slim-Fast French	1 tbsp	20	tr
Ultra Slim-Fast Italian	1 tbsp	6	tr
Ultra Slim-Fast Thousand Island	1 tbsp	18	tr
Walden Farms Italian No Sugar Added	1 tbsp	6	tr
Walden Farms Italian Sodium Free	1 tbsp	9	tr
Walden Farms Ranch	1 tbsp	35	2
Weight Watchers Italian	1 tbsp	6	tr
Weight Watchers Italian Creamy	1 tbsp	50	5
Weight Watchers Russian	1 tbsp	50	5
Weight Watchers Thousand Island	1 tbsp	50	5
Wishbone Ranch Lite	1 tbsp	42	4

SALMON

FOOD	PORTION	CALORIES	FAT
CANNED			
Alaksa Chum (Humpty Dumpty)	½ cup	140	2
Alaska Keta (Deming's)	½ cup	140	5
Alaska Pink (Deming's)	½ cup	140	6
Alaska Pink (Double J)	½ cup	140	6
Alaska Red Sockeye (Deming's)	½ cup	170	9
Bluepack Fancy Diet (S&W)	½ cup	188	11
Keta (Libby's)	½ can (3.8 oz)	140	6
Pink (Bumble Bee)	3 oz	137	7
Pink (Libby's)	½ can (3.8 oz)	150	7

FOOD	PORTION	CALORIES	FAT
Pink Skinless (Bumble Bee)	3.25 oz	120	5
Red (Bumble Bee)	3 oz	154	9
Red Fancy Sockeye Blueback (S&W)	½ cup	190	10
chum w/ bone	3 oz	120	5
chum w/ bone	1 can (13.9 oz)	521	20
pink w/ bone	3 oz	118	5
pink w/ bone	1 can (15.9 oz)	631	27
sockeye w/ bone	3 oz	130	6
sockeye w/ bone	1 can (12.9 oz)	566	27
FRESH			
atlantic, baked	3 oz	155	7
chinook, baked	3 oz	196	11
chum, baked	3 oz	131	4
coho, cooked	3 oz	157	6
coho, cooked	½ fillet (5.4 oz)	286	12
pink, baked	3 oz	127	4
sockeye, cooked	3 oz	183	9
sockeye, cooked	½ fillet (5.4 oz)	334	17
SMOKED			
chinook	3 oz	99	4
chinook	1 oz	33	1
TAKE-OUT			
salmon cake	1 (3 oz)	241	15

SALSA
(*see also* MEXICAN FOOD)

FOOD	PORTION	CALORIES	FAT
Chi Chi's Hot	1 oz	8	tr
Chi Chi's Medium	1 oz	8	0
Chi Chi's Mild	1 oz	9	tr
Ortega Hot Green Chili	1 tbsp	6	0
Ortega Medium Green Chili	1 tbsp	6	0
Ortega Mild Green Chili	1 tbsp	8	0

FOOD	PORTION	CALORIES	FAT
Rosarita Chunky Hot	3 tbsp	25	tr
Rosarita Chunky Medium	3 tbsp	25	tr
Rosarita Chunky Mild	3 tbsp	25	tr
Rosarita Taco Salsa Chunky Medium	3 tbsp	25	tr
Rosarita Taco Salsa Chunky Mild	3 tbsp	25	tr

SALSIFY

FOOD	PORTION	CALORIES	FAT
fresh, cooked, sliced	½ cup	46	tr
fresh, raw, sliced	½ cup	55	tr

SALT/SEASONED SALT
(see also SALT SUBSTITUTES)

FOOD	PORTION	CALORIES	FAT
Garlic (Morton	1 tsp	3	tr
Iodized (Morton)	1 tsp	tr	0
Kosher (Morton)	1 tsp	0	0
Lite (Morton)	1 tsp	tr	0
Nature's Seasons Seasoning Blend (Morton)	1 tsp	3	tr
Non-Iodized (Morton)	1 tsp	0	0
Seasoned (Morton)	1 tsp	4	tr
salt	1 tsp	0	0

SALT SUBSTITUTES

FOOD	PORTION	CALORIES	FAT
Estee Salt-It	⅛ tsp	0	0
Loma Linda Savorex	1 tsp	16	tr
Morton	1 tsp	tr	0
Morton Seasoned	1 tsp	2	tr
Nu-Salt	1 pkg (1g)	0	0
Papa Dash Lite Lite Lite Salt	¼ tsp	1	0
Papa Dash Salt Lover's Blend	¼ tsp	tr	0

FOOD	PORTION	CALORIES	FAT

SAPODILLA

FOOD	PORTION	CALORIES	FAT
fresh	1	140	2
fresh, cut up	1 cup	199	3

SAPOTES

FOOD	PORTION	CALORIES	FAT
fresh	1	301	1

SARDINES

CANNED

FOOD	PORTION	CALORIES	FAT
In Mustard Sauce (Port Clyde Foods)	1 can (3.75 oz)	175	11
In Soybean Oil (Port Clyde Foods)	1 can (3.75 oz)	225	18
In Tomato Sauce (Port Clyde Foods)	1 can (3.75 oz)	170	11
Norwegian Brisling (S&W)	1.5 oz	130	10
Skinless & Boneless Olive Oil (Empress)	1 can (3.8 oz)	420	38
Skinless & Boneless Soy Oil (Empress)	1 can (4.4 oz)	500	45
atlantic in oil w/ bone	2	50	3
atlantic in oil w/ bone	1 can (3.2 oz)	192	11
pacific in tomato sauce w/ bone	1	68	5
pacific in tomato sauce w/ bone	1 can (13 oz)	658	44

FRESH

FOOD	PORTION	CALORIES	FAT
raw	3.5 oz	135	5

SAUCE

(*see also* GRAVY, PIZZA, SPAGHETTI SAUCE, TOMATO)

DRY

FOOD	PORTION	CALORIES	FAT
Au Jus (Knorr)	2 oz	8	tr
Bar-B-Q (Diamond Crystal)	2 oz	35	1
Bearnaise (Knorr)	2 oz	170	17
Brown (Diamond Crystal)	2 oz	15	tr

FOOD	PORTION	CALORIES	FAT
Cheese (Diamond Crystal)	2 oz	50	2
Classic Brown Gravy (Knorr)	2 oz	25	1
Cream (Diamond Crystal)	2 oz	40	1
Demi-Glace (Knorr)	2 oz	30	1
Hollandaise (Knorr)	2 oz	170	18
Hunter (Knorr)	2 oz	25	tr
Italian (Diamond Crystal)	3 oz	50	tr
Lyonnaise (Knorr)	2 oz	20	tr
Marinade for Meat (Kikkoman)	1-oz pkg	64	tr
Mushroom (Knorr)	2 oz	60	3
Napoli (Knorr)	4 oz	100	3
Pepper (Knorr)	2 oz	20	1
Sweet & Sour (Kikkoman)	2.13-oz pkg	228	tr
Sweet 'N Sour Entree Mix (Chun King)	3.8 oz	370	0
Teriyaki (Kikkoman)	1.5-oz pkg	125	tr
bearnaise, as prep w/ milk & butter	1 cup	701	68
cheese, as prep w/ milk	1 cup	307	17
curry, as prep w/ milk	1 cup	270	15
mushroom, as prep w/ milk	1 cup	228	10
sour cream, as prep w/ milk	1 cup	509	30
stroganoff	1 cup	271	11
sweet & sour	1 cup	294	tr
teriyaki	1 cup	131	tr
white	1 cup	241	13
JARRED			
Bandito Diavalo Spicy (Newman's Own)	4 oz	70	2
Barbecue (Estee)	1 tbsp	18	tr
Barbecue (Kraft)	2 tbsp	45	1

FOOD	PORTION	CALORIES	FAT
Barbecue (Maull's)	3.5 oz	123	2
Barbecue (Ott's)	1 tbsp	14	tr
Barbecue Beer Non-Alcoholic (Maull's)	3.5 oz	128	2
Barbecue Country Style (Hunt's)	1 tbsp	20	tr
Barbecue Garlic (Kraft)	2 tbsp	40	0
Barbecue Hickory (Hunt's)	1 tbsp	20	tr
Barbecue Hickory Smoke (Kraft)	2 tbsp	45	1
Barbecue Homestyle (Hunt's)	1 tbsp	20	tr
Barbecue Kansas City Style (Hunt's)	1 tbsp	20	tr
Barbecue Mesquite Smoke (Kraft)	2 tbsp	45	1
Barbecue New Orleans Style (Hunt's)	1 tbsp	20	tr
Barbecue Original (Bull's Eye)	2 tbsp	50	0
Barbecue Original (Hunt's)	1 tbsp	20	tr
Barbecue Select (Heinz)	1 oz	40	0
Barbecue Select Hickory (Heinz)	1 oz	35	0
Barbecue Southern Style (Hunt's)	1 tbsp	20	tr
Barbecue Texas Style (Hunt's)	1 tbsp	25	tr
Barbecue Thick & Rich (Heinz)			
Cajun Style	1 oz	35	0
Chunky	1 oz	30	0
Hawaiian Style	1 oz	40	0
Hickory Smoke	1 oz	35	0
Mesquite Smoke	1 oz	30	0
Mushroom	1 oz	30	0
Old Fashioned	1 oz	35	0
Onion	1 oz	30	0
Original	1 oz	35	0
Texas Hot	1 oz	30	0

FOOD	PORTION	CALORIES	FAT
Barbecue Thick'n Spicy (Kraft)			
Kansas City Style	2 tbsp	60	1
Mesquite Smoke	2 tbsp	50	1
Original	2 tbsp	50	1
With Honey	2 tbsp	60	1
Barbecue Western Style (Hunt's)	1 tbsp	20	tr
Barbecue w/ Onion Bits (Maull's)	3.5 oz	126	2
Cajun Style (Golden Dipt)	1 oz	90	8
Chili 7 Spice Tabasco (McIlhenny)	4 oz	56	0
Cocktail (Sauceworks)	1 tbsp	14	0
Creole (Golden Dipt)	1 oz	20	1
Diable (Escoffier)	1 tbsp	20	0
Dijonnaise (Golden Dipt)	1 oz	52	4
Duck Sauce Sweet & Sour (La Choy)	1 tbsp	25	tr
Enchilada Sauce (Gebhardt)	3 tbsp	25	1
French White (Golden Dipt)	1 oz	55	4
Ginger Teriyaki Marinade (Golden Dipt)	1 oz	120	7
Grilling & Broiling Chardonnay (Knorr)	1.6 oz	50	4
Grilling & Broiling Spicy Plum (Knorr)	1.7 oz	60	2
Grilling & Broiling Tequilla Lime (Knorr)	1.6 oz	50	3
Grilling & Broiling Tuscan Herb (Knorr)	1.6 oz	50	4
Hot Dog (Wolf Brand)	1.25 oz	44	2
Hot Dog Chili Sauce (Gebhardt)	2 tbsp	30	1
Hot Dog Sauce (Just Rite)	2 oz	60	3
Hot Sauce (Gebhardt)	½ tsp	tr	tr
Lemon Butter Dill (Golden Dipt)	1 oz	100	9
Lemon Herb Marinade (Golden Dipt)	1 oz	130	14

FOOD	PORTION	CALORIES	FAT
Manwich Extra Thick & Chunky	2.5 oz	60	tr
Manwich Mexican	2.5 oz	35	1
Microwave Hollandaise (Knorr)	1 oz	50	5
Microwave Mandarin Ginger (Knorr)	1.6 oz	50	4
Microwave Parmesano (Knorr)	1.6 oz	50	4
Microwave Vera Cruz (Knorr)	3.3 oz	70	3
Newburg w/ Sherry (Snow's)	⅓ cup	120	8
Rib (Gold's)	1 oz	60	0
Seafood Cocktail (Golden Dipt)	1 tbsp	20	0
Seafood Cocktail Extra Hot (Golden Dipt)	1 tbsp	20	0
Sloppy Joe (Manwich)	2.5 oz	40	tr
Steak (Estee)	1 tbsp	14	0
Steak (Lea & Perrins)	1 oz	40	tr
Steak (Mrs. Dash)	1 tbsp	17	tr
Stir-Fry (Kikkoman)	1 tbsp	16	tr
Sweet & Sour (Kikkoman)	1 tbsp	19	tr
Sweet & Sour (La Choy)	1 tbsp	25	tr
Sweet 'N Sour (Contadina)	½ cup	150	3
Sweet 'N Sour (Sauceworks)	1 tbsp	25	0
Tabasco (McIlhenny)	¼ tsp	tr	tr
Tartar (Best Foods)	1 tbsp	70	8
Tartar (Bright Day)	1 tbsp	50	5
Tartar (Golden Dipt)	1 tbsp	70	7
Tartar (Hellman's)	1 tbsp	70	8
Tartar (Sauceworks)	1 tbsp	50	5
Tartar (Weight Watchers)	1 tbsp	35	3
Tartar Lite (Golden Dipt)	1 tbsp	50	4
Tartar Natural Lemon & Herb (Kraft)	1 tbsp	70	8
Teriyaki (Kikkoman)	1 tbsp	15	0

FOOD	PORTION	CALORIES	FAT
Welsh Rarebit Cheese (Snow's)	½ cup	170	11
Worcestershire (Heinz)	1 tbsp	6	0
Worcestershire (Lea & Perrins)	1 tsp	5	tr
Worcestershire White Wine (Lea & Perrins)	1 tsp	4	tr
barbecue	1 cup	188	5
teriyaki	1 tbsp	15	0

SAUERKRAUT

CANNED
Claussen	½ cup	17	tr
Libby	½ cup	20	0
S&W	½ cup	25	0
Seneca	½ cup	20	0
SnowFloss Kraut	4 oz	28	0
SnowFloss Kraut Bavarian Style	4 oz	64	0
Vlasic Old Fashioned	1 oz	4	0
canned	½ cup	22	tr

JUICE
S&W	4 oz	14	0

SAUSAGE

(*see also* HOT DOG, SAUSAGE DISHES, SAUSAGE SUBSTITUTES)

Bratwurst Smoked (Oscar Mayer)	1 (2.7 oz)	237	21
Breakfast Links Turkey, cooked (Perdue)	1 (1.3 oz)	40	3
Breakfast Patties Turkey, cooked (Perdue)	1 (1.3 oz)	61	4
Breakfast Sausage Turkey (Bil Mar Foods)	1 oz	58	4
Country Sausage Lower Salt (Armour)	1 oz	110	11

FOOD	PORTION	CALORIES	FAT
Country Sausage Lower Salt Links (Armour)	1 oz	110	11
Country Sausage Lower Salt Patties (Armour)	1.5 oz	160	16
Hot Italian Turkey, cooked (Perdue)	1 (2 oz)	94	6
Italian Smoked Cooked Cured (Oscar Mayer)	1 (2.6 oz)	264	24
Kielbasa (Oscar Mayer)	1 oz	83	8
Knockwurst (Hebrew National)	1 (3 oz)	260	25
Little Friers Pork, cooked (Oscar Mayer)	1 (.7 oz)	82	8
Polish (Oscar Mayer)	1 (2.7 oz)	229	20
Polish Kielbasa (Mr. Turkey)	3 oz	177	13
Pork Breakfast Patties (Jones)	1 (2 oz)	136	11
Pork Brown & Serve Links (Jones)	1 (.8 oz)	55	5
Pork Brown & Serve Patties (Jones)	1 (2 oz)	136	11
Pork Sausage (Armour)	1 oz	110	11
Pork Sausage Links (Armour)	1 oz	110	11
Pork Sausage Patties (Armour)	1.5 oz	160	16
Pork Light Breakfast Links (Jones)	1 (.8 oz)	55	5
Smoked (Oscar Mayer)	1 oz	83	8
Smoked Sausage (Bil Mar Foods)	3 oz	142	10
Smokies Beef (Oscar Mayer)	1 (1.5 oz)	123	11
Smokies Cheese (Oscar Mayer)	1 (1.5 oz)	127	11
Smokies Links (Oscar Mayer)	1 (1.5 oz)	124	11
Smokies Little (Oscar Mayer)	1 (.3 oz)	28	3
Sweet Italian Turkey, cooked (Perdue)	1 (2 oz)	94	6
blutwurst, uncooked	3.5 oz	424	39
bockwurst, pork & veal, raw	1 link (2.3 oz)	200	18
bratwurst pork, cooked	1 link (3 oz)	256	22

FOOD	PORTION	CALORIES	FAT
bratwurst pork & beef	1 link (2.5 oz)	226	19
country-style pork, cooked	1 link (½ oz)	48	4
country-style pork, cooked	1 patty (1 oz)	100	8
gelbwurst, uncooked	3.5 oz	363	33
italian pork, cooked	1 (3 oz)	268	21
italian pork, cooked	1 (2.4 oz)	216	17
kielbasa pork	1 oz	88	8
knockwurst pork & beef	1 oz	87	8
knockwurst pork & beef	1 (2.4 oz)	209	19
mettwurst, uncooked	3.5 oz	483	45
plockwurst, uncooked	3.5 oz	312	45
polish pork	1 oz	92	8
polish pork	1 (8 oz)	739	65
pork & beef, cooked	1 link (½ oz)	52	5
pork & beef, cooked	1 patty (1 oz)	107	10
pork, cooked	1 link (½ oz)	48	4
pork, cooked	1 patty (1 oz)	100	8
regensburger, uncooked	3.5 oz	354	31
smoked pork	1 sm link (½ oz)	62	5
smoked pork	1 link (2.4 oz)	265	22
smoked pork & beef	1 sm link (½ oz)	54	5
smoked pork & beef	1 link (2.4 oz)	229	21
smoked beef, cooked	1 (1.4 oz)	134	12
vienna, canned	1 (½ oz)	45	4
vienna, canned	7 (4 oz)	315	28
weisswurst, uncooked	3.5 oz	305	27
TAKE-OUT			
pork	1 link (½ oz)	48	4
pork	1 patty (1 oz)	100	8

FOOD	PORTION	CALORIES	FAT

SAUSAGE DISHES

FROZEN

FOOD	PORTION	CALORIES	FAT
Ovenstuffs French Roll Italian Sausage	1 (4.75 oz)	390	22
Ovenstuffs French Roll Pepperoni	1 (4.75 oz)	370	20
Sausage Biscuits Microwave (Jimmy Dean)	1	210	14

TAKE-OUT

FOOD	PORTION	CALORIES	FAT
sausage roll	1 (2.3 oz)	311	24

SAUSAGE SUBSTITUTES

FOOD	PORTION	CALORIES	FAT
Grillers, frzn (Morningstar Farms)	3.5 oz	290	19
Linketts (Loma Linda)	2 (2.6 oz)	150	8
Links, frzn (Morningstar Farms)	3.5 oz	237	18
Little Links (Loma Linda)	2 (1.6 oz)	80	5

SAVORY

FOOD	PORTION	CALORIES	FAT
ground	1 tsp	4	tr

SCALLOP

FOOD	PORTION	CALORIES	FAT
fresh, raw	3 oz	75	1

FROZEN

FOOD	PORTION	CALORIES	FAT
Fried (Mrs. Paul's)	2 oz	160	7
Lightly Breaded (King & Prince)	3.5 oz	120	tr

HOME RECIPE

FOOD	PORTION	CALORIES	FAT
breaded & fried	2 lg	67	3

TAKE-OUT

FOOD	PORTION	CALORIES	FAT
breaded & fried	6 (5 oz)	386	19

SCONE

HOME RECIPE

FOOD	PORTION	CALORIES	FAT
apricot scone	1	232	7

FOOD	PORTION	CALORIES	FAT
TAKE-OUT			
cheese	1 (1.75 oz)	182	9
fruit	1 (1.75 oz)	158	5
plain	1 (1.75 oz)	181	7

SCROD

FROZEN			
Microwave Entree Baked (Gorton's)	1 pkg	320	18
Ready-to-Bake (King & Prince)	5 oz	252	16

SCUP

fresh, baked	3 oz	115	3

SEA BASS
(see BASS)

SEA TROUT
(see TROUT)

SEAWEED

DRIED			
agar	1 oz	87	tr
FRESH			
agar	1 oz	tr	tr
irishmoss	1 oz	14	tr
kelp	1 oz	12	tr
kombu	1 oz	12	tr
laver	1 oz	10	tr
nori	1 oz	10	tr
spirulina	1 oz	7	tr
tangle	1 oz	12	tr
wakame	1 oz	13	tr

FOOD	PORTION	CALORIES	FAT
SEMOLINA			
dry	½ cup	303	tr
SESAME			
Sesame Butter (Erewhon)	2 tbsp	190	17
Sesame Seeds (Arrowhead)	1 oz	160	14
Sesame Tahini (Arrowhead)	1 oz	170	17
Sesame Tahini (Erewhon)	2 tbsp	200	18
seeds	1 tsp	16	2
seeds, dried	1 tbsp	52	5
seeds, dried	1 cup	825	72
seeds, roasted & toasted	1 oz	161	14
sesame butter	1 tbsp	95	8
tahini from roasted & toasted kernels	1 tbsp	89	8
tahini from stone ground kernels	1 tbsp	86	7
tahini from unroasted kernels	1 tbsp	85	8
SESBANIA			
flowers	1	1	0
flowers	1 cup	5	tr
flowers, cooked	1 cup	23	tr
SHAD			
american, baked	3 oz	214	15
roe, raw	3½ oz	130	2
SHALLOTS			
dried	1 tbsp	3	0
fresh, raw, chopped	1 tbsp	7	tr

FOOD	PORTION	CALORIES	FAT

SHARK

batter-dipped & fried	3 oz	194	12

SHEEPSHEAD FISH

cooked	3 oz	107	1
cooked	1 fillet (6.5 oz)	234	3

SHELLFISH
(*see individual names*, SHELLFISH SUBSTITUTES)

SHELLFISH SUBSTITUTES

Kibun Sea Pasta w/ dressing	½ pkg	220	7
Kibun Sea Pasta w/o dressing	½ pkg	110	1
Kibun Sea Pasta & Shrimp w/ dressing	½ pkg	210	9
Kibun Sea Pasta & Shrimp w/o dressing	½ pkg	140	1
Kibun Sea Stix Salad Style	4 oz	110	tr
Kibun Sea Stix Whole Leg	4 oz	110	tr
Kibun Sea Tails	4 oz	110	tr
Louis Kemp Crab Delights	2 oz	60	tr
SeaLegs Imitation Lobster Meat	3 oz	80	1
crab, imitation	3 oz	87	1
scallop, imitation	3 oz	84	tr
shrimp, imitation	3 oz	86	1
surimi	1 oz	28	tr
surimi	3 oz	84	1

SHELLIE BEANS

canned shellie beans	½ cup	37	tr

FOOD	PORTION	CALORIES	FAT

SHRIMP

CANNED

FOOD	PORTION	CALORIES	FAT
Canned Shrimp (Robinson)	2 oz	58	1
Deveined Medium Whole Shrimp (S&W)	2 oz	65	0
canned	3 oz	102	2
canned	1 cup	154	3

FRESH

FOOD	PORTION	CALORIES	FAT
cooked	4 large	22	tr
cooked	3 oz	84	1
raw	4 large	30	tr
raw	3 oz	90	1

FROZEN

FOOD	PORTION	CALORIES	FAT
Butterfly Shrimp (Gorton's)	4 oz	160	tr
Cooked in the Shell (King & Prince)	3.5 oz	65	tr
Cooked in the Shell (King & Prince)	4 oz	70	tr
Gourmet Hand Breaded Shrimp Butterfly (King & Prince)	3.5 oz	150	tr
Gourmet Hand Breaded Shrimp Round (King & Prince)	3.5 oz	150	tr
Light Seafood Entrees Shrimp & Clams w/ Linguini (Mrs. Paul's)	10 oz	240	5
Microwave Crunchy Shrimp (Gorton's)	5 oz	380	20
Microwave Entree Shrimp Scampi (Gorton's)	1 pkg	390	30
Shrimp a la Monterey (King & Prince)	2 oz	107	4
Shrimp a la Monterey (King & Prince)	3.5 oz	190	7
Shrimp Crisps (Gorton's)	4 oz	280	15
Shrimp Del Ray (King & Prince)	1.5 oz	43	3

FOOD	PORTION	CALORIES	FAT
Shrimp Del Ray (King & Prince)	3 oz	85	6
Supreme Hand Breaded Shrimp Butterfly (King & Prince)	3.5 oz	130	tr
Supreme Hand Breaded Shrimp Round (King & Prince)	3.5 oz	140	tr
Western Style Breaded Shrimp (King & Prince)	3.5 oz	115	tr
READY-TO-USE Fried Shrimp (American Original Foods)	4 oz	253	12
TAKE-OUT breaded & fried	4 large	73	4
breaded & fried	3 oz	206	10
breaded & fried	6–8 (6 oz)	454	25
jambalaya	¾ cup	188	5

SMELT

FOOD	PORTION	CALORIES	FAT
rainbow, cooked	3 oz	106	3

SNACKS

(*see also* CHIPS; FRUIT SNACKS; NUTS, MIXED; POPCORN; PRETZELS)

FOOD	PORTION	CALORIES	FAT
Apple Chips (Weight Watchers)	¾ oz	70	0
Carrot Lites (Health Valley)	½ oz	75	4
Cheddar Lites (Health Valley)	¼ oz	40	2
Cheddar Lites w/ Green Onion (Health Valley)	¼ oz	40	2
Cheese Balls (Lance)	1 oz	160	11
Cheese Balls (Lance)	1 pkg (1.13 oz)	190	13
Cheese Curls (Weight Watchers)	½ oz	70	2
Cheetos Crunchy Cheese	1 oz	160	10
Cheetos Puffed Balls Cheese	1 oz	160	10
Cheetos Puffs Cheese	1 oz	160	10

FOOD	PORTION	CALORIES	FAT
Cheez Doodles Crunchy	1 oz	160	10
Cheez Doodles Puffed	1 oz	150	9
Cheez Waffles	1 oz	140	8
Chex Snack Mix Barbeque Flavor	⅔ cup	130	5
Chex Snack Mix Cool Sour Cream & Onion	⅔ cup	130	5
Chex Snack Mix Golden Cheddar	⅔ cup	130	5
Chex Snack Mix Traditional	⅔ cup	120	5
Combos Cheddar	1.8 oz	240	9
Combos Nacho	1.8 oz	240	9
Combos Peanut Butter	1.8 oz	240	10
Combos Pizza	1.8 oz	240	9
Cornnuts Barbecue	1 oz	110	4
Cornnuts Nacho Cheese	1 oz	110	4
Cornnuts Original	1 oz	120	4
Cornnuts Unsalted	1 oz	120	4
Crunchy Cheese Twists (Lance)	1 oz	150	9
Crunchy Cheese Twists (Lance)	1 pkg (1.5 oz)	230	13
Doo Dads	1 oz	140	6
Easy Cheddar Nacho (Nabisco)	1 oz	80	6
Easy Cheese American (Nabisco)	1 oz	80	6
Easy Cheese Cheddar (Nabisco)	1 oz	80	6
Easy Cheese Cheese 'N Bacon (Nabisco)	1 oz	80	6
Easy Cheese Sharp Cheddar (Nabisco)	1 oz	80	6
Funyuns (Frito-Lay)	1 oz	140	6
Gold-N-Chee (Lance)	1 oz	130	6
Munchos	1 oz	150	9
Pork Skins (Lance)	½ oz	80	5
Tostada Nacho (Lance)	1 oz	140	7

FOOD	PORTION	CALORIES	FAT
Tostada Regular (Lance)	1 oz	150	8
Ultra Slim-Fast Lite N' Tasty Cheese Curls	1 oz	110	3
Wheat Snax (Estee)	1 oz	100	tr

SNAIL

FOOD	PORTION	CALORIES	FAT
fresh, cooked	3 oz	233	1

SNAP BEANS

FOOD	PORTION	CALORIES	FAT
CANNED			
green	½ cup	13	tr
green low sodium	½ cup	13	tr
italian	½ cup	13	tr
italian low sodium	½ cup	13	tr
yellow	½ cup	13	tr
yellow low sodium	½ cup	13	tr
FRESH			
green, cooked	½ cup	22	tr
green, raw	½ cup	17	tr
yellow, cooked	½ cup	22	tr
yellow, raw	½ cup	17	tr
FROZEN			
green, cooked	½ cup	18	tr
italian, cooked	½ cup	18	tr
yellow, cooked	½ cup	18	tr

SNAPPER

FOOD	PORTION	CALORIES	FAT
fresh, cooked	3 oz	109	1
fresh, cooked	1 fillet (6 oz)	217	3

FOOD	PORTION	CALORIES	FAT

SODA
(*see also* DRINK MIXER)

FOOD	PORTION	CALORIES	FAT
7Up	1 oz	12	0
7Up Cherry	1 oz	13	0
7Up Cherry Diet	1 oz	tr	0
7Up Diet	1 oz	tr	0
7Up Gold	1 oz	13	0
7Up Gold Diet	1 oz	tr	0
Coca-Cola	6 oz	77	0
Coca-Cola Caffeine-Free	6 oz	77	0
Coca-Cola Cherry	6 oz	76	0
Coca-Cola Classic	6 oz	72	0
Coca-Cola Diet Cherry	6 oz	tr	0
Crush Apple	6 oz	90	0
Crush Apple Diet	6 oz	10	0
Crush Cherry	6 oz	100	0
Crush Grape	6 oz	100	0
Crush Orange	6 oz	100	0
Crush Orange Diet	6 oz	12	0
Crush Pineapple	6 oz	100	0
Crush Strawberry	6 oz	90	0
Crystal Geyer Mountain Spring Sparkler			
Cranberry Raspberry	6 oz	65	0
Black Cherry	6 oz	65	0
Kiwi Lemon	6 oz	65	0
Peach	6 oz	65	0
Vanilla Creme	6 oz	65	0
Diet Coke	6 oz	tr	0
Diet Coke Caffeine-Free	6 oz	tr	0
Dr Pepper	1 oz	13	0

FOOD	PORTION	CALORIES	FAT
Dr Pepper Diet	1 oz	tr	0
Fanta Ginger Ale	6 oz	63	0
Fanta Grape	6 oz	86	0
Fanta Orange	6 oz	88	0
Fanta Root Beer	6 oz	78	0
Fresca	6 oz	2	0
Health Valley Ginger Ale	12 oz	153	1
Health Valley Rootbeer Old Fashioned	12 oz	120	1
Health Valley Sarsaparilla Rootbeer	12 oz	153	1
Health Valley Wild Berry	12 oz	142	1
Hires Root Beer	6 oz	90	0
Hires Root Beer Sugar-Free	6 oz	2	0
Jolt	12 oz	167	0
Like Cola	1 oz	13	0
Like Cola Sugar Free	1 oz	tr	0
Lucozade	7 oz	136	0
Manischewitz Seltzer No Salt Added No Calories	8 oz	0	0
Mello Yellow	6 oz	87	0
Minute Maid Lemon-Lime	6 oz	71	0
Minute Maid Lemon-Lime Diet	6 oz	10	0
Minute Maid Orange	6 oz	87	0
Minute Maid Orange Diet	6 oz	4	0
Mr. PIBB	6 oz	71	0
Orangina	9 oz	150	tr
Pepper Free	1 oz	12	0
Pepper Free Diet	1 oz	tr	0
Ramblin' Root Beer	6 oz	88	0
Schweppes Club	6 oz	0	0

FOOD	PORTION	CALORIES	FAT
Schweppes Ginger Ale	6 oz	63	0
Schweppes Ginger Ale Diet	6 oz	tr	0
Schweppes Ginger Beer	6 oz	68	0
Schweppes Grape	6 oz	92	0
Schweppes Grapefruit	6 oz	77	0
Schweppes Lemon Lime	6 oz	71	0
Schweppes Root Beer	6 oz	75	0
Schweppes Seltzer	6 oz	0	0
Schweppes Seltzer, Flavored	6 oz	0	0
Schweppes Sparkling Orange	6 oz	86	0
Shasta Birch Beer Diet	12 oz	4	0
Shasta Black Cherry	12 oz	162	0
Shasta Cherry Cola	12 oz	140	0
Shasta Citrus Mist	12 oz	170	0
Shasta Club	12 oz	0	0
Shasta Cola	8 oz	98	0
Shasta Cola	12 oz	147	0
Shasta Cola Diet	8 oz	0	0
Shasta Collins	12 oz	118	0
Shasta Creme	12 oz	154	0
Shasta Dr. Diablo	12 oz	140	0
Shasta Free Cola	12 oz	151	0
Shasta Fruit Punch	12 oz	173	0
Shasta Ginger Ale	8 oz	80	0
Shasta Ginger Ale	12 oz	120	0
Shasta Ginger Ale Diet	8 oz	0	0
Shasta Grape	12 oz	177	0
Shasta Lemon Lime	8 oz	97	0
Shasta Lemon Lime	12 oz	146	0
Shasta Lemon Lime Diet	8 oz	0	0

FOOD	PORTION	CALORIES	FAT
Shasta Orange	12 oz	177	0
Shasta Red Berry	12 oz	158	0
Shasta Red Pop	12 oz	158	0
Shasta Root Beer	12 oz	154	0
Shasta Strawberry	12 oz	147	0
Shasta Tonic Water	12 oz	0	0
Sprite	6 oz	71	0
Sprite Diet	6 oz	2	0
Sun-Drop	6 oz	90	0
Sun-Drop Diet	6 oz	4	0
TAB	6 oz	tr	0
TAB Caffeine-Free	6 oz	tr	0
Welch's Sparkling Apple	12 oz	180	0
Welch's Sparkling Grape	12 oz	180	0
Welch's Sparkling Orange	12 oz	180	0
Welch's Strawberry Sparkling	12 oz	180	0
club	12 oz	0	0
cola	12 oz	151	tr
cream	12 oz	191	0
diet cola	12 oz	2	0
diet cola w/ Nutrasweet	12 oz	2	0
diet cola w/ saccharin	12 oz	2	0
ginger ale	12 oz	124	0
grape	12 oz	161	0
lemon lime	12 oz	149	0
orange	12 oz	177	0
pepper type	12 oz	151	tr
quinine	12 oz	125	0
root beer	12 oz	152	0
tonic water	12 oz	125	0

FOOD	PORTION	CALORIES	FAT

SOLE

FRESH

raw	3.5 oz	90	1
w/ lemon, raw	3.5 oz	85	1

FROZEN

A La Monterey (King & Prince)	6 oz	221	13
Fishmarket Fresh (Gorton's)	5 oz	110	1
Light Fillets (Mrs. Paul's)	1 fillet	240	10
Lightly Breaded (Van De Kamp's)	5 oz	293	18
Microwave Lightly Breaded (Van De Kamp's)	5 oz	290	18
Microwave Entree in Lemon Butter (Gorton's)	1 pkg	380	24
Microwave Entree in Wine Sauce (Gorton's)	1 pkg	180	8
Today's Catch Baby Sole (Van De Kamp's)	5 oz	100	1

SORGHUM

sorghum	½ cup	325	3

SOUFFLE

HOME RECIPE

cheese	3.5 oz	253	20
cheese	1 cup	308	25
grand marnier	1 cup	109	4
lemon, chilled	1 cup	176	tr
raspberry, chilled	1 cup	173	tr
spinach	1 cup	218	18

FOOD	PORTION	CALORIES	FAT

SOUP

CANNED

FOOD	PORTION	CALORIES	FAT
Bean & Ham (Healthy Choice)	½ can (7.5 oz)	220	4
Bean & Ham Home Cookin' (Campbell)	10.75 oz	210	4
Bean Homestyle, as prep (Campbell)	8 oz	130	1
Bean w/ Bacon, as prep (Campbell)	8 oz	140	4
Bean w/ Bacon Healthy Request, as prep (Campbell)	8 oz	140	4
Beef, as prep (Campbell)	8 oz	80	2
Beef Broth (College Inn)	½ can (7 oz)	16	0
Beef Broth (Health Valley)	7.5 oz	10	tr
Beef Broth (Pritikin)	6.88 oz	20	tr
Beef Broth (Swanson)	7.25 oz	18	1
Beef Broth, as prep (Campbell)	8 oz	16	0
Beef Broth No Salt Added (Health Valley)	7.5 oz	10	tr
Beef Chunky Ready-to-Serve (Campbell)	10.75 oz	200	5
Beef Noodle, as prep (Campbell)	8 oz	70	3
Beef Noodle Homestyle, as prep (Campbell)	8 oz	80	4
Beef Stroganoff Style Chunky Ready-to-Serve (Campbell)	10.75 oz	320	16
Beef w/ Vegetables & Pasta Home Cookin' (Campbell)	10.75 oz	140	2
Beefy Mushroom, as prep (Campbell)	8 oz	60	3
Beefy Noodle Soup w/ Vegetables, Hearty (Lipton)	8 oz	85	tr
Black Bean (Goya)	7.5 oz	160	4
Black Bean (Health Valley)	7.5 oz	150	2

FOOD	PORTION	CALORIES	FAT
Black Bean No Salt Added (Health Valley)	7.5 oz	150	2
Borscht (Gold's)	8 oz	100	0
Borscht Lo-Cal (Gold's)	8 oz	20	tr
Borscht Low Calorie (Manischewitz)	8 oz	20	0
Borscht w/ Beets (Manischewitz)	8 oz	80	0
Cheddar Cheese, as prep (Campbell)	8 oz	110	6
Chicken Alphabet, as prep (Campbell)	8 oz	80	3
Chicken & Stars, as prep (Campbell)	8 oz	60	2
Chicken Barley, as prep (Campbell)	8 oz	70	2
Chicken Broth (College Inn)	½ can (7 oz)	35	3
Chicken Broth (Health Valley)	7.5 oz	35	2
Chicken Broth (Pritikin)	6.86 oz	14	0
Chicken Broth (Swanson)	7.25 oz	30	2
Chicken Broth, as prep (Campbell)	8 oz	30	2
Chicken Broth & Noodles, as prep (Campbell)	8 oz	45	1
Chicken Broth Healthy Request Ready-to-Serve (Campbell)	8 oz	10	0
Chicken Broth Low Sodium Ready-to-Serve (Campbell)	10.5 oz	30	1
Chicken Broth Lower Salt (College Inn)	½ can (7 oz)	20	2
Chicken Broth No Salt Added (Health Valley)	7.5 oz	35	2
Chicken Corn Chowder Chunky Ready-to-Serve (Campbell)	10.75 oz	340	21
Chicken Gumbo (Pritikin)	7.38 oz	60	1
Chicken Gumbo, as prep (Campbell)	8 oz	60	2
Chicken Gumbo w/ Sausage Home Cookin' (Campbell)	10.75 oz	140	4

FOOD	PORTION	CALORIES	FAT
Chicken Minestrone Home Cookin' (Campbell)	10.75 oz	180	6
Chicken Mushroom Creamy, as prep (Campbell)	8 oz	120	8
Chicken 'N Dumplings, as prep (Campbell)	8 oz	80	3
Chicken Noodle (Weight Watchers)	10.5 oz	80	2
Chicken Noodle, as prep (Campbell)	8 oz	60	2
Chicken Noodle Chunky Ready-to-Serve (Campbell)	10.75 oz	200	7
Chicken Noodle Healthy Request (Campbell)	8 oz	60	2
Chicken Noodle, Hearty (Lipton)	8 oz	79	1
Chicken Noodle Homestyle, as prep (Campbell)	8 oz	70	3
Chicken Noodle-O's, as prep (Campbell)	8 oz	70	2
Chicken Nuggets w/ Vegetables & Noodles Chunky Ready-to-Serve (Campbell)	10.75 oz	190	6
Chicken Rice Home Cookin' (Campbell)	10.75 oz	150	6
Chicken Vegetable (Pritikin)	7.25 oz	70	tr
Chicken Vegetable, as prep (Campbell)	8 oz	70	3
Chicken Vegetable Beef Low Sodium Ready-to-Serve (Campbell)	10.75 oz	180	5
Chicken Vegetable Chunky Ready-to-Serve (Campbell)	9.5 oz	170	6
Chicken w/ Ribbon Pasta (Pritikin)	7.25 oz	60	tr
Chicken w/ Noodles Home Cookin' (Campbell)	10.75 oz	140	4
Chicken w/ Noodles Low Sodium Ready-to-Serve (Campbell)	10.75 oz	170	5
Chicken w/ Rice (Healthy Choice)	½ can (7.5 oz)	140	4

FOOD	PORTION	CALORIES	FAT
Chicken w/ Rice, as prep (Campbell)	8 oz	60	3
Chicken w/ Rice Chunky Ready-to-Serve (Campbell)	9.5 oz	140	4
Chicken w/ Rice Healthy Request (Campbell)	8 oz	60	3
Chili Beef, as prep (Campbell)	8 oz	140	5
Chili Beef Chunky Ready-to-Serve (Campbell)	11 oz	290	7
Chunky Beef Vegetable (Healthy Choice)	½ can (7.5 oz)	110	1
Chunky Chicken Noodle & Vegetable (Healthy Choice)	½ can (7.5 oz)	160	4
Chunky Chicken Vegetable (Health Valley)	7.5 oz	125	2
Chunky Five Bean Vegetable (Health Valley)	7.5 oz	110	2
Chunky Five Bean Vegetable No Salt Added (Health Valley)	7.5 oz	110	2
Chunky Vegetable Chicken No Salt Added (Health Valley)	7.5 oz	125	2
Clam Chowder Manhattan Style, as prep (Campbell)	8 oz	70	2
Clam Chowder Manhattan Style Chunky Ready-to-Serve (Campbell)	10.75 oz	160	4
Clam Chowder New England, as prep (Campbell)	8 oz	80	3
Clam Chowder New England, as prep w/ whole milk (Campbell)	8 oz	150	7
Clam Chowder New England Chunky Ready-to-Serve (Campbell)	10.75 oz	290	17
Consomme, as prep (Campbell)	8 oz	25	0
Country Vegetable (Healthy Choice)	½ can (7.5 oz)	120	1
Country Vegetable Home Cookin' (Campbell)	10.75 oz	120	2
Cream of Asparagus, as prep (Campbell)	8 oz	80	4

FOOD	PORTION	CALORIES	FAT
Cream of Broccoli, as prep (Campbell)	8 oz	80	5
Cream of Broccoli, as prep w/ 2% milk (Campbell)	8 oz	140	7
Cream of Celery, as prep (Campbell)	8 oz	100	7
Cream of Chicken, as prep (Campbell)	8 oz	110	7
Cream of Chicken Healthy Request (Campbell)	8 oz	70	2
Cream of Mushroom (Weight Watchers)	10.5 oz	90	2
Cream of Mushroom, as prep (Campbell)	8 oz	100	7
Cream of Mushroom Healthy Request, as prep (Campbell)	8 oz	60	2
Cream of Mushroom Low Sodium Ready-to-Serve (Campbell)	10.5 oz	210	14
Cream of Onion, as prep (Campbell)	8 oz	100	5
Cream of Onion, as prep w/ whole milk & water (Campbell)	8 oz	140	7
Cream of Potato, as prep (Campbell)	8 oz	80	3
Cream of Potato, as prep w/ whole milk & water (Campbell)	8 oz	120	4
Cream of Shrimp, as prep (Campbell)	8 oz	90	6
Cream of Shrimp, as prep w/ whole milk & water (Campbell)	8 oz	160	10
Cream of Tomato Homestyle, as prep (Campbell)	8 oz	110	3
Creamy Chicken Mushroom Chunky Ready-to-Serve (Campbell)	10.5 oz	270	19
Creole Style Chunky Ready-to-Serve (Campbell)	10.75 oz	240	8
Curly Noodle w/ Chicken, as prep (Campbell)	8 oz	80	3

FOOD	PORTION	CALORIES	FAT
French Onion, as prep (Campbell)	8 oz	60	2
Green Pea, as prep (Campbell)	8 oz	160	3
Green Split Pea (Health Valley)	7.5 oz	180	tr
Green Split Pea No Salt Added (Health Valley)	7.5 oz	180	tr
Ham 'N Butter Bean Chunky Ready-to-Serve (Campbell)	10.75 oz	280	10
Hearty Beef (Healthy Choice)	½ can (7.5 oz)	120	2
Hearty Chicken (Healthy Choice)	½ can (7.5 oz)	150	5
Hearty Chicken Noodle Healthy Request Ready-to-Serve (Campbell)	8 oz	80	2
Hearty Chicken Rice Healthy Request Ready-to-Serve (Campbell)	8 oz	110	2
Hearty Lentil Home Cookin' (Campbell)	10.75 oz	170	2
Hearty Minestrone Healthy Request Ready-to-Serve (Campbell)	8 oz	90	3
Hearty Vegetable Beef Healthy Request Ready-to-Serve (Campbell)	8 oz	120	3
Hearty Vegetable Healthy Request Ready-to-Serve (Campbell)	8 oz	110	3
Lentil (Health Valley)	7.5 oz	220	4
Lentil (Pritikin)	7.38 oz	100	0
Lentil No Salt Added	7.5 oz	220	4
Manhattan Clam Chowder (Health Valley)	7.5 oz	110	2
Manhattan Clam Chowder (Pritikin)	7.38 oz	70	tr
Manhattan Clam Chowder, as prep w/ water (Snow's)	7.5 oz	70	2
Manhattan Clam Chowder No Salt Added (Health Valley)	7.5 oz	110	2
Mediterranean Vegetable Chunky Ready-to-Serve (Campbell)	9.5 oz	170	6
Minestrone (Health Valley)	7.5 oz	130	3

FOOD	PORTION	CALORIES	FAT
Minestrone (Healthy Choice)	½ can (7.5 oz)	160	2
Minestrone (Pritikin)	7.38 oz	110	tr
Minestrone, as prep (Campbell)	8 oz	80	2
Minestrone Chunky Ready-to-Serve (Campbell)	9.5 oz	160	4
Minestrone Home Cookin' (Campbell)	10.75 oz	140	3
Minestrone No Salt Added (Health Valley)	7.5 oz	130	3
Mushroom (Pritikin)	7.38 oz	60	tr
Mushroom Barley (Health Valley)	7.5 oz	100	2
Mushroom Barley No Salt Added (Health Valley)	7.5 oz	100	2
Mushroom Golden, as prep (Campbell)	8 oz	70	3
Nacho Cheese, as prep (Campbell)	8 oz	110	8
Nacho Cheese, as prep w/ milk (Campbell)	8 oz	180	12
Natural Goodness Clear Chicken Broth (Swanson)	7.5 oz	20	1
Navy Bean (Pritikin)	7.38 oz	130	tr
New England Chowder (American Original Foods)	4 oz	64	1
New England Chowder, as prep w/ milk (American Original Foods)	4 oz	145	6
New England Clam Chowder (Pritikin)	7.38 oz	118	tr
New England Clam Chowder, as prep w/ milk (Snow's)	7.5 oz	140	6
New England Clam Chowder, as prep w/ whole milk (Gorton's)	¼ can	140	5
New England Corn Chowder, as prep w/ milk (Snow's)	7.5 oz	150	6

FOOD	PORTION	CALORIES	FAT
New England Fish Chowder, as prep w/ milk (Snow's)	7.5 oz	130	6
New England Seafood Chowder, as prep w/ milk (Snow's)	7.5 oz	130	6
Noodles & Ground Beef, as prep (Campbell)	8 oz	90	4
Old Fashioned Bean w/ Ham Chunky Ready-to-Serve (Campbell)	11 oz	290	9
Old Fashioned Chicken Chunky Ready-to-Serve (Campbell)	10.75 oz	180	5
Old Fashioned Chicken Noodle (Healthy Choice)	½ can (7.5 oz)	90	3
Old Fashioned Vegetable Beef Chunky Ready-to-Serve (Campbell)	10.75 oz	190	6
Oyster Stew, as prep (Campbell)	8 oz	70	5
Oyster Stew, as prep w/ whole milk (Campbell)	8 oz	140	9
Pepper Pot, as prep (Campbell)	8 oz	90	4
Pepper Steak Chunky Ready-to-Serve (Campbell)	10.75 oz	180	3
Potato Leek (Health Valley)	7.5 oz	130	2
Potato Leek No Salt Added (Health Valley)	7.5 oz	130	2
Schav (Gold's)	8 oz	25	0
Schav (Manischewitz)	1 cup	11	tr
Scotch Broth, as prep (Campbell)	8 oz	80	3
Seafood, Spicy (Port Clyde Foods)	7.5 oz	68	1
Sirloin Burger Chunky Ready-to-Serve (Campbell)	10.75 oz	220	9
Split Pea (Pritikin)	7.5 oz	130	tr
Split Pea & Ham (Healthy Choice)	½ can (7.5 oz)	170	3
Split Pea Low Sodium Ready-to-Serve (Campbell)	10.75 oz	230	4

FOOD	PORTION	CALORIES	FAT
Split Pea w/ Bacon, as prep (Campbell)	8 oz	160	4
Split Pea w/ Ham Chunky Ready-to-Serve (Campbell)	10.75 oz	230	6
Split Pea w/ Ham Home Cookin' (Campbell)	10.75 oz	230	1
Steak & Potato Chunky Ready-to-Serve (Campbell)	10.75 oz	200	5
Teddy Bear, as prep (Campbell)	8 oz	70	2
Tomato (Health Valley)	7.5 oz	130	3
Tomato, as prep (Campbell)	8 oz	90	2
Tomato, as prep w/ 2% milk (Campbell)	8 oz	150	4
Tomato Bisque, as prep (Campbell)	8 oz	120	3
Tomato Garden (Healthy Choice)	½ can (7.5 oz)	130	3
Tomato Garden Home Cookin' (Campbell)	10.75 oz	150	3
Tomato Healthy Request, as prep (Campbell)	8 oz	90	2
Tomato Healthy Request, as prep w/ Skim Milk (Campbell)	8 oz	130	2
Tomato No Salt Added (Health Valley)	7.5 oz	130	3
Tomato Rice Old Fashioned, as prep (Campbell)	8 oz	110	2
Tomato w/ Tomato Pieces (Pritikin)	7.5 oz	70	0
Tomato w/ Tomato Pieces Low Sodium Ready-to-Serve (Campbell)	10.5 oz	190	6
Tomato Zesty, as prep (Campbell)	8 oz	100	2
Turkey Noodle, as prep (Campbell)	8 oz	70	2
Turkey Vegetable, as prep (Campbell)	8 oz	70	3
Turkey Vegetable Chunky Ready-to-Serve (Campbell)	9.38 oz	150	6

FOOD	PORTION	CALORIES	FAT
Turkey Vegetable w/ Ribbon Pasta (Pritikin)	7.38 oz	50	tr
Vegetable (Health Valley)	7.5 oz	110	1
Vegetable (Pritikin)	7.38 oz	70	0
Vegetable, as prep (Campbell)	8 oz	90	2
Vegetable Beef (Healthy Choice)	½ can (7.5 oz)	130	1
Vegetable Beef, as prep (Campbell)	8 oz	70	2
Vegetable Beef Healthy Request, as prep (Campbell)	8 oz	70	2
Vegetable Chunky Ready-to-Serve (Campbell)	10.75 oz	160	4
Vegetable Healthy Request, as prep (Campbell)	8 oz	90	2
Vegetable Homestyle, as prep (Campbell)	8 oz	60	2
Vegetable No Salt Added (Health Valley)	7.5 oz	110	1
Vegetable Beef Home Cookin' (Campbell)	10.75 oz	140	3
Vegetable Old Fashioned, as prep (Campbell)	8 oz	60	2
Vegetarian Vegetable, as prep (Campbell)	8 oz	80	2
Won Ton, as prep (Campbell)	8 oz	40	1
asparagus, cream of, as prep w/ milk	1 cup	161	8
asparagus, cream of, as prep w/ water	1 cup	87	4
beef broth, ready-to-serve	1 cup	16	1
beef noodle, as prep w/ water	1 cup	84	3
black bean, as prep w/ water	1 cup	116	2
black bean turtle soup	1 cup	218	1
celery, cream of, as prep w/ milk	1 cup	165	10

FOOD	PORTION	CALORIES	FAT
celery, cream of, as prep w/ water	1 cup	90	6
cheese, as prep w/ milk	1 cup	230	15
cheese, as prep w/ water	1 cup	155	10
chicken broth, as prep w/ water	1 cup	39	1
chicken, cream of, as prep w/ milk	1 cup	191	11
chicken, cream of, as prep w/ water	1 cup	116	7
chicken gumbo, as prep w/ water	1 cup	56	1
chicken noodle, as prep w/ water	1 cup	75	2
chicken rice, as prep w/ water	1 cup	251	2
chicken vegetable, as prep w/ water	1 cup	74	3
clam chowder, Manhattan, as prep w/ water	1 cup	77	2
clam chowder, New England, as prep w/ milk	1 cup	163	7
clam chowder, New England, as prep w/ water	1 cup	95	3
consomme w/ gelatin, as prep w/ water	1 cup	29	0
escarole, ready-to-serve	1 cup	27	2
french onion, as prep w/ water	1 cup	57	2
gazpacho, ready-to-serve	1 cup	57	2
minestrone, as prep w/ water	1 cup	83	3
mushroom, cream of, as prep w/ milk	1 cup	203	14
mushroom, cream of, as prep w/ water	1 cup	129	9
oyster stew, as prep w/ milk	1 cup	134	8
oyster stew, as prep w/ water	1 cup	59	4
pepperpot, as prep w/ water	1 cup	103	5
potato, cream of, as prep w/ milk	1 cup	148	6
potato, cream of, as prep w/ water	1 cup	73	2
scotch broth, as prep w/ water	1 cup	80	3

FOOD	PORTION	CALORIES	FAT
split pea w/ ham, as prep w/ water	1 cup	189	4
tomato, as prep w/ milk	1 cup	160	6
tomato, as prep w/ water	1 cup	86	2
vegetarian vegetable, as prep w/ water	1 cup	72	2
vichyssoise	1 cup	148	6
DRY			
Asparagus, as prep (Knorr)	8 oz	80	3
Bean w/ Bacon 'N Ham Microwave Soup (Campbell)	7.5 oz	230	5
Beef, as prep (Diamond Crystal)	6 oz	30	1
Beef Bouillon, as prep w/ water (Knorr)	8 oz	15	1
Beef Bouillon Instant (Wylers)	1 tsp	6	tr
Beef Bouillon Instant Cube (Wylers)	1	6	tr
Beef Bouillon Instant Low Sodium (Lite Line)	1 tsp	12	tr
Beef Broth Instant (Weight Watchers)	1 pkg	8	0
Beef Flavor Bouillon, as prep (Diamond Crystal)	6 oz	17	tr
Beef Flavor Low Fat Ramen Noodle, as prep	8 oz	160	1
Beef Flavor Noodle Campbell's Cup	1 (1.35 oz)	130	2
Beef Flavor Ramen Noodle, as prep	8 oz	190	8
Beef Flavor w/ Vegetables Cup-A-Ramen, as prep	8 oz	270	10
Beef Flavor w/ Vegetables Low Fat Cup-A-Ramen, as prep	8 oz	220	2
Beef Mushroom (Lipton)	8 oz	38	1
Beef Noodle (Ultra Slim-Fast)	6 oz	45	tr
Beefy Onion (Lipton)	8 oz	27	1

FOOD	PORTION	CALORIES	FAT
Broth & Brown Seasoning (George Washington)	1 serving	6	0
Broth & Golden Seasoning (George Washington)	1 serving	6	0
Broth & Onion Seasoning (George Washington)	1 serving	12	0
Broth & Vegetable Seasoning (George Washington)	1 serving	12	0
Cauliflower, as prep (Knorr)	8 oz	100	3
Chick 'N Pasta, as prep (Knorr)	8 oz	90	2
Chicken, as prep (Diamond Crystal)	6 oz	30	1
Chicken Bouillon, as prep w/ water (Knorr)	8 oz	16	1
Chicken Bouillon Instant (Wylers)	1 tsp	8	tr
Chicken Bouillon Instant Cube (Wylers)	1	8	tr
Chicken Bouillon Instant Low Sodium (Lite Line)	1 tsp	12	tr
Chicken Broth Instant (Weight Watchers)	1 pkg	8	0
Chicken Flavor Bouillon, as prep (Diamond Crystal)	6 oz	20	1
Chicken Flavor Low Fat Ramen Noodle, as prep	8 oz	160	1
Chicken Flavor Noodle Campbell's Cup	1 (1.35 oz)	140	3
Chicken Flavor Ramen Noodle, as prep	8 oz	190	8
Chicken Flavor w/ Vegetables Cup-A-Ramen, as prep	8 oz	270	10
Chicken Flavor w/ Vegetables Low Fat Cup-A-Ramen, as prep	8 oz	220	2
Chicken Leek (Ultra Slim-Fast)	6 oz	50	tr
Chicken Noodle (Lipton)	8 oz	82	2

FOOD	PORTION	CALORIES	FAT
Chicken Noodle (Ultra Slim-Fast)	6 oz	45	tr
Chicken Noodle (Weight Watchers)	7.5 oz	90	1
Chicken Noodle, as prep (Campbell)	8 oz	100	2
Chicken Noodle, as prep (Knorr)	8 oz	100	2
Chicken Noodle Hearty (Lipton)	8 oz	81	4
Chicken Noodle Microwave (Campbell)	7.5 oz	100	4
Chicken Noodle w/ White Meat Campbell's Cup, as prep	6 oz	90	2
Chicken w/ Rice Microwave Soup (Campbell)	7.5 oz	100	4
Chili Beef Microwave Soup (Campbell)	7.5 oz	190	4
Chunky Beef Stew (Weight Watchers)	7.5 oz	120	2
Country Barley, as prep (Knorr)	8 oz	120	2
Country Vegetable (Lipton)	8 oz	80	1
Creamy Broccoli (Ultra Slim-Fast)	6 oz	75	tr
Creamy Chicken w/ White Meat Campbell's Cup, as prep	6 oz	90	4
Creamy Tomato (Ultra Slim-Fast)	6 oz	60	tr
Fines Herb, as prep (Knorr)	8 oz	130	6
Fish Bouillon, as prep w/ water (Knorr)	8 oz	10	tr
French Onion, as prep (Knorr)	8 oz	50	1
Giggle Noodle (Lipton)	8 oz	72	2
Hearty Minestrone, as prep (Knorr)	10 oz	130	2
Hearty Noodle, as prep (Campbell)	8 oz	90	1
Hearty Noodle w/ Vegetable (Lipton)	8 oz	75	2
Hearty Noodle w/ Vegetables Campbell's Cup	1 (1.7 oz)	180	2
Hearty Vegetable (Ultra Slim-Fast)	6 oz	50	tr

FOOD	PORTION	CALORIES	FAT
Leek, as prep (Knorr)	8 oz	110	4
Lobster Bisque (Golden Dipt)	¼ pkg	30	1
Manhattan Clam Chowder (Golden Dipt)	¼ pkg	80	2
Minestrone Soup Mix, as prep (Manischewitz)	6 oz	50	tr
Mushroom, as prep (Knorr)	8 oz	100	4
New England Clam Chowder (Golden Dipt)	¼ pkg	24	2
New England Clam Chowder (Weight Watchers)	7.5 oz	90	0
Noodle, as prep (Campbell)	8 oz	110	2
Noodle w/ Chicken Broth Campbell's Cup	1 (1.35 oz)	130	2
Noodle w/ Chicken Broth Campbell's Cup, as prep	6 oz	90	2
Onion (Lipton)	8 oz	20	tr
Onion (Ultra Slim-Fast)	6 oz	45	tr
Onion, as prep (Campbell)	8 oz	30	0
Onion Bouillon Instant (Wylers)	1 tsp	10	tr
Onion Golden (Lipton)	8 oz	62	2
Onion Mushroom (Lipton)	8 oz	41	1
Oriental Flavor Low Fat Ramen Noodle, as prep	8 oz	150	1
Oriental Flavor Ramen Noodle, as prep	8 oz	190	8
Oriental Flavor w/ Vegetables Cup-A-Ramen, as prep	8 oz	270	10
Oriental Flavor w/ Vegetables Low Fat Cup-A-Ramen, as prep	8 oz	220	2
Oriental Hot & Sour, as prep (Knorr)	8 oz	80	3
Oxtail Hearty Beef, as prep (Knorr)	8 oz	70	2

FOOD	PORTION	CALORIES	FAT
Pork Flavor Low Fat Ramen Noodle, as prep	8 oz	150	1
Pork Flavor Ramen Noodle, as prep	8 oz	200	8
Potato Leek (Ultra Slim-Fast)	6 oz	80	tr
Potato Leek, as prep (Nile Spice)	10 oz	160	6
Potato Romano, as prep (Nile Spice)	10 oz	150	6
Potato Tomato, as prep (Nile Spice)	10 oz	160	6
Ring-O-Noodle (Lipton)	8 oz	67	2
Seafood Chowder (Golden Dipt)	¼ pkg	70	2
Shrimp Bisque (Golden Dipt)	¼ pkg	30	1
Shrimp Flavor w/ Vegetables Cup-A-Ramen, as prep	8 oz	280	10
Shrimp Flavor w/ Vegetables Low Fat Cup-A-Ramen, as prep	8 oz	230	2
Split Pea Soup Mix, as prep (Manischewitz)	6 oz	45	tr
Spring Vegetable w/ Herbs, as prep (Knorr)	8 oz	30	tr
Tomato, as prep (Diamond Crystal)	6 oz	70	2
Tomato Basil, as prep (Knorr)	8 oz	90	3
Tortellini in Brodo, as prep (Knorr)	8 oz	60	1
Vegetable (Lipton)	8 oz	37	1
Vegetable, as prep (Campbell)	8 oz	40	0
Vegetable, as prep (Knorr)	8 oz	35	1
Vegetable Bouillon Instant (Wylers)	1 tsp	6	tr
Vegetable Beef (Weight Watchers)	7.5 oz	90	1
Vegetable Beef Microwave Soup (Campbell)	7.5 oz	100	2
Vegetable Soup Mix, as prep (Manischewitz)	6 oz	50	tr
Vegetarian Vegetable Bouillon, as prep w/ water (Knorr)	8 oz	16	2

FOOD	PORTION	CALORIES	FAT
asparagus, cream of, as prep w/ water	1 cup	59	2
beef broth, as prep w/ water	1 cup	19	1
beef broth, not prep	1 pkg (.2 oz)	14	1
beef broth, not prep	1 cube (3.6 g)	6	tr
celery, cream of, as prep w/ water	1 cup	63	2
chicken broth, as prep w/ water	1 cup	21	1
chicken broth, not prep	1 cube (4.8 g)	9	tr
chicken broth, not prep	1 pkg (.2 oz)	16	1
chicken, cream of, as prep w/ water	1 cup	107	5
chicken noodle, as prep w/ water	1 cup	53	1
french onion, not prep	1 pkg (1.4 oz)	115	2
leek, as prep w/ water	1 cup	71	2
onion, as prep w/ water	1 cup	28	1
onion, not prep	1 pkg (1.4 oz)	115	2
tomato, as prep w/ water	1 cup	102	2
FROZEN			
Barley & Mushroom (Jaclyn's)	7.5 oz	90	1
Boston Clam Chowder (Kettle Ready)	8 oz	199	11
Split Pea (Jaclyn's)	7.5 oz	180	2
Split Pea w/ Ham (Kettle Ready)	8 oz	189	5
Vegetable (Jaclyn's)	7.5 oz	90	1
HOME RECIPE			
black bean turtle soup	1 cup	241	1
corn & cheese chowder	¾ cup	215	12
greek	¾ cup	63	2
hot & sour	1 cup	74	2
SHELF STABLE			
Chunky Beef Vegetable (Healthy Choice)	7.5 oz cup	110	1

FOOD	PORTION	CALORIES	FAT
Chunky Chicken Noodle & Vegetable (Healthy Choice)	7.5 oz cup	160	4
TAKE-OUT			
gazpacho	1 cup	46	tr
oxtail	5 oz	64	3

SOUR CREAM
(*see also* SOUR CREAM SUBSTITUTES)

FOOD	PORTION	CALORIES	FAT
Breakstone's	1 tbsp	30	3
Breakstone's Light Choice Cultured Half & Half	1 tbsp	25	2
Cabot	1 oz	60	6
Cabot Light	1 oz	33	2
Friendship	2 tbsp	55	5
Friendship Lite Delite	2 tbsp	35	2
Knudsen Hampshire	1 oz	60	6
Knudsen Light N'Lively Light	1 oz	40	3
Land O'Lakes Light	2 tbsp	40	2
Land O'Lakes Light w/ Chives	2 tbsp	40	2
Sealtest	1 tbsp	30	3
Sealtest Light Cultured Half & Half	1 tbsp	25	2
Weight Watchers Light Sour	2 tbsp	35	2
sour cream	1 tbsp	26	3
sour cream	1 cup	493	48

SOUR CREAM SUBSTITUTES

FOOD	PORTION	CALORIES	FAT
Formagg	1 oz	40	3
nondairy	1 cup	479	45
nondairy	1 oz	59	6

FOOD	PORTION	CALORIES	FAT
SOURSOP			
fresh	1	416	2
fresh, cut up	1 cup	150	1
SOY			
(*see also* TOFU)			
Soo Moo Beverage (Health Valley)	1 cup	120	6
Soy Sauce (Kikkoman)	1 tbsp	12	0
Soy Sauce (La Choy)	½ tsp	2	tr
Soy Sauce Lite (Kikkoman)	1 tbsp	13	0
Soy Sauce Lite (La Choy)	½ tsp	1	tr
Soy Sauce Mix (Diamond Crystal)	1 tsp	5	tr
Soybean Flakes (Arrowhead)	2 oz	250	11
Soybeans (Arrowhead)	2 oz	230	10
lecithin	1 tbsp	104	14
milk	1 cup	79	5
soy sauce	1 tbsp	7	tr
soy sauce, shoyu	1 tbsp	9	tr
soy sauce, tamari	1 tbsp	11	tr
soya cheese	1.4 oz	128	11
soybean sprouts, raw	½ cup	43	2
soybean sprouts, steamed	½ cup	38	2
soybean sprouts, stir-fried	1 cup	125	7
soybeans, dry-roasted	½ cup	387	19
soybeans, roasted	½ cup	405	22
soybeans, roasted & toasted	1 oz	129	7
soybeans, roasted & toasted	1 cup	490	26
soybeans, salted, roasted & toasted	1 oz	129	7
soybeans, salted, roasted & toasted	1 cup	490	26

FOOD	PORTION	CALORIES	FAT
soybeans, cooked	1 cup	298	15
soybeans, dried	1 cup	774	37

SPAGHETTI
(*see* PASTA, SPAGHETTI SAUCE)

SPAGHETTI SAUCE
(*see also* PIZZA, TOMATO)

JARRED			
Chef Boyardee Meatless	4 oz	60	1
Chef Boyardee w/ Ground Beef	4 oz	90	3
Chef Boyardee w/ Mushrooms	4 oz	70	2
Estee Sauce	4 oz	60	1
Hunt's Chunky	4 oz	70	2
Hunt's Homestyle	4 oz	70	2
Hunt's Homestyle w/ Meat	4 oz	60	2
Hunt's Homestyle w/ Mushrooms	4 oz	50	1
Hunt's Traditional	4 oz	70	2
Hunt's w/ Meat	4 oz	70	2
Hunt's w/ Mushrooms	4 oz	70	2
Newman's Own	4 oz	70	2
Newman's Own Sockarooni	4 oz	70	2
Newman's Own w/ Mushrooms	4 oz	70	2
Prego Chunky Sausage & Green Peppers	4 oz	160	8
Prego Extra Chunky Garden Combination	4 oz	80	2
Prego Extra Chunky Mushroom & Green Pepper	4 oz	100	4
Prego Extra Chunky Mushroom & Onion	4 oz	100	4

FOOD	PORTION	CALORIES	FAT
Prego Extra Chunky Mushroom & Tomato	4 oz	110	5
Prego Extra Chunky Mushroom w/ Extra Spice	4 oz	100	3
Prego Extra Chunky Tomato & Onion	4 oz	110	5
Prego Marinara	4 oz	100	6
Prego Meat Flavored	4 oz	140	6
Prego Mushroom	4 oz	130	5
Prego Onion & Garlic	4 oz	110	4
Prego Regular	4 oz	130	5
Prego Three Cheese	4 oz	100	2
Prego Tomato & Basil	4 oz	100	2
Pritikin	4 oz	60	0
Pritikin w/ Mushrooms	4 oz	60	0
Ragu Chunky Gardenstyle Extra Tomatoes, Garlic & Onions	4 oz	70	3
Ragu Chunky Gardenstyle Green & Red Peppers	4 oz	70	3
Ragu Chunky Gardenstyle Italian Garden Combination	4 oz	70	3
Ragu Chunky Gardenstyle Mushrooms & Onions	4 oz	70	3
Ragu Homestyle w/ Meat	4 oz	110	5
Ragu Homestyle w/ Mushrooms	4 oz	110	5
Ragu Homestyle w/ Tomato & Herbs	4 oz	110	5
Ragu Italian Cooking Sauce	4 oz	70	2
Ragu Joe	3.5 oz	50	0
Ragu Old World Style Marinara	4 oz	80	5
Ragu Old World Style Pizza	1.6 oz	25	1
Ragu Old World Style Plain	4 oz	80	4
Ragu Old World Style w/ Meat	4 oz	80	5

FOOD	PORTION	CALORIES	FAT
Ragu Old World Style w/ Mushrooms	4 oz	80	4
Ragu Thick & Hearty Plain	4 oz	100	3
Ragu Thick & Hearty w/ Meat	4 oz	120	5
Ragu Thick & Hearty w/ Mushrooms	4 oz	100	3
Weight Watchers Flavored w/ Meat	⅓ cup	45	1
Weight Watchers Flavored w/ Mushrooms	⅓ cup	35	0
marinara sauce	1 cup	171	8
spaghetti sauce	1 cup	272	12
TAKE-OUT			
bolognese	5 oz	195	15

SPARE RIBS
(see PORK)

SPICES
(see HERBS/SPICES)

SPINACH

CANNED			
Libby	½ cup	25	0
S&W Northwest Premium	½ cup	25	0
Seneca	½ cup	25	0
spinach	½ cup	25	1
FRESH			
Dole	3 oz	9	tr
cooked	½ cup	21	tr
mustard, chopped, cooked	½ cup	14	tr
mustard, raw, chopped	½ cup	17	tr
new zealand, chopped, cooked	½ cup	11	tr

FOOD	PORTION	CALORIES	FAT
new zealand, raw	½ cup	4	tr
raw, chopped	½ cup	6	tr
raw, chopped	1 pkg (10 oz)	46	1
FROZEN			
Birds Eye Chopped	⅓ cup	22	tr
Birds Eye Creamed	⅓ cup	59	4
Birds Eye Leaf	⅓ cup	22	tr
Green Giant	½ cup	25	0
Green Giant Creamed	½ cup	70	3
Green Giant Cut Leaf in Butter Sauce	½ cup	40	2
Green Giant Harvest Fresh	½ cup	25	0
cooked	½ cup	27	tr
JUICE			
spinach juice	3.5 oz	7	0

SPOT

FOOD	PORTION	CALORIES	FAT
fresh, baked	3 oz	134	5

SQUAB

FOOD	PORTION	CALORIES	FAT
breast w/o skin, raw	1 (3.5 oz)	135	5
w/ skin, raw	1 squab (6.9 oz)	584	47
w/o skin, raw	1 squab (5.9 oz)	239	13

SQUASH
(*see also* ZUCCHINI)

FOOD	PORTION	CALORIES	FAT
CANNED			
crookneck, sliced	½ cup	14	tr
FRESH			
acorn, cooked, mashed	½ cup	41	tr

FOOD	PORTION	CALORIES	FAT
acorn, cubed, baked	½ cup	57	tr
butternut, baked	½ cup	41	tr
crookneck, sliced, cooked	½ cup	18	tr
crookneck, raw, sliced	½ cup	12	tr
hubbard, baked	½ cup	51	tr
hubbard, cooked, mashed	½ cup	35	tr
scallop, raw, sliced	½ cup	12	tr
scallop, sliced, cooked	½ cup	14	tr
spaghetti, cooked	½ cup	23	tr
FROZEN			
Butternut (Southland)	4 oz	45	0
Prepared Squash (Southland)	3.6 oz	80	2
Winter Cooked (Birds Eye)	⅓ cup	45	tr
butternut, cooked, mashed	½ cup	47	tr
crookneck, sliced, cooked	½ cup	24	tr
SEEDS			
dried	1 oz	154	13
dried	1 cup	747	63
roasted	1 oz	148	12
roasted	1 cup	1184	96
salted & roasted	1 oz	148	12
salted & roasted	1 cup	1184	96
whole, roasted	1 oz	127	6
whole, roasted	1 cup	285	12
whole, salted & roasted	1 oz	127	6
whole, salted & roasted	1 cup	285	12

SQUID

FOOD	PORTION	CALORIES	FAT
fresh, fried	3 oz	149	6

FOOD	PORTION	CALORIES	FAT

SQUIRREL

FOOD	PORTION	CALORIES	FAT
roasted	3 oz	147	4

STRAWBERRIES

FOOD	PORTION	CALORIES	FAT
CANNED			
in heavy syrup	½ cup	117	tr
FRESH			
Dole	8	50	0
strawberries	1 cup	45	1
strawberries	1 pint	97	1
FROZEN			
Halved in Lite Syrup (Birds Eye)	½ cup	87	tr
Halved Quick Thaw (Birds Eye)	½ cup	119	tr
Whole in Lite Syrup (Birds Eye)	½ cup	81	tr
sweetened, sliced	1 cup	245	tr
sweetened, sliced	1 pkg (10 oz)	273	tr
unsweetened	1 cup	52	tr
whole, sweetened	1 cup	200	tr
whole, sweetened	1 pkg (10 oz)	223	tr
JUICE			
Juice Works	6 oz	100	0
Kern's Nectar	6 oz	110	0
Libby's Nectar	6 oz	110	0
Libby's Ripe Nectar	8 oz	150	0
Smucker's Juice	8 oz	130	0
Wyler's Wild Strawberry	8 oz	80	tr

STUFFING/DRESSING

FOOD	PORTION	CALORIES	FAT
HOME RECIPE			
bread, as prep w/ water & fat	½ cup	251	15

FOOD	PORTION	CALORIES	FAT
bread, as prep w/ water, egg & fat	½ cup	107	7
sausage	½ cup	292	11
MIX			
Golden Grain Bread Stuffing			
Chicken	½ cup	180	9
Corn Bread	½ cup	180	9
Herb & Butter	½ cup	180	9
With Wild Rice	½ cup	180	9
Pepperidge Farm			
Corn Bread	1 oz	110	1
Country Style	1 oz	100	1
Cube	1 oz	110	1
Distinctive Apple Raisin	1 oz	110	1
Distinctive Classic Chicken	1 oz	110	1
Distinctive Country Garden Herb	1 oz	120	4
Distinctive Vegetable & Almond	1 oz	110	3
Distinctive Wild Rice & Mushroom	1 oz	130	5
Herb Seasoned	1 oz	110	1
Stove Top			
Chicken	½ cup	181	9
Chicken w/ Rice	½ cup	184	9
Cornbread	½ cup	163	8
Flexible Serve Chicken	½ cup	180	9
Flexible Serve Cornbread	½ cup	180	9
Flexible Serve Herb Homestyle	½ cup	180	9
Long Grain & Wild Rice	½ cup	184	9
Pork	½ cup	179	9
Savory Herbs	½ cup	180	9
Select Chicken Florentine	½ cup	203	12
Select Garden Herb	½ cup	219	13
Select Vegetable & Almond	½ cup	227	15

FOOD	PORTION	CALORIES	FAT
Stove Top *(cont.)*			
Select Wild Rice & Mushroom	½ cup	172	9
Turkey	½ cup	179	9
bread, dry	1 cup	500	31

STURGEON

FRESH			
cooked	3 oz	115	4
SMOKED			
sturgeon	1 oz	48	1
sturgeon	3 oz	147	4

SUCKER

white, baked	3 oz	101	3

SUGAR
(*see also* FRUCTOSE, HONEY, SUGAR SUBSTITUTES, SYRUP)

C&H White	1 tsp	16	0
brown	1 cup	820	0
powdered, sifted	1 cup	385	0
white	1 pkt (6 g)	25	0
white	1 tbsp	45	0
white	1 cup	770	0

SUGAR SUBSTITUTES
(*see also* FRUCTOSE)

Equal	1 pkt	4	0
Estee Swiss Sweet Packet	6	4	0
Estee Swiss Sweet Tablet	1	0	0
S&W Liquid Table Sweetener	⅛ tsp	0	0
Spoon for Spoon	1 tsp	2	0

FOOD	PORTION	CALORIES	FAT
Sprinkle Sweet	1 tsp	2	0
SugarTwin	1 tsp	2	0
SugarTwin	1 pkt	3	0
SugarTwin Brown	1 tsp	2	0
Sweet 'N Low Brown	1/10 tsp	2	0
Sweet 'N Low Granulated	1 pkt (1 g)	4	0
Sweet 'N Low Liquid	10 drops	0	0
Sweet One	1 pkt	4	0
Sweet*10	1/8 tsp	0	0
Weight Watchers Sweet'ner	1 pkt	4	0

SUGAR-APPLE

fresh	1	146	tr
fresh, cut up	1 cup	236	1

SUNDAE TOPPINGS
(*see* ICE CREAM TOPPINGS)

SUNFISH

pumpkinseed, baked	3 oz	97	1

SUNFLOWER SEEDS

Arrowhead	1 oz	160	13
Planters	1 oz	160	14
Sunflower Butter (Erewhon)	2 tbsp	200	18
Sunflower Nuts Dry Roasted	1 oz	170	15
dried	1 oz	162	14
dried	1 cup	821	71
dry roasted	1 oz	165	14
dry roasted	1 cup	745	64
dry roasted, salted	1 oz	165	14

FOOD	PORTION	CALORIES	FAT
dry roasted, salted	1 cup	745	64
oil roasted	1 cup	830	78
oil roasted, salted	1 oz	175	16
oil roasted, salted	1 cup	830	78
sunflower butter	1 tbsp	93	8
sunflower butter w/o salt	1 tbsp	93	8
toasted	1 oz	176	16
toasted	1 cup	826	76
toasted, salted	1 oz	176	16
toasted, salted	1 cup	826	76

SURF

CANNED American Original Foods	4 oz	100	tr
FRESH American Original Foods	4 oz	90	tr

SWAMP CABBAGE

chopped, cooked	½ cup	10	tr
raw, chopped	1 cup	11	tr

SWEET POTATO
(see also YAM)

CANNED in syrup	½ cup	106	tr
pieces	1 cup	183	tr
FRESH baked w/ skin	1 (3.5 oz)	118	tr
leaves, cooked	½ cup	11	tr
mashed	½ cup	172	tr

FOOD	PORTION	CALORIES	FAT
FROZEN			
Candied Sweet Potatoes (Mrs. Paul's)	4 oz	170	0
Candied Sweets 'N Apples (Mrs. Paul's)	4 oz	160	0
cooked	½ cup	88	tr
HOME RECIPE			
candied	3.5 oz	144	3

SWEETBREADS

beef, braised	3 oz	230	15
lamb, braised	3 oz	199	13
veal, braised	3 oz	218	12

SWISS CHARD

fresh, cooked	½ cup	18	tr
fresh, raw, chopped	½ cup	3	tr

SWORDFISH

cooked	3 oz	132	4

SYRUP
(*see also* ICE CREAM TOPPINGS, PANCAKE/WAFFLE SYRUP)

Blueberry (Estee)	1 tbsp	8	0
Blueberry Diet (S&W)	1 tbsp	4	0
Corn Syrup Dark (Karo)	1 tbsp	60	0
Corn Syrup Dark (Karo)	1 cup	975	0
Corn Syrup Light (Karo)	1 tbsp	60	0
Corn Syrup Light (Karo)	1 cup	960	0
Fruit Syrup, All Flavors (Smuckers)	2 tbsp	100	0
Maple Flavored Diet (S&W)	1 tbsp	4	0
Maple Rich (Home Brands)	1 oz	110	0

FOOD	PORTION	CALORIES	FAT
Strawberry Diet (S&W)	1 tbsp	4	0
corn	2 tbsp	122	0
raspberry	3.5 oz	267	0

TAHINI
(*see* SESAME)

TAMARIND

FRESH			
cut up	1 cup	287	1
tamarind	1	5	tr

TANGERINE

CANNED			
in light syrup	½ cup	76	tr
juice pack	½ cup	46	tr
FRESH			
Dole	2	70	1
sections	1 cup	86	tr
tangerine	1	37	tr
JUICE			
Dole Pure & Light	6 oz	100	tr
canned, sweetened	1 cup	125	1
fresh	1 cup	106	tr
frzn, sweetened, as prep	1 cup	110	tr
frzn, sweetened, as prep	6 oz	344	1

TAPIOCA

Minute Tapioca (General Foods)	1 tbsp	35	tr
pearl dry	⅓ cup	174	0
starch	3.5 oz	344	tr

FOOD	PORTION	CALORIES	FAT
TARO			
chips	10	110	6
chips	½ cup	57	3
leaves, cooked	½ cup	18	tr
raw, sliced	½ cup	56	tr
shoots, sliced, cooked	½ cup	10	tr
sliced, cooked	½ cup	94	tr
tahitian, sliced, cooked	½ cup	30	tr
TARRAGON			
ground	1 tsp	5	tr
TEA/HERBAL TEA			
HERBAL			
Almond Orange (Bigelow)	5 oz	tr	tr
Almond Sunset (Celestial Seasonings)	1 cup	3	tr
Apple Orchard (Bigelow)	1 cup	5	tr
Apple Spice (Bigelow)	5 oz	tr	tr
Chamomile (Bigelow)	5 oz	tr	tr
Chamomile (Celestial Seasonings)	1 cup	2	tr
Chamomile Mint (Bigelow)	5 oz	tr	tr
Cinnamon Apple Spice (Celestial Seasonings)	1 cup	3	tr
Cinnamon Orange (Bigelow)	5 oz	tr	tr
Cinnamon Rose (Celestial Seasonings)	1 cup	2	tr
Country Peach Spice (Celestial Seasonings)	1 cup	3	tr
Cranberry Cove (Celestial Seasonings)	1 cup	3	tr
Early Riser (Bigelow)	1 cup	3	3

FOOD	PORTION	CALORIES	FAT
Emperor's Choice (Celestial Seasonings)	1 cup	4	tr
Feeling Free (Bigelow)	1 cup	1	1
Fruit & Almond (Bigelow)	1 cup	1	tr
Ginseng Plus (Celestial Seasonings)	1 cup	3	tr
Grandma's Tummy Mints (Celestial Seasonings)	1 cup	2	tr
Hibiscus & Rose Hips (Bigelow)	5 oz	1	1
I Love Lemon (Bigelow)	1 cup	1	1
Lemon & C (Bigelow)	5 oz	tr	tr
Lemon Mist (Celestial Seasonings)	1 cup	2	tr
Lemon Zinger (Celestial Seasonings)	1 cup	4	tr
Looking Good (Bigelow)	1 cup	1	tr
Mandarin Orange Spice (Celestial Seasonings)	1 cup	5	tr
Mellow Mint (Celestial Seasonings)	1 cup	2	tr
Mint Blend (Bigelow)	5 oz	tr	1
Mint Magic (Celestial Seasonings)	1 cup	1	tr
Mint Medley (Bigelow)	1 cup	1	1
Mo's 24 (Celestial Seasonings)	1 cup	2	tr
Nice Over Ice (Bigelow)	1 cup	1	tr
Orange & C (Bigelow)	5 oz	tr	tr
Orange & Spice (Bigelow)	1 cup	1	tr
Orange Zinger (Celestial Seasonings)	1 cup	5	tr
Peppermint (Bigelow)	5 oz	tr	tr
Peppermint (Celestial Seasonings)	1 cup	2	tr
Raspberry Patch (Celestial Seasonings)	1 cup	4	tr
Red Zinger (Celestial Seasonings)	1 cup	4	tr
Roastaroma (Celestial Seasonings)	1 cup	11	tr
Roasted Grain & Carob (Bigelow)	5 oz	3	2

FOOD	PORTION	CALORIES	FAT
Sleepytime (Celestial Seasonings)	1 cup	5	tr
Spearmint (Bigelow)	5 oz	tr	tr
Spearmint (Celestial Seasonings)	1 cup	5	tr
Strawberry Fields (Celestial Seasonings)	1 cup	4	tr
Sunburst C (Celestial Seasonings)	1 cup	3	tr
Sweets Dreams (Bigelow)	1 cup	1	2
Take-a-Break (Bigelow)	1 cup	3	2
Wild Forest Blueberry (Celestial Seasonings)	1 cup	2	tr
REGULAR			
Amaretto Nights (Celestial Seasonings)	1 cup	3	tr
Apple Spice & Tea (Celestial Seasonings)	1 cup	tr	tr
Bavarian Chocolate Orange (Celestial Seasonings)	1 cup	7	tr
Caffeine-Free (Celestial Seasonings)	1 cup	4	tr
Chinese Fortune (Bigelow)	1 cup	1	tr
Cinnamon Stick (Bigelow)	1 cup	1	tr
Cinnamon Vienna (Celestial Seasonings)	1 cup	2	tr
Classic English Breakfast (Celestial Seasonings)	1 cup	3	tr
Constant Comment (Bigelow)	1 cup	1	1
Darjeeling Blend (Bigelow)	1 cup	1	tr
Darjeeling Gardens (Celestial Seasonings)	1 cup	3	tr
Earl Gray (Bigelow)	1 cup	1	tr
English Teatime (Bigelow)	1 cup	1	tr
Extraordinary Earl Grey (Celestial Seasonings)	1 cup	3	tr

FOOD	PORTION	CALORIES	FAT
Fruit Tea Fruit Cooler, as prep (Lipton)	8 oz	87	0
Iced Berry Tea, as prep (Crystal Light)	8 oz	3	0
Iced Tea (Shasta)	12 oz	124	0
Iced Tea (SIPPS)	8.45 oz	100	0
Irish Cream Mist (Celestial Seasonings)	1 cup	3	tr
Lemon Lift (Bigelow)	1 cup	1	tr
Lemons & Tea (Celestial Seasonings)	1 cup	tr	tr
Morning Thunder (Celestial Seasonings)	1 cup	3	tr
Nestea 100% Instant, as prep	8 oz	2	0
Nestea Decaffeinated 100% Instant, as prep	8 oz	0	0
Nestea Ice Teasers Citrus	8 oz	6	0
Nestea Ice Teasers Lemon	8 oz	6	0
Nestea Ice Teasers Orange	8 oz	6	0
Nestea Ice Teasers Tropical	8 oz	6	0
Nestea Ice Teasers Wild Cherry	8 oz	6	0
Nestea Iced Tea Mix w/ Sugar & Lemon, as prep	8 oz	70	0
Nestea Lemon	8 oz	6	0
Nestea Ready-to-Drink Iced Tea w/ Sugar & Lemon	8 oz	70	0
Nestea Ready-to-Drink Sugarfree Iced Tea w/ Lemon	8 oz	2	0
Nestea Sugarfree Decaffeinated Iced Tea Mix	2 tsp	6	0
Nestea Sugarfree Iced Tea Mix	8 oz	4	0
Nestea Tea Bag, as prep	6 oz	0	0
Orange Pekoe (Bigelow)	1 cup	1	tr

FOOD	PORTION	CALORIES	FAT
Orange Spice & Tea (Celestial Seasonings)	1 cup	tr	tr
Peppermint Stick (Bigelow)	1 cup	1	tr
Plantation Mint (Bigelow)	1 cup	1	tr
Raspberries & Tea (Celestial Seasonings)	1 cup	2	tr
Raspberry Royale (Bigelow)	1 cup	1	tr
Swiss Mint (Celestial Seasonings)	1 cup	tr	tr
brewed tea	6 oz	2	0
instant artificially sweetened, lemon flavor	8 oz	5	0
instant sweetened, lemon flavor	9 oz	87	tr
instant unsweetened	8 oz	2	0
instant unsweetened, lemon flavor	8 oz	4	0

TEFF

Arrowhead Teff Seeds	2 oz	200	1

TEMPEH

tempeh	½ cup	165	6

THYME

ground	1 tsp	4	tr

TILEFISH

fresh, cooked	3 oz	125	4
fresh, cooked	½ fillet (5.3 oz)	220	7

TOFU

Baked Barbecue (Spring Creek)	2 oz	88	4
Baked Cajun (Spring Creek)	2 oz	87	4
Baked Teriyaki (Spring Creek)	2 oz	84	4

FOOD	PORTION	CALORIES	FAT
Blue Label (Azumaya)	3.5 oz	46	1
Great Balls of Tofu! (Spring Creek)	2 (3 oz)	107	5
Green Label (Azumaya)	3.5 oz	68	2
Grilled in Black Bean Sauce (Jaclyn's)	10.75 oz	270	8
Grilled in Peanut Sauce (Jaclyn's)	10.75 oz	260	9
Mori-Nu Silken Extra-Firm	½ box (5.25 oz)	90	3
Mori-Nu Silken Firm	½ box (5.25 oz)	90	4
Mori-Nu Silken Soft	½ box (5.25 oz)	80	4
Name Age Fried (Azumaya)	3.5 oz	144	4
Nigari Firm (Spring Creek)	4 oz	140	8
Red Label (Azumaya)	3.5 oz	68	1
Tofu Salads Missing Egg (Spring Creek)	2 oz	49	14
Tofu Salads Onion Dip (Spring Creek)	2 oz	46	14
Tofu Salads Taco Dip (Spring Creek)	2 oz	46	14
firm	¼ block (3 oz)	118	7
firm	½ cup	183	11
fresh, fried	1 piece (½ oz)	35	3
fuyu, salted & fermented	1 block (⅓ oz)	13	1
koyadofu, dried, frozen	1 piece (½ oz)	82	5
okara	½ cup	47	1
regular	¼ block (4 oz)	88	6
regular	½ cup	94	6
YOGURT Stir Fruity Black Cherry	6 oz	141	2
Stir Fruity Blueberry	6 oz	140	1
Stir Fruity Lemon Chiffon	6 oz	152	3

FOOD	PORTION	CALORIES	FAT
Stir Fruity Mixed Berry	6 oz	149	2
Stir Fruity Orange	6 oz	143	2
Stir Fruity Peach	6 oz	160	3
Stir Fruity Pina Colada	6 oz	162	3
Stir Fruity Raspberry	6 oz	155	2
Stir Fruity Spiced Apple	6 oz	167	2
Stir Fruity Strawberry	6 oz	140	2
Stir Fruity Tropical Fruit	6 oz	170	2

TOFUTTI
(see ICE CREAM AND FROZEN DESSERTS)

TOMATILLO

fresh	1 (1.2 oz)	11	tr
fresh, chopped	½ cup	21	1

TOMATO
(see also PIZZA, SPAGHETTI SAUCE)

CANNED

Claussen Kosher	1	9	tr
Contadina California Sliced	½ cup	40	tr
Contadina Crushed in Tomato Puree	½ cup	30	tr
Contadina Italian Paste	2 oz	65	1
Contadina Italian Style	½ cup	25	tr
Contadina Italian Style Stewed	½ cup	35	tr
Contadina Paste	2 oz	50	tr
Contadina Puree	½ cup	40	0
Contadina Stewed	½ cup	35	tr
Contadina Thick & Zesty Sauce	½ cup	40	0
Contadina Whole Peeled	½ cup	25	tr
Health Valley Sauce	1 cup	70	1

FOOD	PORTION	CALORIES	FAT
Hunt's Crushed Angela Mia	4 oz	35	tr
Hunt's Crushed Italian	4 oz	40	tr
Hunt's Italian Pear Shaped	4 oz	20	tr
Hunt's Paste	2 oz	45	tr
Hunt's Paste Italian Style	2 oz	50	tr
Hunt's Paste No Salt Added	2 oz	45	tr
Hunt's Paste w/ Garlic	2 oz	50	tr
Hunt's Peeled Choice-Cut	4 oz	20	tr
Hunt's Puree	4 oz	45	tr
Hunt's Sauce	4 oz	30	tr
Hunt's Sauce Herb	4 oz	70	2
Hunt's Sauce Italian	4 oz	60	2
Hunt's Sauce Meatloaf Fixin's	4 oz	20	tr
Hunt's Sauce No Salt Added	4 oz	35	tr
Hunt's Sauce Special	4 oz	35	tr
Hunt's Sauce w/ Bits	4 oz	30	tr
Hunt's Sauce w/ Garlic	4 oz	70	2
Hunt's Sauce w/ Mushrooms	4 oz	25	tr
Hunt's Stewed	4 oz	35	tr
Hunt's Stewed Italian	4 oz	40	tr
Hunt's Stewed No Salt Added	4 oz	35	tr
Hunt's Whole	4 oz	20	tr
Hunt's Whole Italian	4 oz	25	tr
Hunt's Whole No Salt Added	4 oz	20	tr
S&W Aspic Supreme	½ cup	60	0
S&W Diced in Rich Puree	½ cup	35	0
S&W Italian Stewed Sliced	½ cup	35	0
S&W Italian Style w/ Basil	½ cup	25	0
S&W Mexican Style Stewed	½ cup	40	0
S&W Paste	6 oz	150	0

FOOD	PORTION	CALORIES	FAT
S&W Peeled Ready Cut	½ cup	25	0
S&W Puree	½ cup	60	0
S&W Sauce	½ cup	40	0
S&W Sauce Chunky	½ cup	45	0
S&W Stewed 50% Salt Reduced	½ cup	35	0
S&W Stewed Sliced	½ cup	35	0
S&W Whole Diet	½ cup	25	0
S&W Whole Peeled	½ cup	25	0
paste	½ cup	110	1
puree	1 cup	102	tr
puree w/o salt	1 cup	102	tr
red whole	½ cup	24	tr
sauce	½ cup	37	tr
sauce spanish style	½ cup	40	tr
sauce w/ mushrooms	½ cup	42	tr
sauce w/ onion	½ cup	52	tr
stewed	½ cup	34	tr
tomato w/ green chiles	½ cup	18	tr
wedges in tomato juice	½ cup	34	tr
DRIED			
sun dried	1 piece	5	tr
sun dried	1 cup	140	2
sun dried in oil	1 piece	6	tr
sun dried in oil	1 cup	235	15
FRESH			
cooked	½ cup	32	1
green	1	30	tr
red	1 (4.5 oz)	26	tr
red, chopped	1 cup	35	tr

FOOD	PORTION	CALORIES	FAT
JUICE			
Campbell	6 oz	40	0
Hunt's	6 oz	30	tr
Hunt's No Salt Added	6 oz	35	tr
Libby's	6 oz	35	0
Mott's Beefamato	6 oz	80	0
Mott's Clamato	6 oz	96	0
S&W California	6 oz	35	0
S&W Diet	½ cup	35	0
beef broth & tomato	5.5 oz	61	tr
clam & tomato	1 can (5.5 oz)	77	tr
juice	6 oz	32	tr
juice	½ cup	21	tr
TAKE-OUT			
stewed	1 cup	80	3

TONGUE

FOOD	PORTION	CALORIES	FAT
beef, simmered	3 oz	241	18
lamb, braised	3 oz	234	17
pork, braised	3 oz	230	16

TOPPINGS
(*see* ICE CREAM TOPPINGS)

TORTILLA CHIPS
(*see* CHIPS)

TREE FERN

FOOD	PORTION	CALORIES	FAT
chopped, cooked	½ cup	28	tr

FOOD	PORTION	CALORIES	FAT

TRITICALE
(*see also* FLOUR)

dry	½ cup	323	2

TROUT

FRESH

baked	3 oz	162	7
rainbow, cooked	3 oz	129	4
sea trout, baked	3 oz	113	4

TRUFFLES

fresh	3½ oz	25	1

TUNA
(*see also* TUNA DISHES)

CANNED

Bumble Bee Chunk Light in Oil	3 oz	200	15
Bumble Bee Chunk Light in Water	3 oz	90	2
Bumble Bee Chunk White in Oil	3 oz	200	15
Bumble Bee Chunk White in Water	3 oz	90	2
Bumble Bee Solid White in Oil	3 oz	190	10
Bumble Bee Solid White in Water	3 oz	90	2
Empress Chunk Light	2 oz	60	1
Empress Chunk Light Tongol	2 oz	50	1
Empress Solid White	2 oz	70	2
S&W Chunk Light Fancy in Oil	2 oz	140	10
S&W Chunk Light Fancy in Water	2 oz	60	1
S&W Fancy White Albacore in Oil	2 oz	160	12
light in oil	3 oz	169	7
light in oil	1 can (6 oz)	399	14
light in water	3 oz	99	1

FOOD	PORTION	CALORIES	FAT
light in water	1 can (5.8 oz)	192	1
white in oil	3 oz	158	7
white in oil	1 can (6.2 oz)	331	14
white in water	3 oz	116	2
white in water	1 can (6 oz)	234	4
FRESH			
bluefin, cooked	3 oz	157	5
skipjack, baked	3 oz	112	1
yellowfin, baked	3 oz	118	1

TUNA DISHES

FROZEN			
Microwave Tuna Sandwich (Mrs. Paul's)	1	200	6
Tuna Melt (Chefwich)	5 oz	360	14
MIX			
Tuna Mix-ins Garden Herb (Bumble Bee)	2 oz	25	0
READY-TO-USE			
Tuna Salad (The Spreadables)	¼ can	90	6
Tuna Salad (Wampler Longacre)	1 oz	61	13
TAKE-OUT			
tuna salad	3 oz	159	8
tuna salad	1 cup	383	19
tuna salad submarine sandwich w/ lettuce & oil	1	584	28

TURBOT

fresh european, baked	3 oz	104	3

FOOD	PORTION	CALORIES	FAT

TURKEY
(*see also* DINNER, HOT DOG, TURKEY DISHES, TURKEY SUBSTITUTES)

FOOD	PORTION	CALORIES	FAT
CANNED			
White (Swanson)	2.5 oz	80	1
w/ broth	1 can (5 oz)	231	10
w/ broth	½ can (2.5 oz)	116	5
FRESH			
Breast (Louis Rich)	1 oz	50	2
Breast Cutlets Thin-Sliced Skinless & Boneless (Perdue)	1 oz	28	tr
Breast Fillets Skinless & Boneless, Fit 'N Easy (Perdue)	1 oz	28	tr
Breast Hen w/ Wing (Louis Rich)	1 oz	53	2
Breast Hen w/o Back (Louis Rich)	1 oz	47	2
Breast Hen w/o Wing (Louis Rich)	1 oz	53	2
Breast Hotel Style Prime w/ skin (Perdue)	1 oz	43	2
Breast Prime Young (Shady Brook)	3 oz	140	7
Breast Roast (Louis Rich)	1 oz	41	tr
Breast Skinless & Boneless, Fit 'N Easy (Perdue)	1 oz	28	tr
Breast Slices (Louis Rich)	1 oz	44	1
Breast Steaks (Louis Rich)	1 oz	40	tr
Breast Tenderloins (Louis Rich)	1 oz	41	tr
Breast Tenderloins Skinless & Boneless (Perdue)	1 oz	29	tr
Breast Fresh Young w/ skin (Perdue)	1 oz	44	2
Drumsticks (Louis Rich)	1 oz	55	3
Drumsticks Fresh Young w/ skin, cooked (Perdue)	1 oz	36	2
Ground Breast Meat (Perdue)	1 oz	28	tr

FOOD	PORTION	CALORIES	FAT
Ground Lean 90% Fat Free (Louis Rich)	1 oz	51	8
Ground Lean 90% Fat Free (Louis Rich)	3.5 oz	183	9
Ground (Bil Mar Foods)	3 oz	163	12
Ground (Louis Rich)	1 oz	61	4
Ground (Louis Rich)	3.5 oz	217	13
Ground (Perdue)	1 oz	35	2
Thighs (Louis Rich)	1 oz	65	4
Thighs Fresh Young w/ skin (Perdue)	1 oz	48	3
Thighs Skinless & Boneless, Fit 'N Fresh (Perdue)	1 oz	36	2
Whole (Louis Rich)	3.5 oz	200	10
Whole (Louis Rich)	1 oz	56	3
Whole Dark Meat w/ skin (Perdue)	1 oz	48	3
Whole White Meat Fresh Young w/ skin (Perdue)	1 oz	44	2
Wing Drumettes (Louis Rich)	1 oz	52	2
Wing Drummettes Fresh Young w/ skin (Perdue)	1 oz	43	2
Wing Portions Fresh Young w/ skin (Perdue)	1 oz	51	3
Wings (Louis Rich)	1 oz	54	3
Wings (Shady Brook)	3 oz	130	6
Wings Fresh Young w/ skin (Perdue)	1 oz	45	2
back w/ skin, roasted	½ back (9 oz)	637	38
breast w/ skin, roasted	4 oz	212	8
dark meat w/ skin, roasted	3.6 oz	230	12
dark meat w/o skin, roasted	3 oz	170	7
dark meat w/o skin, roasted	1 cup (5 oz)	262	10
ground, cooked	3 oz	188	11
leg w/ skin, roasted	2.5 oz	147	7

FOOD	PORTION	CALORIES	FAT
leg w/ skin, roasted	1 (1.2 lbs)	1133	54
light meat w/ skin, roasted	4.7 oz	268	11
light meat w/ skin, roasted	from ½ turkey (2.3 lbs)	2069	87
light meat w/o skin, roasted	4 oz	183	4
neck, simmered	1 (5.3 oz)	274	11
skin, roasted	1 oz	141	13
skin, roasted	from ½ turkey (9 oz)	1096	98
w/ skin, neck & giblets, roasted	½ turkey (8.8 lbs)	4123	190
w/ skin, roasted	8.4 oz	498	23
w/ skin, roasted	½ turkey (4 lbs)	3857	181
w/o skin, roasted	1 cup (5 oz)	238	7
w/o skin, roasted	7.3 oz	354	10
wing w/ skin, roasted	1 (6.5 oz)	426	23
FROZEN			
roast boneless seasoned light & dark meat, roasted	1 pkg (1.7 lbs)	1213	45
READY-TO-USE			
Bil Mar Foods			
Breast	1 slice (1 oz)	31	tr
Buffet Style Smoked Ham	1 oz	32	1
Cheese Patties	3 oz	213	13
Ham Smoked	1 oz	32	1
Ham Square Chopped	1 slice (1 oz)	37	2
Luncheon Loaf Square Spiced	1 slice (1 oz)	51	4
Smoked Breast	1 oz	31	tr
Smoked Sliced Breast	1 oz	31	tr
Carl Buddig	1 oz	50	3
Carl Buddig Turkey Ham	1 oz	40	2
Deli Chef Breast & White	1 oz	39	6

FOOD	PORTION	CALORIES	FAT
Hansel 'N Gretel			
Doubledecker Turkey-Corned Beef	1 oz	30	1
Doubledecker Turkey Ham	1 oz	30	1
Gourmet Breast	1 oz	28	1
Gourmet Smoked Breast	1 oz	31	1
Honey Breast	1 oz	28	1
Lessalt Cooked Breast	1 oz	25	1
Oven Cooked Breast	1 oz	26	tr
Louis Rich			
Barbecued Breast	1 oz	36	1
Bologna	1 slice (28 g)	59	5
Breakfast Sausage, cooked	1 (1 oz)	59	4
Chopped Ham	1 slice (28 g)	42	2
Cotto Salami	1 slice (28 g)	52	4
Cured Thigh Meat Ham	1 slice (28 g)	34	1
Cured Thigh Meat Square Ham	1 slice (28 g)	24	tr
Cured Thigh Meat Water Added Ham	1 slice (28 g)	34	1
Hickory Smoked Breast	1 oz	31	tr
Honey Cured Ham	1 slice (21 g)	25	tr
Honey Roasted Breast	1 slice (28 g)	29	tr
Luncheon Loaf	1 slice (28 g)	43	3
Mild Bologna	1 slice (28 g)	61	5
Oven Roasted Breast	1 oz	30	tr
Oven Roasted Breast	1 slice (28 g)	31	tr
Salami	1 slice (28 g)	52	4
Smoked	1 slice (28 g)	33	1
Smoked Chunk Breast	1 oz	34	1
Smoked Sausage, cooked	1 (1 oz)	55	4
Smoked Sausage w/ Cheese, cooked	1 (1 oz)	58	4

FOOD	PORTION	CALORIES	FAT
Smoked Sliced Breast	1 slice (21 g)	21	tr
Square Pastrami	1 slice (23 g)	23	tr
Summer Sausage	1 slice (28 g)	52	4
Mr. Turkey			
BBQ Breast Quarter	1 oz	34	1
Bologna	1 oz	63	5
Bologna Red Rind	1 oz	63	5
Breakfast Smoked Ham	1 oz	33	1
Cotto Salami	1 oz	45	3
Diced White Meat	2 oz	84	2
Nuggets	1 nugget	33	2
Oven Roasted Quarter Breast	1 oz	34	1
Patties	3 oz	195	11
Smoked Breast Quarter	1 oz	35	1
Sticks	1 stick	65	4
Oscar Mayer Oven Roasted Breast	1 slice (21 g)	22	tr
Oscar Mayer Smoked Breast	1 slice (21 g)	20	tr
Perdue Done It! Nuggets	1 (.67 oz)	54	3
Wampler Longacre			
Baked Ham	1 oz	38	6
Baked Ham w/ 12% Water	1 oz	33	5
Baked Ham w/ 20% Water	1 oz	39	6
Bologna	1 oz	56	16
Breaded Nuggets	1 oz	87	20
Chunk Ham w/ 12% Water	1 oz	36	6
Chunk Ham w/ 20% Water	1 oz	39	6
Chunk Pastrami	1 oz	35	5
Combination Roll	1 oz	43	10
Dark Smoked Cured	1 oz	45	10
Diced Combination Roll	1 oz	43	10

FOOD	PORTION	CALORIES	FAT
Wampler Longacre *(cont.)*			
Diced Ham w/ 20% Water	1 oz	39	6
Diced White Roll	1 oz	43	10
Gourmet Breast	1 oz	31	2
Gourmet Brown & Glazed Breast	1 oz	28	2
Gourmet Brown & Roasted Breast	1 oz	35	3
Gourmet High Yield Skinless Breast	1 oz	28	tr
Gourmet Mini Breast	1 oz	35	4
Gourmet Skinless Brown & Roasted Breast	1 oz	31	1
Gourmet Smoked Breast	1 oz	37	3
Ham w/ 20% Water	1 oz	39	6
Lean-Lite Ham	1 oz	36	5
Lean-Lite Smoked Ham	1 oz	38	4
Mini Gourmet Smoked Breast	1 oz	37	3
Oven Roasted Oven Lite Breast	1 oz	35	3
Pastrami	1 oz	35	5
Premium Breast	1 oz	29	2
Premium Brown & Glazed Breast	1 oz	29	2
Premium Skinless Breast	1 oz	26	1
Premium Skinless Brown & Roasted Breast	1 oz	26	1
Roasted Thighs	1 oz	38	6
Roll Sliced Breast	1 oz	37	5
Roll White	1 oz	43	10
Salami	1 oz	45	8
Salt Watchers Breast	1 oz	35	tr
Sliced Bologna	1 oz	57	16
Sliced Ham	1 oz	37	5
Sliced Pastrami	1 oz	34	5

FOOD	PORTION	CALORIES	FAT
Sliced Salami	1 oz	46	9
Smoked Sliced Breast	1 oz	27	tr
Smoked Whole	1 oz	40	4
Turkey Deli Chef Breast & White	1 oz	35	5
Turkey No Skin Breast & White	1 oz	39	5
Weight Watchers			
Oven Roasted Breast	2 slices (¾ oz)	25	1
Oven Roasted Turkey Ham	2 slices (¾ oz)	25	1
Roasted & Smoked Breast	2 slices (¾ oz)	25	1
Smoked Deli Thin Breast	5 slices (⅓ oz)	10	tr
bologna	1 oz	57	4
breast	1 slice (¾ oz)	23	tr
diced light & dark, seasoned	1 oz	39	2
diced light & dark, seasoned	½ lb	313	14
ham thigh meat	2 oz	73	3
ham thigh meat	1 pkg (8 oz)	291	12
pastrami	2 oz	80	4
pastrami	1 pkg (8 oz)	320	14
patties, battered & fried	1 (3.3 oz)	266	17
poultry salad sandwich spread	1 tbsp	109	2
poultry salad sandwich spread	1 oz	238	4
prebasted breast w/ skin, roasted	½ breast (1.9 lbs)	1087	30
prebasted breast w/ skin, roasted	1 breast (3.8 lbs)	2175	60
prebasted thigh w/ skin, roasted	1 thigh (11 oz)	494	27
roll, light & dark meat	1 oz	42	2
roll, light meat	1 oz	42	2
salami, cooked	2 oz	111	8
salami, cooked	1 pkg (8 oz)	446	31
turkey loaf breast meat	2 slices (1.5 oz)	47	1

FOOD	PORTION	CALORIES	FAT
turkey loaf breast meat	1 pkg (6 oz)	187	3
turkey sticks, battered & fried	1 stick (2.3 oz)	178	11

TURKEY DISHES
(*see also* DINNER, TURKEY SUBSTITUTES)

FROZEN

Banquet Family Entrees Gravy & Sliced Turkey	6 oz	120	6
Banquet Entree Gravy & Turkey w/ Dressing	7 oz	220	8
Healthy Choice Roasted Turkey & Mushroom Gravy	8.5 oz	200	3
Kibun Turkey Pasta Salad w/ Dressing	½ pkg	250	12
Kibun Turkey Pasta Salad w/o Dressing	½ pkg	140	2
Le Menu Entree LightStyle Glazed Turkey	8.25 oz	260	6
Le Menu Entree LightStyle Traditional Turkey	8 oz	200	5
Ovenstuffs Turkey Turnover	1 (4.75 oz)	350	16
gravy & turkey	1 pkg (5 oz)	95	4
gravy & turkey	1 cup (8.4 oz)	160	6
READY-TO-USE			
Turkey Salad (The Spreadables)	¼ can	100	6
Turkey Salad (Wampler Longacre)	1 oz	71	17

TURKEY SUBSTITUTES

Meatless Turkey (Loma Linda)	2 slices (2 oz)	95	3
Smoked Turkey, frzn (Worthington)	3.5 oz	239	15

TURMERIC

ground	1 tsp	8	tr

FOOD	PORTION	CALORIES	FAT

TURNIPS

CANNED

Turnip Greens w/ Diced Turnips Seasoned w/ Pork (Luck's)	7.5 oz	90	6
greens	½ cup	17	tr

FRESH

cooked, mashed	½ cup	21	tr
greens, chopped, cooked	½ cup	15	tr
greens, raw, chopped	½ cup	7	tr
raw, cubed	½ cup	18	tr

FROZEN

Mashed (Southland)	3.6 oz	90	6
Rutabaga Yellow Turnips (Southland)	4 oz	50	0
greens, cooked	½ cup	24	tr

TURTLE

raw	3.5 oz	85	1

TUSK FISH

raw	3.5 oz	79	tr

VANILLA EXTRACT

Pure Vanilla Extract (Virginia Dare)	1 tsp	10	0

VEAL
(see also BEEF, VEAL DISHES)

FRESH

cubed, lean only, raw	1 oz	31	1
cutlet, lean only, braised	3 oz	172	4
cutlet, lean only, fried	3 oz	156	4
ground, broiled	3 oz	146	6

FOOD	PORTION	CALORIES	FAT
loin chop w/ bone, lean & fat, braised	1 (2.8 oz)	227	14
loin chop w/ bone, lean only, braised	1 (2.4 oz)	155	6
shoulder w/ bone, lean only, braised	3 oz	169	5
sirloin w/ bone, lean & fat, roasted	3 oz	171	9
sirloin w/ bone, lean only, roasted	3 oz	143	5

VEAL DISHES

TAKE-OUT

parmigiana	4.2 oz	279	18

VEGETABLES, MIXED
(*see also individual vegetables*)

FOOD	PORTION	CALORIES	FAT
CANNED			
Hanover	½ cup	110	0
Libby	½ cup	40	0
Seneca	½ cup	40	0
Chop Suey Vegetables (La Choy)	½ cup	10	tr
Cut Tomatoes & Corn (Trappey's)	½ cup	25	0
Cut w/ Tomatoes (Trappey's)	½ cup	25	0
Garden Medley (Green Giant)	½ cup	40	tr
Garden Salad Marinated (S&W)	½ cup	60	0
Peas & Carrots (Libby)	½ cup	50	0
Peas & Carrots (Seneca)	½ cup	50	0
Peas & Carrots Water Pack (S&W)	½ cup	35	0
Succotash Country Style (S&W)	½ cup	80	1
Sweet Peas w/ Tiny Pearl Onions (S&W)	½ cup	60	1
Vegetable Salad (Hanover)	½ cup	90	0
mixed vegetables	½ cup	39	tr

FOOD	PORTION	CALORIES	FAT
peas & carrots	½ cup	48	tr
peas & carrots, low sodium	½ cup	48	tr
peas & onions	½ cup	30	tr
succotash	½ cup	102	1
FROZEN			
American Mixtures (Green Giant)			
California	½ cup	25	0
Heartland	½ cup	25	0
New England	½ cup	70	1
San Francisco	½ cup	25	0
Santa Fe	½ cup	70	1
Seattle	½ cup	25	0
Breaded Medley (Ore Ida)	3 oz	160	9
Broccoli & Cauliflower, Cut (Hanover)	½ cup	20	0
Broccoli, Baby Carrots & Water Chestnuts Farm Fresh Mixtures (Birds Eye)	¾ cup	45	tr
Broccoli, Carrots & Pasta Twists in Lightly Seasoned Sauce (Birds Eye)	⅔ cup	87	11
Broccoli, Cauliflower & Carrots Farm Fresh Mixtures (Birds Eye)	¾ cup	33	tr
Broccoli, Cauliflower & Carrots in Butter Sauce (Green Giant)	½ cup	30	1
Broccoli, Cauliflower & Carrots in Cheese Sauce (Green Giant)	½ cup	60	2
Broccoli, Cauliflower, Carrots w/ Cheese Sauce (Birds Eye)	½ cup	99	5
Broccoli, Cauliflower w/ Creamy Italian Cheese Sauce (Birds Eye)	½ cup	89	6
Broccoli, Corn & Red Peppers Farm Fresh Mixtures (Birds Eye)	⅔ cup	60	tr

FOOD	PORTION	CALORIES	FAT
Brussels Sprouts, Cauliflower & Carrots Farm Fresh Mixtures (Birds Eye)	¾ cup	40	tr
Caribbean Blend (Hanover)	½ cup	20	0
Cauliflower, Baby Whole Carrots & Snow Peas Farm Fresh Mixtures (Birds Eye)	⅔ cup	38	tr
Carrots, Baby Whole Sweet Peas & Onions Deluxe Vegetable (Birds Eye)	½ cup	48	tr
Chinese Style International Recipe (Birds Eye)	½ cup	68	4
Chinese Style Stir Fry Vegetable (Birds Eye)	½ cup	36	tr
Chow Mein Style International Recipe (Birds Eye)	½ cup	89	4
Corn, Green Beans & Pasta Curls in Light Cream Sauce (Birds Eye)	½ cup	107	5
Garden Medley (Hanover)	½ cup	20	0
Green Peas & Pearl Onions (Birds Eye)	½ cup	71	tr
Harvest Fresh Mixed Vegetables (Green Giant)	½ cup	40	0
Italian Style International Recipe (Birds Eye)	½ cup	101	5
Japanese Style International Recipe (Birds Eye)	½ cup	88	4
Japanese Style Stir Fry Vegetable (Birds Eye)	½ cup	29	tr
Mandarin Style International Recipe (Birds Eye)	½ cup	86	4
Mandarin Vegetables (Budget Gourmet)	1 pkg	160	11
Mixed Fancy (La Choy)	½ cup	12	tr
Mixed Vegetables (Birds Eye)	½ cup	58	tr
Mixed Vegetables (Green Giant)	½ cup	40	0

FOOD	PORTION	CALORIES	FAT
Mixed Vegetables (Hanover)	½ cup	50	0
Mixed Vegetables in Butter Sauce (Green Giant)	½ cup	60	2
Mixed Vegetables w/ Onion Sauce (Birds Eye)	⅓ cup	97	5
New England Recipe Vegetables (Budget Gourmet)	1 pkg	230	14
New England Style International Recipe (Birds Eye)	½ cup	124	6
One Serve Broccoli, Carrots & Rotini in Cheese Sauce (Green Giant)	1 pkg	120	3
One Serve Broccoli, Cauliflower & Carrots (Green Giant)	1 pkg	25	0
Oriental Blend (Hanover)	½ cup	25	0
Pasta Primavera Style International Recipe (Birds Eye)	½ cup	121	5
Peas & Cauliflower in Cream Sauce (Budget Gourmet)	1 pkg	150	8
Peas & Pearl Onions w/ Cream Sauce (Birds Eye)	½ cup	137	5
Peas & Potatoes w/ Cream Sauce (Birds Eye)	½ cup	126	6
Peas & Water Chestnuts Oriental (Budget Gourmet)	1 pkg	110	4
Peppers & Onions (Southland)	2 oz	15	0
San Francisco Style International Recipe (Birds Eye)	½ cup	90	4
Soup Mix Vegetables (Southland)	3.2 oz	50	0
Spring Vegetables in Cheese Sauce (Budget Gourmet)	1 pkg	150	9
Stew Vegetables (Ore Ida)	3 oz	50	tr
Stew Vegetables (Southland)	4 oz	60	0
Succotash (Hanover)	½ cup	80	0
Summer Vegetables (Hanover)	½ cup	35	0

FOOD	PORTION	CALORIES	FAT
Valley Combinations Broccoli & Cauliflower (Green Giant)	½ cup	60	2
Vegetables for Soup (Hanover)	½ cup	60	0
mixed vegetables, cooked	½ cup	54	tr
peas & carrots, cooked	½ cup	38	tr
peas & onions, cooked	½ cup	40	tr
succotash, cooked	½ cup	79	1
HOME RECIPE			
succotash	½ cup	111	1
JUICE			
Smucker's Vegetable Juice Hearty	8 oz	58	tr
Smucker's Vegetable Juice Hot & Spicy	8 oz	58	tr
V8	6 oz	35	0
V8 No Salt Added	6 oz	35	0
V8 Spicy Hot	6 oz	35	0
vegetable juice cocktail	6 oz	34	tr
SHELF STABLE			
Corn, Green Beans, Carrots & Pasta in Tomato Sauce (Pantry Express)	½ cup	80	2
Green Beans, Potatoes & Mushrooms in a Seasoned Sauce (Pantry Express)	½ cup	50	2
Mixed Vegetables (Pantry Express)	½ cup	35	tr
TAKE-OUT			
caponata	¼ cup	28	1
curry	7.7 oz	398	33
pakoras	1 (2 oz)	108	5
ratatouille	8.8 oz	190	16
samosa	2 (4 oz)	519	46

FOOD	PORTION	CALORIES	FAT

VENISON

roasted	3 oz	134	3

VINEGAR

Apple Cider (White House)	2 tbsp	2	0
Red Wine (Regina)	1 oz	4	0
Red Wine (White House)	2 tbsp	4	0
cider	1 tbsp	tr	0

WAFFLES

FROZEN

Apple Cinnamon (Aunt Jemima)	2.5 oz	176	6
Apple Cinnamon (Eggo)	1	130	5
Belgian (Weight Watchers)	1 (1.5 oz)	120	4
Belgian Chef	1	90	2
Belgian Waffles & Sausage (Great Starts)	2.85 oz	280	19
Belgian Waffles w/ Strawberries & Sausage (Great Starts)	3.5 oz	210	8
Blueberry (Aunt Jemima)	2.5 oz	175	5
Blueberry (Eggo)	1	130	5
Blueberry Batter, as prep (Aunt Jemima)	3.6 oz	204	4
Buttermilk (Aunt Jemima)	2.5 oz	179	6
Buttermilk (Eggo)	1	130	5
Homestyle (Eggo)	1	130	5
Minis (Eggo)	4	90	3
Multi-Bran (Nutri-Grain)	1	120	5
Multi-Grain Belgian (Weight Watchers)	1 (1.5 oz)	120	4
Nut & Honey (Eggo)	1	130	5

FOOD	PORTION	CALORIES	FAT
Oat Bran (Common Sense)	1	110	4
Oat Bran w/ Fruit & Nut (Common Sense)	1	120	5
Original (Aunt Jemima)	2.5 oz	173	6
Plain (Nutri-Grain)	1	120	5
Raisin & Bran (Nutri-Grain)	1	120	5
Special K (Kellogg's)	1	80	0
Strawberry (Eggo)	1	130	5
Waffle (Kid Cuisine)	3.6 oz	160	3
Waffle w/ Bacon (Great Starts)	2.2 oz	230	14
Waffles (Roman Meal)	2	280	14
Wholegrain Wheat/Oat Bran (Aunt Jemima)	2.5 oz	154	3
HOME RECIPE waffle	7" diam	245	13
MIX as prep w/ egg & milk	1 waffle (2.6 oz)	205	8

WALNUTS

Black (Planters)	1 oz	180	17
English Halves (Planters)	1 oz	190	20
black, dried	1 oz	172	16
black, dried, chopped	1 cup	759	71
english, dried	1 oz	182	18
english, dried, chopped	1 cup	770	74

WATER
(*see* MINERAL/BOTTLED WATER)

FOOD	PORTION	CALORIES	FAT

WATER CHESTNUTS

CANNED

Empress Sliced	2 oz	14	0
Empress Whole	2 oz	14	0
La Choy Sliced	¼ cup	18	tr
La Choy Whole	4	14	tr
chinese sliced	½ cup	35	tr

FRESH

| sliced | ½ cup | 66 | tr |

WATERCRESS
(see also CRESS*)*

| raw, chopped | ½ cup | 2 | tr |

WATERMELON

| cut up | 1 cup | 50 | 1 |
| wedge | 1/16 | 152 | 2 |

SEEDS

| dried | 1 oz | 158 | 13 |
| dried | 1 cup | 602 | 51 |

WAX BEANS

CANNED

Libby	½ cup	20	0
Owatonna Cut	½ cup	20	0
S&W Golden Cut Premium	½ cup	20	0
Seneca	½ cup	20	0

WHALE

| raw | 3.5 oz | 134 | 3 |

FOOD	PORTION	CALORIES	FAT

WHEAT
(*see also* BULGUR, BRAN, COUSCOUS, CEREAL, FLOUR, WHEAT GERM)

FOOD	PORTION	CALORIES	FAT
Hard Red Spring (Arrowhead)	2 oz	190	1
Hard Red Winter (Arrowhead)	2 oz	190	1
Soft Red (Arrowhead)	2 oz	190	1
Vital Wheat Gluten	2 oz	200	1
Wheat Flakes (Arrowhead)	2 oz	210	1
sprouted	⅓ cup	71	tr
starch	3.5 oz	348	tr

WHEAT GERM

FOOD	PORTION	CALORIES	FAT
Arrowhead Raw	2 oz	210	6
Kretschmer	¼ cup	103	3
Kretschmer Honey Crunch	¼ cup	105	3
plain, toasted	¼ cup	108	3
plain, toasted	1 cup	431	12
plain, untoasted	¼ cup	104	3
w/ brown sugar & honey, toasted	1 oz	107	2
w/ brown sugar & honey, toasted	1 cup	426	9

WHIPPED TOPPINGS
(*see also* CREAM)

FOOD	PORTION	CALORIES	FAT
Cool Whip Extra Creamy Dairy	1 tbsp	16	1
Cool Whip Non Dairy	1 tbsp	11	tr
Diamond Crystal	1 tbsp	7	tr
Dream Whip	1 tbsp	9	tr
D-Zerta w/ Nutrasweet	1 tbsp	7	tr
Estee Whipped Topping	1 tbsp	4	tr
Kraft Real Cream Topping	¼ cup	30	2
Kraft Whipped Topping	¼ cup	35	3
cream, pressurized	1 tbsp	8	tr

FOOD	PORTION	CALORIES	FAT
cream, pressurized	1 cup	154	13
nondairy, powdered, as prep w/ whole milk	1 tbsp	8	tr
nondairy, powdered, as prep w/ whole milk	1 cup	151	10
nondairy, pressurized	1 tbsp	11	1
nondairy, pressurized	1 cup	184	16
nondairy, frzn	1 tbsp	13	1

WHITE BEANS

CANNED			
Spanish Style (Goya)	7.5 oz	130	1
white beans	1 cup	306	1

DRIED			
regular, cooked	1 cup	249	1
regular, raw	1 cup	674	2
small, cooked	1 cup	253	1
small, raw	1 cup	723	3

WHITEFISH

fresh, baked	3 oz	146	6
smoked whitefish	1 oz	39	tr
smoked whitefish	3 oz	92	1

WHITING

fresh, cooked	3 oz	98	1

WILD RICE
(see also RICE)

cooked	½ cup	83	tr

FOOD	PORTION	CALORIES	FAT
WINE			
(*see also* WINE COOLERS)			
red	3.5 oz	74	0
rose	3.5 oz	73	0
sherry	2 oz	84	0
sweet dessert	2 oz	90	0
vermouth, dry	3.5 oz	105	0
vermouth, sweet	3.5 oz	167	0
white	3.5 oz	70	0
WINE COOLERS			
Bartles & Jaymes			
Berry	6 oz	107	0
Black Cherry	6 oz	104	0
Blush	6 oz	94	0
Light Berry	6 oz	71	0
Original	6 oz	99	0
Peach	6 oz	107	0
Premium Light	6 oz	65	0
Red Sangria	6 oz	107	0
Tropical	6 oz	115	0
WINGED BEANS			
dried, cooked	1 cup	252	10
dried, raw	1 cup	745	30
WOLFFISH			
fresh atlantic, baked	3 oz	105	3

FOOD	PORTION	CALORIES	FAT

YAM
(see also SWEET POTATO)

CANNED

Candied (S&W)	½ cup	180	0
Golden Cut in Syrup (Sugary Sam)	½ cup	110	0
Golden Whole in Heavy Syrup (Trappey's)	½ cup	130	0
Southern Whole in Extra Heavy Syrup (S&W)	½ cup	139	1

FRESH

mountain yam, hawaiian, cooked	½ cup	59	tr
yam, cubed, cooked	½ cup	79	tr

YAM BEAN

cooked	¾ cup	38	tr

YARDLONG BEANS

dried, cooked	1 cup	202	1
dried, raw	1 cup	580	2

YEAST

baker's, dry, active	1 pkg (7 g)	20	tr
brewer's, dry	1 tbsp	25	tr

YELLOW BEANS

dried, cooked	1 cup	254	2
dried, raw	1 cup	676	5

YELLOW-EYE BEANS

CANNED

Yellow Eye Baked Beans (B&M)	⅞ cup	290	7

FOOD	PORTION	CALORIES	FAT

YELLOWTAIL

FOOD	PORTION	CALORIES	FAT
fresh, baked	3 oz	159	6

YOGURT
(*see also* TOFU; YOGURT, FROZEN)

FOOD	PORTION	CALORIES	FAT
All Flavors (Cabot)	8 oz	220	3
All Flavors Ultimate 90 (Weight Watchers)	1 cup	90	0
All Flavors w/ Fruit Lowfat (Friendship)	8 oz	230	3
Amaretto Almond Yo Creme (Yoplait)	5 oz	240	10
Apple (La Yogurt)	6 oz	190	4
Apple Cinnamon Breakfast Yogurt (Yoplait)	6 oz	220	4
Apple Crisp Lowfat (New Country)	6 oz	150	2
Apple Original (Yoplait)	4 oz	120	2
Apple Original (Yoplait)	6 oz	190	3
Apples 'N Spice Nonfat Lite (Colombo)	8 oz	190	tr
Banana Custard Style	6 oz	190	4
Banana Fruit on Bottom (Dannon)	8 oz	240	3
Banana Strawberry Classic (Colombo)	8 oz	250	6
Banana Strawberry Nonfat Lite (Colombo)	8 oz	190	tr
Banana Strawberry Nonfat Lite Swiss Style (Colombo)	4.4 oz	100	0
Bavarian Chocolate Yo Creme	5 oz	270	11
Berries Breakfast Yogurt (Yoplait)	6 oz	230	4
Black Cherry 100 Calorie w/ Aspartame (Light N'Lively)	8 oz	100	0
Black Cherry Classic (Colombo)	8 oz	230	6

FOOD	PORTION	CALORIES	FAT
Black Cherry Lowfat (Breyers)	8 oz	260	3
Black Cherry Lowfat (Light N'Lively)	8 oz	230	2
Black Cherry w/ Aspartame (Knudsen Cal 70)	8 oz	70	0
Blueberry (Dannon)	8 oz	200	4
Blueberry (La Yogurt)	6 oz	190	4
Blueberry (La Yogurt 25)	8 oz	200	0
Blueberry (Mountain High)	1 cup	220	6
Blueberry (Yoplait 150)	6 oz	150	0
Blueberry 100 Calorie w/ Aspartame (Light N'Lively)	8 oz	90	0
Blueberry Classic (Colombo)	8 oz	230	6
Blueberry Custard Style (Yoplait)	6 oz	190	4
Blueberry Fruit on Bottom (Dannon)	4.4 oz	130	2
Blueberry Fruit on Bottom (Dannon)	8 oz	240	3
Blueberry Lowfat (Breyers)	8 oz	250	2
Blueberry Lowfat (Light N'Lively)	4.4 oz	130	1
Blueberry Lowfat (Light N'Lively)	8 oz	240	2
Blueberry Nonfat (Dannon)	6 oz	140	0
Blueberry Nonfat Light (Dannon)	4.4 oz	60	0
Blueberry Nonfat Light (Dannon)	8 oz	100	0
Blueberry Nonfat Lite (Colombo)	8 oz	190	tr
Blueberry Nonfat Lite Swiss Style (Colombo)	4.4 oz	100	0
Blueberry Original (Yoplait)	4 oz	120	2
Blueberry Original (Yoplait)	6 oz	190	3
Blueberry Supreme Lowfat (New Country)	6 oz	150	2
Blueberry w/ Aspartame (Knudsen Cal 70)	8 oz	70	0
Blueberry w/ Aspartame (Light N'Lively Free)	8 oz	50	0

FOOD	PORTION	CALORIES	FAT
Boysenberry Fruit on Bottom (Dannon)	8 oz	240	3
Boysenberry Lowfat (Knudsen)	8 oz	240	4
Boysenberry Original (Yoplait)	4 oz	120	2
Cherries Jubilee (Yoplait)	5 oz	220	8
Cherry (La Yogurt)	6 oz	190	4
Cherry (La Yogurt 25)	8 oz	200	0
Cherry (Yoplait 150)	6 oz	150	0
Cherry Custard Style (Yoplait)	6 oz	180	4
Cherry Fruit on Bottom (Dannon)	4.4 oz	130	2
Cherry Fruit on Bottom (Dannon)	8 oz	240	3
Cherry Lowfat (Knudsen)	8 oz	240	4
Cherry Lowfat (Light N'Lively)	4.4 oz	140	1
Cherry Nonfat Lite (Colombo)	8 oz	190	tr
Cherry Original (Yoplait)	4 oz	120	2
Cherry Supreme Lowfat (New Country)	6 oz	150	2
Cherry Vanilla (La Yogurt)	6 oz	190	4
Cherry Vanilla (Lite Line)	1 cup	240	2
Cherry Vanilla Nonfat Light (Dannon)	8 oz	100	0
Cherry w/ Almonds Breakfast Yogurt (Yoplait)	6 oz	210	3
Coffee Lowfat (Dannon)	8 oz	200	3
Coffee Lowfat (Friendship)	8 oz	210	3
Coffee Nonfat Lite (Colombo)	8 oz	190	tr
Dutch Apple Fruit on Bottom (Dannon)	8 oz	240	3
Exotic Fruit Fruit on Bottom (Dannon)	8 oz	240	3
French Vanilla Classic (Colombo)	8 oz	215	7
French Vanilla Lowfat (New Country)	6 oz	150	2

FOOD	PORTION	CALORIES	FAT
Fruit Cocktail Nonfat Lite (Colombo)	8 oz	190	tr
Fruit Crunch Lowfat (New Country)	6 oz	150	2
Grape Lowfat (Light N'Lively)	4.4 oz	130	1
Hawaiian Salad Lowfat (New Country)	6 oz	150	2
Key Lime (La Yogurt)	6 oz	190	4
Lemon 100 Calorie w/ Aspartame (Light N'Lively)	8 oz	100	0
Lemon Custard Style (Yoplait)	6 oz	190	4
Lemon Lowfat (Dannon)	8 oz	200	3
Lemon Lowfat (Knudsen)	8 oz	240	4
Lemon Nonfat Lite (Colombo)	8 oz	190	tr
Lemon Original (Yoplait)	4 oz	120	2
Lemon Supreme Lowfat (New Country)	6 oz	150	2
Lemon w/ Aspartame (Knudsen Cal 70)	8 oz	70	0
Lime Lowfat (Knudsen)	8 oz	240	4
Mixed Berries Fruit on Bottom (Dannon)	4.4 oz	130	2
Mixed Berries Fruit on Bottom (Dannon)	8 oz	240	3
Mixed Berries Lowfat (New Country)	6 oz	150	2
Mixed Berries Lowfat (Dannon)	8 oz	240	3
Mixed Berry (La Yogurt)	6 oz	190	4
Mixed Berry Custard Style (Yoplait)	6 oz	180	4
Mixed Berry Lowfat (Breyers)	8 oz	250	4
Mixed Berry Original (Yoplait)	4 oz	120	2
Orange Original (Yoplait)	4 oz	120	2
Orange Supreme Lowfat (New Country)	6 oz	150	2
Peach (La Yogurt)	6 oz	190	4

FOOD	PORTION	CALORIES	FAT
Peach (Lite Line)	1 cup	230	2
Peach (Yoplait 150)	6 oz	150	0
Peach 100 Calorie w/ Aspartame (Light N'Lively)	8 oz	100	0
Peach Fruit Mousette (Colombo)	3.5 oz	80	tr
Peach Fruit on Bottom (Dannon)	8 oz	240	3
Peach Lowfat (Breyers)	8 oz	250	2
Peach Lowfat (Knudsen)	8 oz	240	4
Peach Lowfat (Light N'Lively)	4.4 oz	130	1
Peach Lowfat (Light N'Lively)	8 oz	240	2
Peach Lowfat Blended w/ Fruit (Dannon)	4 oz	110	2
Peach Melba Classic (Colombo)	8 oz	230	6
Peach Nonfat (Dannon)	6 oz	140	0
Peach Nonfat Light (Dannon)	8 oz	100	0
Peach Nonfat Lite (Colombo)	8 oz	190	tr
Peach Nonfat Lite Swiss Style (Colombo)	4.4 oz	100	0
Peach Original (Yoplait)	4 oz	120	2
Peach w/ Aspartame (Knudsen Cal 70)	8 oz	70	0
Peaches 'N Cream Lowfat (New Country)	6 oz	150	2
Pina Colada (La Yogurt)	6 oz	190	4
Pina Colada Fruit on Bottom (Dannon)	8 oz	240	3
Pina Colada Original (Yoplait)	4 oz	120	2
Pineapple Lowfat (Breyers)	8 oz	250	2
Pineapple Lowfat (Light N'Lively)	4.4 oz	130	1
Pineapple Lowfat (Light N'Lively)	8 oz	230	2
Pineapple Original (Yoplait)	4 oz	120	2

FOOD	PORTION	CALORIES	FAT
Pineapple w/ Aspartame (Knudsen Cal 70)	8 oz	70	0
Plain (Cabot)	8 oz	140	4
Plain (Friendship)	8 oz	170	8
Plain (Knudsen)	8 oz	200	9
Plain (La Yogurt)	6 oz	140	6
Plain (Mountain High)	1 cup	200	9
Plain (Yoplait)	4 oz	80	2
Plain (Yoplait)	6 oz	120	3
Plain Classic (Colombo)	8 oz	150	7
Plain Extra Mild Sweetened (Colombo)	8 oz	200	7
Plain Lowfat (Breyers)	8 oz	140	3
Plain Lowfat (Dannon)	8 oz	140	4
Plain Lowfat (Knudsen)	8 oz	160	5
Plain Lowfat (Meadow Gold)	1 cup	160	5
Plain Lowfat Swiss Style (Lite Line)	1 cup	140	2
Plain Nonfat (Colombo)	8 oz	110	tr
Plain Nonfat (Dannon)	8 oz	110	0
Plain Nonfat (Weight Watchers)	1 cup	90	0
Raspberries & Cream (Yoplait)	5 oz	230	9
Raspberry (La Yogurt 25)	8 oz	200	0
Raspberry (Yoplait 150)	6 oz	150	0
Raspberry Classic (Colombo)	8 oz	230	6
Raspberry Custard Style (Yoplait)	6 oz	190	4
Raspberry Fruit Mousette (Colombo)	3.5 oz	80	tr
Raspberry Fruit on Bottom (Dannon)	4.4 oz	120	1
Raspberry Fruit on Bottom (Dannon)	8 oz	240	3
Raspberry Lowfat (Knudsen)	8 oz	240	4
Raspberry Lowfat Blended w/ Fruit (Dannon)	4 oz	110	2

FOOD	PORTION	CALORIES	FAT
Raspberry Nonfat (Dannon)	6 oz	140	0
Raspberry Nonfat (Dannon)	8 oz	200	4
Raspberry Nonfat Light (Dannon)	8 oz	100	0
Raspberry Nonfat Lite (Colombo)	8 oz	190	tr
Raspberry Nonfat Lite Swiss Style (Colombo)	4.4 oz	100	0
Raspberry Original (Yoplait)	4 oz	120	2
Raspberry Sundae Style (Meadow Gold)	1 cup	250	4
Raspberry Supreme Lowfat (New Country)	6 oz	150	2
Red Raspberry 100 Calorie w/ Aspartame (Light N'Lively)	8 oz	90	0
Red Raspberry Lowfat (Breyers)	8 oz	250	2
Red Raspberry Lowfat (Light N'Lively)	4.4 oz	130	1
Red Raspberry Lowfat (Light N'Lively)	8 oz	230	2
Red Raspberry w/ Aspartame (Knudsen Cal 70)	8 oz	70	0
Red Raspberry w/ Aspartame (Light N'Lively)	8 oz	50	0
Strawberries Romanoff (Yoplait)	5 oz	220	8
Strawberry (La Yogurt)	6 oz	190	4
Strawberry (La Yogurt 25)	8 oz	200	0
Strawberry (Lite Line)	1 cup	240	2
Strawberry (Yoplait 150)	6 oz	150	0
Strawberry 100 Calorie w/ Aspartame (Light N'Lively)	8 oz	90	0
Strawberry Banana (La Yogurt)	6 oz	190	4
Strawberry Banana (La Yogurt 25)	8 oz	200	0
Strawberry Banana (Yoplait 150)	6 oz	150	0

FOOD	PORTION	CALORIES	FAT
Strawberry Banana 100 Calorie w/ Aspartame (Light N'Lively)	8 oz	90	0
Strawberry Banana Breakfast Yogurt (Yoplait)	6 oz	240	4
Strawberry Banana Fruit on Bottom (Dannon)	4.4 oz	130	2
Strawberry Banana Lowfat (Breyers)	8 oz	250	2
Strawberry Banana Lowfat (Dannon)	8 oz	200	4
Strawberry Banana Lowfat (Knudsen)	8 oz	250	4
Strawberry Banana Lowfat (Light N'Lively)	4.4 oz	140	1
Strawberry Banana Lowfat (Light N'Lively)	8 oz	260	2
Strawberry Banana Lowfat (New Country)	6 oz	150	2
Strawberry Banana Lowfat Blended w/ Fruit (Dannon)	4 oz	110	2
Strawberry Banana Nonfat Light (Dannon)	8 oz	100	0
Strawberry Banana Original (Yoplait)	4 oz	120	2
Strawberry Banana w/ Aspartame (Knudsen Cal 70)	8 oz	70	0
Strawberry Banana w/ Aspartame (Light N'Lively Free)	8 oz	50	0
Strawberry Classic (Colombo)	8 oz	230	6
Strawberry Custard Style (Yoplait)	6 oz	190	4
Strawberry Fruit Cup Nonfat Light (Dannon)	8 oz	100	0
Strawberry Fruit Cup w/ Aspartame (Light N'Lively Free)	8 oz	50	0
Strawberry Fruit Mousette (Colombo)	3.5 oz	80	tr
Strawberry Fruit on Bottom (Dannon)	4.4 oz	130	2

FOOD	PORTION	CALORIES	FAT
Strawberry Fruit on Bottom (Dannon)	8 oz	240	3
Strawberry Lowfat (Breyers)	8 oz	250	2
Strawberry Lowfat (Dannon)	8 oz	200	4
Strawberry Lowfat (Knudsen)	8 oz	250	4
Strawberry Lowfat (Light N'Lively)	4.4 oz	130	1
Strawberry Lowfat (Light N'Lively)	8 oz	240	2
Strawberry Lowfat Blended w/ Fruit (Dannon)	4 oz	110	2
Strawberry Nonfat (Dannon)	6 oz	140	0
Strawberry Nonfat Light (Dannon)	4.4 oz	60	0
Strawberry Nonfat Light (Dannon)	8 oz	100	0
Strawberry Nonfat Lite (Colombo)	8 oz	190	tr
Strawberry Nonfat Lite Swiss Style (Colombo)	4.4 oz	100	0
Strawberry Original (Yoplait)	4 oz	120	2
Strawberry Rhubarb Original (Yoplait)	4 oz	120	2
Strawberry Supreme Lowfat (New Country)	6 oz	150	2
Strawberry w/ Almonds Breakfast Yogurt (Yoplait)	6 oz	210	3
Strawberry w/ Aspartame (Knudsen Cal 70)	8 oz	70	0
Strawberry w/ Aspartame (Light N'Lively Free)	8 oz	50	0
Strawberry Fruit Basket w/ Aspartame (Knudsen Cal 70)	8 oz	70	0
Strawberry Fruit Cup (La Yogurt)	6 oz	190	4
Strawberry Fruit Cup Lowfat (Light N'Lively)	4.4 oz	130	1
Strawberry Fruit Cup Lowfat (Light N'Lively)	8 oz	240	2

FOOD	PORTION	CALORIES	FAT
Strawberry Fruit Cup Lowfat (New Country)	6 oz	150	2
Sunrise Peach Breakfast Yogurt (Yoplait)	6 oz	230	3
Tropical Fruits Breakfast Yogurt (Yoplait)	6 oz	230	4
Tropical Orange (La Yogurt)	6 oz	190	4
Vanilla (La Yogurt)	6 oz	160	4
Vanilla Bean Lowfat (Breyers)	8 oz	230	3
Vanilla Custard Style (Yoplait)	6 oz	180	4
Vanilla Lowfat (Dannon)	8 oz	200	3
Vanilla Lowfat (Friendship)	8 oz	210	3
Vanilla Lowfat (Knudsen)	8 oz	240	4
Vanilla Nonfat Light (Dannon)	8 oz	100	0
Vanilla Nonfat Lite (Colombo)	8 oz	160	tr
Vanilla Nonfat Lite Swiss Style (Colombo)	4.4 oz	100	0
Vanilla w/ Aspartame (Knudsen Cal 70)	8 oz	70	0
coffee lowfat	8 oz	194	3
fruit lowfat	4 oz	113	1
fruit lowfat	8 oz	225	3
plain	8 oz	139	7
plain lowfat	8 oz	144	4
plain nonfat	8 oz	127	tr
vanilla lowfat	8 oz	194	3

YOGURT, FROZEN

All Flavors Gourmet Yogurt (Bresler's)	5 oz	145	2
All Flavors Just 10	1 oz	10	0

FOOD	PORTION	CALORIES	FAT
All Flavors Lite Yogurt (Bresler's)	5 oz	135	0
Banana Strawberry (Edy's)	3 oz	80	1
Black Cherry (Sealtest Free)	½ cup	110	0
Blueberry (Edy's)	3 oz	80	1
Blueberry (Elan)	4 oz	130	3
Blueberry Softy (Dannon)	4 oz	110	2
Butter Pecan Softy (Dannon)	4 oz	110	2
Cappuccino Softy (Dannon)	4 oz	110	2
Caramel Almond Praline (Elan)	4 oz	150	4
Cheesecake Softy (Dannon)	4 oz	110	2
Cherry (Ben & Jerry's)	4 oz	160	5
Cherry (Edy's)	3 oz	80	1
Chocolate (Ben & Jerry's)	4 oz	121	4
Chocolate (Edy's)	3 oz	80	1
Chocolate (Elan)	4 oz	130	3
Chocolate (Haagen-Dazs)	3 oz	130	3
Chocolate (Sealtest Free)	½ cup	110	0
Chocolate Almond (Elan)	4 oz	160	6
Chocolate Bee-Lite	4 oz	100	tr
Chocolate Chip (Edy's)	3 oz	100	1
Chocolate Fi-Bar	1	190	7
Chocolate Kissed w/ Honey	3.5 oz	100	3
Chocolate Kissed w/ Honey Nonfat	3.5 oz	85	tr
Chocolate Nonfat Softy (Dannon)	4 oz	110	0
Chocolate Softy (Dannon)	4 oz	140	2
Chocolate Yogurt Bar (Dole)	1	70	tr
Chocolate Yogurt Shake (Weight Watchers)	7.5 oz	220	1
Citrus Heights (Edy's)	3 oz	80	1
Coffee (Elan)	4 oz	130	3

FOOD	PORTION	CALORIES	FAT
Cookies 'N' Cream (Edy's)	3 oz	100	1
Decaffeinated Coffee (Elan)	4 oz	130	3
Dutch Chocolate Deserve	4 oz	80	0
Golden Vanilla Nonfat Softy (Dannon)	4 oz	100	0
Lemon Meringue Softy (Dannon)	4 oz	110	2
Marble Fudge (Edy's)	3 oz	100	1
Peach (Ben & Jerry's)	4 oz	133	2
Peach (Elan)	4 oz	130	3
Peach (Haagen-Dazs)	3 oz	120	3
Peach (Sealtest Free)	½ cup	100	0
Peach Softy (Dannon)	4 oz	110	2
Peanut Butter Softy (Dannon)	4 oz	130	3
Perfectly Peach (Edy's)	3 oz	80	1
Pina Colada Softy (Dannon)	4 oz	110	2
Plain Softy (Dannon)	4 oz	90	1
Raspberry (Ben & Jerry's)	4 oz	133	2
Raspberry (Edy's)	3 oz	80	1
Raspberry Softy (Dannon)	4 oz	110	2
Raspberry Vanilla Swirl (Edy's)	3 oz	80	1
Red Raspberry (Sealtest Free)	½ cup	100	0
Red Raspberry Nonfat Softy (Dannon)	4 oz	100	0
Rum Raisin (Elan)	4 oz	135	3
Rum Raisin Nonfat Softy (Dannon)	4 oz	100	0
Strawberry (Borden)	½ cup	100	2
Strawberry (Edy's)	3 oz	80	1
Strawberry (Elan)	4 oz	125	3
Strawberry (Haagen-Dazs)	3 oz	120	3
Strawberry (Meadow Gold)	½ cup	100	2

FOOD	PORTION	CALORIES	FAT
Strawberry (Sealtest Free)	½ cup	100	0
Strawberry Banana Yogurt Bar (Dole)	1	60	tr
Strawberry Banana Softy (Dannon)	4 oz	110	2
Strawberry Fi-Bar	1	190	7
Strawberry Nonfat (Dannon)	6 oz	140	0
Strawberry Nonfat Softy (Dannon)	4 oz	100	0
Strawberry Softy (Dannon)	4 oz	110	2
Strawberry Yogurt Bar (Dole)	1	70	tr
Sweet Cream (Ben & Jerry's)	4 oz	130	3
Vanilla (Edy's)	3 oz	80	1
Vanilla (Elan)	4 oz	130	3
Vanilla (Haagen-Dazs)	3 oz	130	3
Vanilla (Sealtest Free)	½ cup	100	0
Vanilla Almond Crunch (Haagen-Dazs)	3 oz	150	5
Vanilla Bee-Lite	4 oz	110	tr
Vanilla Desserve	4 oz	70	0
Vanilla Fi-Bar	1	190	7
Vanilla Kissed w/ Honey	3.5 oz	100	3
Vanilla Kissed w/ Honey Nonfat	3.5 oz	85	tr
Vanilla Softy (Dannon)	4 oz	110	2

ZABAGLIONE
(*see* CUSTARD)

ZUCCHINI

CANNED
S&W Italian Style | ½ cup | 45 | 1 |

| italian style | ½ cup | 33 | tr |

FOOD	PORTION	CALORIES	FAT
FRESH			
baby, raw	1 (½ oz)	3	tr
raw, sliced	½ cup	9	tr
sliced, cooked	½ cup	14	tr
FROZEN			
Breaded Zucchini (Ore Ida)	3 oz	150	8
Zucchini Sliced (Southland)	3.2 oz	15	0
cooked	½ cup	19	tr

PART II
Restaurant, Take-Out and Fast-Food Chains

PART II

Restaurant, Take-Out and Fast-Food Chains

FOOD	PORTION	CALORIES	FAT

ARBY'S

BEVERAGES

FOOD	PORTION	CALORIES	FAT
7UP	12 oz	144	0
Coca-Cola Classic	12 oz	141	0
Coffee, Black	8 oz	3	0
Diet 7UP	12 oz	4	0
Diet Coke	12 oz	1	0
Hot Chocolate	8 oz	110	1
Iced Tea	16 oz	6	0
Milk, 2%	8 oz	121	4
Nehi Orange	12 oz	190	0
Orange Juice	6 oz	82	0
Pepsi-Cola	12 oz	159	0
R.C. Cola	12 oz	173	0
R.C. Diet Rite	12 oz	1	0
R.C. Root Beer	12 oz	173	0
Upper Ten	12 oz	169	0

BREAKFAST SELECTIONS

FOOD	PORTION	CALORIES	FAT
Biscuit, Bacon	1	318	18
Biscuit, Ham	1	323	17
Biscuit, Plain	1	280	14
Biscuit, Sausage	1	460	32
Blueberry Muffin	1	200	6
Cinnamon Nut Danish	1	340	10
Croissant, Bacon & Egg	1	389	26
Croissant, Ham & Cheese	1	345	21
Croissant, Mushroom & Cheese	1	493	38
Croissant, Plain	1	260	16
Croissant, Sausage & Egg	1	519	39

FOOD	PORTION	CALORIES	FAT
Maple Syrup	1.5 oz	120	tr
Platter, Bacon	1	860	32
Platter, Egg	1	460	24
Platter, Ham	1	518	26
Platter, Sausage	1	640	41
Toastix	1 serving	420	25
DESSERTS			
Butterfinger Polar Swirl	1	457	18
Cheese Cake	1 serving	306	23
Chocolate Chip Cookie	1	130	4
Chocolate Shake	12 oz	451	12
Heath Polar Swirl	1	543	22
Jamocha Shake	11.5 oz	368	11
Oreo Polar Swirl	1	482	20
P'nut Butter Cup Polar Swirl	1	517	24
Snickers Polar Swirl	1	511	19
Turnover, Apple	1	303	18
Turnover, Blueberry	1	320	19
Turnover, Cherry	1	280	18
Vanilla Shake	11 oz	330	12
MAIN MENU SELECTIONS			
Arby's Sauce	½ oz	15	tr
Au Jus	4 oz	7	0
Bac N'Cheddar Deluxe Sandwich	1	532	33
Baked Potato, Broccoli 'N Cheddar	1	417	18
Baked Potato, Deluxe	1	621	36
Baked Potato, Mushroom & Cheese	1	515	27
Baked Potato, Plain	1	240	2
Baked Potato w/ Butter/Margarine & Sour Cream	1	463	25

FOOD	PORTION	CALORIES	FAT
Beef N'Cheddar Sandwich	1	451	20
Cheddar Fries	1 serving (5 oz)	399	22
Chicken Breast Sandwich	1	489	46
Chicken Cordon Bleu Sandwich	1	658	37
Chicken Fajita Pita	1	272	9
Curly Fries	1 serving (3.5 oz)	337	18
Fish Fillet Sandwich	1	537	29
French Dip	1	345	12
French Dip 'N Swiss	1	425	18
French Fries	1 serving	246	13
Grilled Chicken Barbeque Sandwich	1	378	14
Grilled Chicken Deluxe Sandwich	1	426	21
Ham 'N Cheese Sandwich	1	330	15
Horsey Sauce	½ oz	55	5
Ketchup	½ oz	16	0
Light Ham Deluxe	1	255	6
Light Roast Beef Deluxe	1	294	10
Light Roast Chicken Deluxe	1	263	6
Light Roast Turkey Deluxe	1	260	5
Mayonnaise, Cholesterol Free	½ oz	90	10
Mustard	½ oz	11	1
Philly Beef N' Swiss Sandwich	1	498	26
Potato Cakes	1 serving	204	12
Roast Beef Sandwich, Giant	1	530	27
Roast Beef Sandwich, Junior	1	218	11
Roast Beef Sandwich, Regular	1	353	15
Roast Beef Sandwich, Super	1	529	28
Roast Chicken Club	1	513	29
Roast Chicken Deluxe Sandwich	1	373	20

FOOD	PORTION	CALORIES	FAT
Roast Chicken Salad	1	184	7
Sub Deluxe	1	482	26
Sugar Substitute	⅓ oz	4	0
Turkey Deluxe Sandwich	1	399	20
SALADS AND DRESSINGS			
Blue Cheese	2 oz	295	31
Buttermilk Ranch	2 oz	349	39
Cashew Chicken Salad	1	590	37
Chef Salad	1	210	11
Croutons	½ oz	59	2
Garden Salad	1	149	9
Honey French	2 oz	322	27
Italian Light	2 oz	23	1
Thousand Island	2 oz	298	29
Weight Watchers Creamy French	1 oz	48	3
Weight Watchers Creamy Italian	1 oz	29	3
SOUPS			
Beef w/ Vegetables & Barley	8 oz	96	3
Boston Clam Chowder	8 oz	207	11
Cream of Broccoli	8 oz	180	8
French Onion	8 oz	67	3
Lumberjack Mixed Vegetable	8 oz	89	4
Old Fashioned Chicken Noodle	8 oz	99	2
Pilgrim's Corn Chowder	5 oz	193	11
Split Pea w/ Ham	8 oz	200	10
Tomato Florentine	8 oz	244	2
Wisconsin Cheese	8 oz	287	19

FOOD	PORTION	CALORIES	FAT

AU BON PAIN

BREAD AND ROLLS

FOOD	PORTION	CALORIES	FAT
3-Seed Raisin	1 roll	250	4
Alpine	1 roll	220	3
Baguette	1 loaf	810	2
Cheese	1 loaf	1670	29
Country Seed	1 roll	220	4
Four Grain	1 loaf	1420	11
French	1 roll	320	tr
Hearth	1 roll	250	2
Hearth Sandwich Roll	1	370	3
Onion Herb	1 loaf	1430	13
Parisienne	1 loaf	1490	4
Petit Pain	1 roll	220	tr
Pumpernickel	1 roll	210	2
Rye	1 roll	230	2
Sandwich Croissant	1	300	14
Soft Roll	1	310	8
Vegetable	1 roll	230	5

COOKIES

FOOD	PORTION	CALORIES	FAT
Chocolate Chip	1	280	15
Chocolate Chunk Pecan	1	290	17
Oatmeal Raisin	1	250	9
Peanut Butter	1	290	15
White Chocolate Chunk Pecan	1	300	17

CROISSANTS

FOOD	PORTION	CALORIES	FAT
Almond	1	420	25
Apple	1	250	10
Blueberry Cheese	1	380	20
Chocolate	1	400	24

FOOD	PORTION	CALORIES	FAT
Chocolate Hazelnut	1	480	28
Cinnamon Raisin	1	390	13
Coconut Pecan	1	440	23
Ham & Cheese	1	370	20
Plain	1	220	10
Raspberry Cheese	1	400	20
Spinach & Cheese	1	290	16
Strawberry Cheese	1	400	20
Sweet Cheese	1	420	23
Turkey & Cheddar	1	410	22
Turkey & Harvati	1	410	21
MUFFINS			
Blueberry	1	390	11
Bran	1	390	11
Carrot	1	450	22
Corn	1	460	17
Cranberry Walnut	1	350	13
Oat Bran Apple	1	400	10
Pumpkin	1	410	16
Whole Grain	1	440	16
SALADS			
Chicken Cracked Pepper	1	100	2
Chicken Grilled	1	110	2
Chicken Tarragon	1	310	15
Garden, Large	1	40	tr
Garden, Small	1	20	tr
Shrimp	1	102	2
Tuna	1	350	25
SANDWICH FILLINGS			
Boursin	1 serving	290	18

FOOD	PORTION	CALORIES	FAT
Brie	1 serving	300	24
Chicken Cracked Pepper	1 serving	120	2
Chicken Grilled	1 serving	130	4
Chicken Tarragon	1 serving	270	15
Country Ham	1 serving	150	7
Roast Beef	1 serving	180	8
Smoked Turkey	1 serving	100	1
Swiss	1 serving	330	24
Tuna Salad	1 serving	310	24
SOUPS			
Beef Barley	1 cup	80	2
Beef Barley	1 bowl	125	3
Chicken Noodle	1 cup	80	2
Chicken Noodle	1 bowl	125	2
Clam Chowder	1 cup	270	17
Clam Chowder	1 bowl	390	25
Cream of Broccoli	1 cup	250	18
Cream of Broccoli	1 bowl	380	15
Garden Vegetarian	1 cup	50	tr
Garden Vegetarian	1 bowl	70	tr
Minestrone	1 cup	120	2
Minestrone	1 bowl	190	3
Split Pea	1 cup	250	3
Split Pea	1 bowl	380	3
Tomato Florentine	1 cup	90	2
Tomato Florentine	1 bowl	120	2
Vegetarian Chili	1 cup	180	4
Vegetarian Chili	1 bowl	280	7

FOOD	PORTION	CALORIES	FAT
BASKIN-ROBBINS			
Chocolate Raspberry Truffle	1 scoop	310	17
Daiquiri Ice	1 scoop	140	0
Fat Free Chocolate Vanilla Twist	½ cup	100	0
Fat Free Just Peachy	½ cup	100	0
Light Chocolate w/ Caramel Ribbon Bar	1	150	5
Light Praline Dream	½ cup	130	6
Light Strawberry Royal	½ cup	110	3
Pralines 'N Cream Ice Cream Bar	1	310	13
Rainbow Sherbet	1 scoop	160	2
Strawberry Low Fat Frozen Yogurt	½ cup	120	1
Strawberry Nonfat Frozen Yogurt	½ cup	110	0
Sugar Cone	1	60	1
Sugar Free Jamoca Swiss Almond	½ cup	90	2
Sugar Free Strawberry	½ cup	80	1
Vanilla Chilly Burger	1	240	11
Vanilla Ice Cream	1 scoop	240	14
Very Berry Strawberry Ice Cream	1 scoop	220	10
Waffle Cone	1	140	2
World Class Chocolate Ice Cream	1 scoop	280	14
BURGER KING			
BEVERAGES			
7UP	1 reg	144	0
Coffee, Black	6 oz	2	0
Diet Pepsi	1 reg	1	0
Milk, 2%	8 oz	121	5
Milk, Whole	8 oz	157	9
Orange Juice	6 oz	80	0

FOOD	PORTION	CALORIES	FAT
Pepsi-Cola	1 reg	159	0
Shake, Chocolate	1 reg	320	12
Shake, Vanilla	1 reg	321	10
BREAKFAST SELECTIONS			
Breakfast Croissan'wich, Bacon	1	355	21
Breakfast Croissan'wich, Ham	1	335	20
Breakfast Croissan'wich, Sausage	1	538	41
French Toast Sticks	1 serving	499	29
Scrambled Egg Platter	1	468	30
Scrambled Egg Platter w/ Bacon	1	536	36
Scrambled Egg Platter w/ Sausage	1	702	52
DESSERTS			
Apple Pie	1	305	12
Great Danish	1	500	36
MAIN MENU SELECTIONS			
Bacon Double Cheeseburger	1	510	31
Cheeseburger	1	317	15
Chicken Specialty Sandwich	1	688	40
Chicken Tenders	6 pieces	204	10
French Fries	1 reg	227	13
Ham & Cheese Specialty Sandwich	1	471	23
Hamburger	1	275	12
Onion Rings	1 reg	274	16
Whaler Fish Sandwich	1	488	27
Whopper Double Beef	1	863	53
Whopper Double Beef w/ Cheese	1	946	60
Whopper Jr. Sandwich	1	322	17
Whopper Jr. Sandwich w/ Cheese	1	364	20
Whopper Sandwich	1	628	36
Whopper Sandwich w/ Cheese	1	711	43

FOOD	PORTION	CALORIES	FAT
SALADS AND DRESSINGS			
1000 Island	3 tbsp	117	12
Bleu Cheese	3 tbsp	156	16
House	3 tbsp	130	13
Italian, Reduced Calorie	3 tbsp	14	0
Salad w/o Dressing	1 reg	28	0

CARL'S JR.

FOOD	PORTION	CALORIES	FAT
BAKERY SELECTIONS			
Chocolate Chip Cookies	2.5 oz	330	17
Cinnamon Roll	1	460	18
Danish	1	520	16
Fudge Brownie	1	430	19
Fudge Moussecake	1 slice	400	23
Muffin, Blueberry	1	340	9
Muffin, Bran	1	310	6
Raspberry Cheesecake	1 slice	310	17
BEVERAGES			
Iced Tea	1 reg	2	0
Milk, 2%	10 oz	180	6
Orange Juice	1 sm	90	tr
Shake	1 reg	330	7
Soda	1 reg	240	0
Soda, Diet	1 reg	2	0
BREAKFAST SELECTIONS			
Bacon	2 strips	45	4
Breakfast Burrito	1	430	26
English Muffin w/ Margarine	1	190	5
French Toast Dips w/o Syrup	1 serving	490	26
Hash Brown Nuggets	1 serving	270	17

FOOD	PORTION	CALORIES	FAT
Hot Cakes w/ Margarine w/o Syrup	1 serving	510	24
Sausage	1 patty	190	18
Scrambled Eggs	1 serving	120	9
Sunrise Sandwich	1	300	13
MAIN MENU SELECTIONS			
All Star Chili Dog	1	720	47
All Star Hot Dog	1	540	35
American Cheese	½ oz	60	5
Carl's Catch Fish Sandwich	1	560	30
Cheeseburger, Double Western Bacon	1	1030	63
Cheeseburger, Western Bacon	1	730	39
Chicken Club Charbroiler	1	570	29
Chicken Charbroiler BBQ Sandwich	1	310	6
Chicken Santa Fe Sandwich	1	540	13
Country Fried Steak Sandwich	1	720	45
CrissCut Fries	1 serving	330	22
French Fries	1 reg	420	20
Guacamole	1 oz	50	1
Hamburger	1	220	14
Hamburger, Famous Star	1	610	38
Hamburger, Old Time Star	1	460	20
Hamburger, Super Star	1	820	53
Jr. Crisp Burrito	1	140	7
Onion Rings	1 serving	520	26
Potato, Bacon & Cheese	1	730	43
Potato, Broccoli & Cheese	1	590	31
Potato, Fiesta	1	720	38
Potato, Lite	1	250	1
Potato, Sour Cream & Chives	1	470	19

FOOD	PORTION	CALORIES	FAT
Potato w/ Cheese	1	690	36
Roast Beef Club	1	620	34
Roast Beef Deluxe Sandwich	1	540	26
Salsa	1 oz	8	0
Swiss Cheese	½ oz	60	4
Taco Sauce	1 oz	8	0
Zucchini	1 serving	390	23
SALADS AND DRESSINGS			
1000 Island	1 oz	110	11
Blue Cheese	1 oz	150	15
French Reduced Calorie	1 oz	40	2
House	1 oz	110	11
Italian	1 oz	120	13
Salad-to-Go Chicken	1	200	8
Salad-to-Go Garden	1 sm	50	3

CARVEL

FOOD	PORTION	CALORIES	FAT
Lo-Yo Vanilla Frozen Yogurt	1 oz	34	1

CHICK-FIL-A

FOOD	PORTION	CALORIES	FAT
BEVERAGES			
Iced Tea, Unsweetened	9 oz	3	tr
Lemonade	10 oz	124	tr
DESSERTS			
Fudge Brownie w/ Nuts	1	369	19
Icedream	4.5 oz	134	5
Lemon Pie	1 slice	329	5
MAIN MENU SELECTIONS			
Carrot-Raisin Salad	1 serving	116	5
Chargrilled Chicken	3.6 oz	128	2

FOOD	PORTION	CALORIES	FAT
Chargrilled Chicken Deluxe Sandwich	1	266	5
Chargrilled Chicken Garden Salad	10.4 oz	126	2
Chargrilled Chicken Sandwich	1	258	5
Chick-fil-A Chicken	1 piece (3.6 oz)	219	7
Chick-fil-A Chicken Deluxe Sandwich	1	368	9
Chick-fil-A Nuggets	8 pack	287	15
Chick-fil-A Nuggets	12 pack	430	23
Chick-fil-A Sandwich	1	360	9
Chick-n-Q Sandwich	1	206	7
Chicken Salad Cup	3.4 oz	309	28
Chicken Salad Plate	1 (11.8 oz)	579	45
Chicken Salad Sandwich w/ Wheat Bread	1	449	26
Cole Slaw	1 serving	175	14
Hearty Breast of Chicken Soup	8.5 oz	152	3
Potato Salad	1 serving	198	15
Tossed Salad	4.5 oz	21	tr
Tossed Salad w/ Honey French	6 oz	246	24
Tossed Salad w/ Lite Italian	6 oz	46	2
Tossed Salad w/ Ranch	6 oz	177	16
Tossed Salad w/ Thousand Island	6 oz	231	22
Waffle Potato Fries	1 reg	270	14

CHURCH'S FRIED CHICKEN

Breast	4.3 oz	278	17
Corn w/ Butter Oil	1 ear	237	9
French Fries	1 reg	138	6
Leg	2.9 oz	147	9
Thigh	4.2 oz	306	22
Wing & Breast	4.8 oz	303	20

FOOD	PORTION	CALORIES	FAT

D'ANGELO SANDWICH SHOPS

DESSERTS

FOOD	PORTION	CALORIES	FAT
Frozen Banana Yogurt	5 oz	125	3
Frozen Banana Yogurt w/ Cone	5 oz	215	4
Frozen Peach Yogurt	5 oz	130	3
Frozen Peach Yogurt w/ Cone	5 oz	220	3

SALADS

FOOD	PORTION	CALORIES	FAT
Beef	1 serving (3.25 oz)	350	5
Chicken	1 serving (3.25 oz)	325	4
Tuna	1 serving (2 oz)	305	2
Turkey	1 serving (3.25 oz)	375	4

SANDWICHES

FOOD	PORTION	CALORIES	FAT
D'Lite Pocket, Chicken Stir Fry	1	340	4
D'Lite Pocket, Roast Beef	1	325	5
D'Lite Pocket, Steak	1	415	11
D'Lite Pocket, Steak & Mushroom	1	420	11
D'Lite Pocket, Steak & Pepper	1	420	11
D'Lite Pocket, Turkey	1	350	4
D'Lite Pocket, Vegetarian	1	350	11
D'Lite Small Sub, Roast Beef	1	365	7
D'Lite Small Sub, Turkey	1	390	6

DAIRY QUEEN/BRAZIER

FOOD SELECTION

FOOD	PORTION	CALORIES	FAT
¼-lb Super Dog	1	590	38
Baked Chicken Fillet Sandwich w/ Cheese	1	480	25
BBQ Beef Sandwich	1	225	4

FOOD	PORTION	CALORIES	FAT
Breaded Chicken Fillet Sandwich	1	430	20
Double Hamburger	1	460	25
Double Hamburger w/ Cheese	1	570	34
DQ Homestyle Ultimate Burger	1	700	47
Fish Fillet Sandwich	1	370	16
Fish Fillet Sandwich w/ Cheese	1	420	21
French Dressing, Reduced Calorie	2 oz	90	5
French Fries	1 sm	210	10
French Fries	1 reg	300	14
French Fries	1 lg	390	18
Garden Salad	1	200	13
Grilled Chicken Fillet Sandwich	1	300	8
Hot Dog	1	280	16
Hot Dog w/ Cheese	1	330	21
Hot Dog w/ Chili	1	320	19
Lettuce	½ oz	2	0
Onion Rings	1 reg	240	12
Side Salad	1	25	0
Single Hamburger	1	310	13
Single Hamburger w/ Cheese	1	365	18
Thousand Island Dressing	2 oz	225	21
Tomato	½ oz	3	0
ICE CREAM			
Banana Split	1	510	11
Blizzard, Strawberry	1 sm	500	12
Blizzard, Strawberry	1 reg	740	16
Breeze, Strawberry	1 sm	400	tr
Breeze, Strawberry	1 reg	590	1
Buster Bar	1	450	29
Cone, Chocolate	1 reg	230	7

FOOD	PORTION	CALORIES	FAT
Cone, Chocolate	1 lg	350	11
Cone, Dipped Chocolate	1 reg	330	16
Cone, Vanilla	1 sm	140	4
Cone, Vanilla	1 reg	230	7
Cone, Vanilla	1 lg	340	10
Cone, Yogurt	1 reg	180	tr
Cone, Yogurt	1 lg	260	tr
Cup, Yogurt	1 reg	170	tr
Cup, Yogurt	1 lg	230	tr
Dilly Bar	1	210	13
DQ Frozen Cake Slice Undecorated	1	380	18
DQ Sandwich	1	140	4
Heath Blizzard	1 sm	560	23
Heath Blizzard	1 reg	820	36
Heath Breeze	1 sm	450	12
Heath Breeze	1 reg	680	21
Hot Fudge Brownie Delight	1	710	29
Malt, Vanilla	1 reg	610	14
Mr. Misty	1 reg	250	0
Nutty Double Fudge	1	580	22
Peanut Buster Parfait	1	710	32
QC Big Scoop, Chocolate	1	310	14
QC Big Scoop, Vanilla	1	300	14
Shake, Chocolate	1 reg	540	14
Shake, Vanilla	1 reg	520	14
Shake, Vanilla	1 lg	600	16
Sundae, Chocolate	1 reg	300	7
Sundae, Strawberry Yogurt	1 reg	200	tr
Sundae, Strawberry Waffle Cone	1	350	12

FOOD	PORTION	CALORIES	FAT

DOMINO'S PIZZA
(see also GODFATHER'S, PIZZA, PIZZA HUT, SHAKEY'S)

10″ PIZZA

FOOD	PORTION	CALORIES	FAT
Double Cheese	2 slices	284	11
Double Cheese & Pepperoni	2 slices	331	15
Ground Beef	2 slices	250	8
Ground Beef & Pepperoni	2 slices	297	13
Mushroom & Sausage	2 slices	248	9
Pepperoni	2 slices	265	10
Pepperoni & Mushroom	2 slices	267	11
Pepperoni & Sausage	2 slices	293	13
Plain Cheese	2 slices	218	6
Sausage	2 slices	246	8

14″ PIZZA

FOOD	PORTION	CALORIES	FAT
Double Cheese	2 slices	365	14
Double Cheese & Pepperoni	2 slices	427	19
Ground Beef	2 slices	321	11
Ground Beef & Pepperoni	2 slices	382	13
Mushroom & Sausage	2 slices	322	11
Pepperoni	2 slices	343	13
Pepperoni & Mushroom	2 slices	346	13
Pepperoni & Sausage	2 slices	380	17
Plain Cheese	2 slices	281	7
Sausage	2 slices	318	11

LARGE PIZZA

FOOD	PORTION	CALORIES	FAT
Double Cheese	2 slices	700	19
Double Cheese & Pepperoni	2 slices	778	26
Ground Beef	2 slices	527	14
Ground Beef & Pepperoni	2 slices	605	22
Mushroom & Sausage	2 slices	532	15

FOOD	PORTION	CALORIES	FAT
Pepperoni	2 slices	556	18
Pepperoni & Mushroom	2 slices	550	17
Pepperoni & Sausage	2 slices	606	20
Plain Cheese	2 slices	478	10
Sausage	2 slices	528	15
SMALL PIZZA			
Double Cheese	2 slices	480	16
Double Cheese & Pepperoni	2 slices	453	22
Ground Beef	2 slices	361	12
Ground Beef & Pepperoni	2 slices	431	16
Mushroom & Sausage	2 slices	365	13
Pepperoni	2 slices	384	15
Pepperoni & Mushroom	2 slices	388	15
Pepperoni & Sausage	2 slices	431	19
Plain Cheese	2 slices	314	9
Sausage	2 slices	360	13

DUNKIN' DONUTS
(*see also* DOUGHNUT, WINCHELL'S)

FOOD	PORTION	CALORIES	FAT
CROISSANTS			
Almond	1	420	27
Chocolate	1	440	29
Plain	1	310	19
DOUGHNUTS			
Apple-Filled w/ Cinnamon Sugar	1	250	11
Bavarian-Filled w/ Chocolate Frosting	1	240	11
Blueberry-Filled	1	210	8
Chocolate Frosted Yeast Ring	1	200	10
Glazed Buttermilk Ring	1	290	14
Glazed Chocolate Ring	1	324	21

FOOD	PORTION	CALORIES	FAT
Glazed Coffee Roll	1	280	12
Glazed French Cruller	1	140	8
Glazed Whole Wheat Ring	1	330	18
Glazed Yeast Ring	1	200	9
Jelly-Filled	1	220	9
Lemon-Filled	1	260	12
Plain Cake Ring	1	270	17
MISCELLANEOUS			
Chocolate Chunk Cookie	1	200	10
Chocolate Chunk Cookie w/ Nuts	1	210	11
Oatmeal Pecan Raisin Cookie	1	200	9
MUFFINS			
Apple N'Spice	1	300	8
Banana Nut	1	310	10
Blueberry	1	280	8
Bran w/ Raisins	1	310	9
Corn	1	340	12
Cranberry Nut	1	290	9
Oat Bran	1	330	11

EL POLLO LOCO

FOOD	PORTION	CALORIES	FAT
Beans	3.5 oz	110	1
Chicken	2 pieces	310	18
Coleslaw	2.8 oz	80	6
Combo Meal	1	720	28
Corn	3.3 oz	110	2
Corn Tortillas	3.3 oz	210	2
Dolewhip	4.5 oz	90	0
Flour Tortillas	3.3 oz	280	7
Potato Salad	4.3 oz	140	8

FOOD	PORTION	CALORIES	FAT
Rice	2.5 oz	100	1
Salsa	1.8 oz	10	0

GODFATHER'S PIZZA

FOOD	PORTION	CALORIES	FAT
Golden Crust Cheese	1/6 sm	213	8
Golden Crust Cheese	1/8 med	229	9
Golden Crust Cheese	1/10 lg	261	11
Golden Crust Combo	1/6 sm	273	12
Golden Crust Combo	1/8 med	283	13
Golden Crust Combo	1/10 lg	322	15
Original Crust Cheese	1/4 mini	138	4
Original Crust Cheese	1/6 sm	239	7
Original Crust Cheese	1/8 med	242	7
Original Crust Cheese	1/10 lg	271	8
Original Crust Combo	1/4 mini	164	5
Original Crust Combo	1/6 sm	299	11
Original Crust Combo	1/8 med	318	12
Original Crust Combo	1/10 lg	332	12

HAAGEN-DAZS

FOOD	PORTION	CALORIES	FAT
Banana Nonfat Soft Yogurt	1 oz	25	0
Blueberry Sorbet & Cream	4 oz	190	8
Butter Pecan	4 oz	390	24
Caramel Almond Crunch Bar	1	240	18
Caramel Nut Sundae	4 oz	310	21
Chocolate	4 oz	270	17
Chocolate Chocolate Chip	4 oz	290	20
Chocolate Chocolate Mint	4 oz	300	20
Chocolate Dark Chocolate Bar	1	390	27
Chocolate Frozen Yogurt	3 oz	130	3

FOOD	PORTION	CALORIES	FAT
Chocolate Nonfat Soft Yogurt	1 oz	30	0
Chocolate Soft Yogurt	1 oz	30	1
Coffee	4 oz	270	17
Coffee Soft Yogurt	1 oz	28	1
Deep Chocolate	4 oz	290	14
Deep Chocolate Fudge	4 oz	290	14
Fudge Pop Bar	1	210	14
Honey Vanilla	4 oz	250	16
Keylime Sorbet & Cream	4 oz	190	7
Lemon Sorbet	4 oz	140	0
Macadamia Brittle	4 oz	280	18
Orange & Cream Pop	1	130	6
Orange Sorbet	4 oz	113	0
Orange Sorbet & Cream	4 oz	190	8
Peach Frozen Yogurt	3 oz	120	3
Peanut Butter Crunch Bar	1	270	21
Raspberry Soft Yogurt	1 oz	30	1
Raspberry Sorbet	4 oz	93	0
Raspberry Sorbet & Cream	4 oz	180	8
Rum Raisin	4 oz	250	17
Strawberry	4 oz	250	15
Strawberry Frozen Yogurt	3 oz	120	3
Strawberry Nonfat Soft Yogurt	1 oz	25	0
Vanilla	4 oz	260	17
Vanilla Almond Crunch Frozen Yogurt	3 oz	150	5
Vanilla Crunch Bar	1	220	16
Vanilla Frozen Yogurt	3 oz	130	3
Vanilla Fudge	4 oz	270	17
Vanilla Milk Chocolate Almond Bar	1	370	27

FOOD	PORTION	CALORIES	FAT
Vanilla Milk Chocolate Bar	1	360	27
Vanilla Milk Chocolate Brittle Bar	1	370	25
Vanilla Peanut Butter Swirl	4 oz	280	21
Vanilla Soft Yogurt	1 oz	28	1
Vanilla Swiss Almond	4 oz	290	19

HARDEE'S

FOOD	PORTION	CALORIES	FAT
BEVERAGES			
Shake, Chocolate	12 oz	460	8
Shake, Strawberry	12 oz	440	8
Shake, Vanilla	12 oz	400	9
BREAKFAST SELECTIONS			
Bacon & Egg Biscuit	1	410	24
Bacon Biscuit	1	360	21
Bacon, Egg & Cheese Biscuit	1	460	28
Big Country Breakfast, Bacon	1	660	40
Big Country Breakfast, Country Ham	1	670	38
Big Country Breakfast, Ham	1	620	33
Big Country Breakfast, Sausage	1	850	57
Biscuit 'N' Gravy	1	440	24
Canadian Rise 'N' Shine Biscuit	1	470	27
Chicken Biscuit	1	430	22
Cinnamon 'N' Raisin Danish	1	320	17
Country Ham Biscuit	1	350	18
Country Ham & Egg Biscuit	1	400	22
Ham & Egg Biscuit	1	370	19
Ham Biscuit	1	320	16
Ham, Egg & Cheese Biscuit	1	420	23
Hash Rounds	1 serving	230	14
Margarine/Butter Blend	1 tsp	35	4

FOOD	PORTION	CALORIES	FAT
Rise 'N' Shine Biscuit	1	320	18
Sausage & Egg Biscuit	1	490	31
Sausage Biscuit	1	440	28
Steak & Egg Biscuit	1	550	32
Steak Biscuit	1	500	39
Syrup	1.5 oz	120	tr
Three Pancakes	1 serving	280	28
Three Pancakes w/ 1 Sausage Pattie	1 serving	430	16
Three Pancakes w/ 2 Bacon Strips	1 serving	350	9
DESSERTS			
Apple Turnover	1	270	12
Big Cookie	1	250	13
Cool Twist Sundae, Caramel	1	330	10
Cool Twist Sundae, Hot Fudge	1	320	12
Cool Twist Sundae, Strawberry	1	260	8
Cool Twist Cone, Chocolate	1	200	6
Cool Twist Cone, Vanilla/Chocolate	1	190	6
MAIN MENU SELECTIONS			
All Beef Hot Dog	1	300	17
Bacon Cheeseburger	1	610	39
Big Deluxe Burger	1	500	30
Big Fry	1 serving	500	23
Big Roast Beef	1	300	11
Big Twin	1	450	25
Cheeseburger	1	320	14
Chef Salad	1	240	9
Chicken Fillet	1	370	13
Chicken 'N' Pasta Salad	1	414	3
Chicken Stix	6 pieces	210	9
Chicken Stix	9 pieces	310	14

FOOD	PORTION	CALORIES	FAT
Crispy Curls	1 serving	300	16
Fisherman's Fillet	1	500	24
French Fries	1 reg	230	11
French Fries	1 lg	360	17
Garden Salad	1	210	14
Grilled Chicken Sandwich	1	310	9
Hamburger	1	270	10
Hot Ham 'N' Cheese	1	330	12
Mushroom 'N' Swiss Burger	1	490	27
Quarter-Pound Cheeseburger	1	500	29
Regular Roast Beef	1	260	9
Side Salad	1	20	tr
Turkey Club	1	390	16

JACK IN THE BOX

BEVERAGES

Coca-Cola Classic	12 oz	144	0
Coffee, Black	8 oz	2	0
Diet Coke	12 oz	1	0
Dr Pepper	12 oz	144	0
Iced Tea	12 oz	3	0
Milk, 2%	8 oz	122	5
Milk Shake, Chocolate	11 oz	330	7
Milk Shake, Strawberry	11 oz	320	7
Milk Shake, Vanilla	11 oz	320	6
Orange Juice	6 oz	80	0
Ramblin' Root Beer	12 oz	176	0
Sprite	12 oz	144	0

BREAKFAST SELECTIONS

Breakfast Jack	1	307	13

FOOD	PORTION	CALORIES	FAT
Country Crock Spread	1 pat	25	3
Grape Jelly	1 pkg	38	0
Hash Browns	1 serving	156	11
Pancake Platter	1	612	22
Pancake Syrup	1 pkg	121	0
Sausage Crescent	1	584	43
Scrambled Egg Platter	1	559	32
Scrambled Egg Pocket	1	431	21
Sourdough Breakfast Sandwich	1	381	20
Supreme Crescent	1	547	40
DESSERTS			
Cheesecake	1	309	18
Double Fudge Cake	1 slice	288	9
Hot Apple Turnover	1	354	19
MAIN MENU SELECTIONS			
Bacon Cheeseburger	1	705	45
BBQ Sauce	1 oz	44	tr
Cheeseburger	1	315	14
Chicken & Mushroom Sandwich	1	438	18
Chicken Fajita Pita	1	292	8
Chicken Strips	4 pieces	285	13
Chicken Strips	6 pieces	451	20
Chicken Supreme	1	641	39
Double Cheeseburger	1	467	27
Egg Rolls	3	437	24
Egg Rolls	5	753	41
Fish Supreme	1	510	27
French Fries	1 sm	219	11
French Fries	1 reg	351	17
French Fries	1 jumbo	396	19

FOOD	PORTION	CALORIES	FAT
Grilled Chicken Fillet	1	431	19
Grilled Sourdough Burger	1	712	50
Guacamole	1 oz	55	5
Ham & Turkey Melt	1	592	36
Hamburger	1	267	11
Jumbo Jack	1	584	34
Jumbo Jack w/ Cheese	1	677	40
Old Fashioned Patty Melt	1	713	46
Onion Rings	1 serving	380	23
Pastrami Melt	1	556	27
Salsa	1 oz	8	tr
Seasoned Curly French Fries	1 serving	358	20
Sesame Breadsticks	1	70	2
Super Taco	1	281	17
Sweet & Sour Sauce	1 oz	40	tr
Taco	1	187	11
Taquitos	7 pieces	511	21
Tortilla Chips	1 oz	139	6
Ultimate Cheeseburger	1	942	69
SALADS AND DRESSINGS			
Bleu Cheese	1 pkg	262	22
Buttermilk House	1 pkg	362	36
Chef Salad	1	325	18
Italian Low Calorie	1 pkg	25	2
Side Salad	1	51	3
Taco Salad	1	503	31
Thousand Island	1 pkg	312	30

FOOD	PORTION	CALORIES	FAT

KENTUCKY FRIED CHICKEN

CHICKEN DISHES

FOOD	PORTION	CALORIES	FAT
Chicken Little Sandwich	1	169	10
Colonel's Chicken Sandwich	1	482	27
Extra Crispy Center Breast	1	342	20
Extra Crispy Drumstick	1	204	14
Extra Crispy Thigh	1	406	30
Extra Crispy Wing	1	254	19
Kentucky Nuggets	1	46	3
Original Center Breast	1	283	15
Original Drumstick	1	146	9
Original Side Breast	1	267	17
Original Wing	1	178	12

SIDE DISHES

FOOD	PORTION	CALORIES	FAT
Buttermilk Biscuit	1	235	12
Cole Slaw	1 serving	119	7
Corn-on-the-Cob	1 ear	176	3
French Fries	1 reg	244	12
Mashed Potatoes & Gravy	1 serving	71	2
Sauce, Barbecue	1 oz	35	1
Sauce, Honey	½ oz	49	0
Sauce, Mustard	1 oz	36	1
Sauce, Sweet & Sour	1 oz	58	1

LONG JOHN SILVER'S

CHILDREN'S MENU SELECTIONS

FOOD	PORTION	CALORIES	FAT
Chicken Planks, 2 Pieces & Fryes	7.8 oz	510	22
Fish & Fryes, 1 Piece	6.9 oz	450	21
Fish, Chicken & Fryes	8.9 oz	580	27

FOOD	PORTION	CALORIES	FAT
DESSERTS			
Apple Pie	1 slice	320	13
Cherry Pie	1 slice	360	13
Chocolate Chip Cookie	1	230	9
Lemon Pie	1 slice	340	9
Oatmeal Raisin Cookie	1	160	10
Walnut Brownie	1	440	22
MAIN MENU SELECTIONS			
Batter Dipped Fish, 1 Piece	3.1 oz	210	12
Batter Dipped Fish, 2 Pieces	6.2 oz	410	24
Chicken	17.3 oz	620	16
Chicken Plank, 1 Piece	2 oz	130	6
Chicken Planks, 2 Pieces & Fryes	6.9 oz	440	18
Chicken Planks, 2 pieces	4 oz	270	13
Chicken Planks, 3 Pieces	5.9 oz	400	20
Chicken Planks, 3 Pieces w/ Fryes & Slaw	14.1 oz	860	37
Chicken Planks, 4 Pieces w/ Fryes & Slaw	16 oz	990	44
Clams w/ Fryes & Slaw	12.7 oz	910	44
Cole Slaw	3.4 oz	140	6
Corn Cobbette	1 piece	140	8
Fish & Chicken w/ Fryes & Slaw	15.2 oz	930	11
Fish & Fryes, 2 Pieces	9.2 oz	580	30
Fish & Fryes, 3 Pieces	14 oz	930	47
Fish & More, 2 Pieces	14 oz	860	11
Fish & More, 3 Pieces w/ Fryes & Slaw	17.5 oz	1070	53
Fish Light Portion w/ Lemon Crumb, 2 Pieces	10.3 oz	320	4
Fish Light Portion w/ Paprika, 2 Pieces	10 oz	300	2

FOOD	PORTION	CALORIES	FAT
Fish w/ Lemon Crumb, 3 Pieces	18.4 oz	640	14
Fish w/ Paprika, 3 Pieces	18.2 oz	610	12
Fish w/ Scampi Sauce, 3 Pieces	18.6 oz	660	18
Fryes	1 reg	170	6
Green Beans	4 oz	113	tr
Homestyle Fish, 1 Piece	1.6 oz	125	7
Homestyle Fish, 2 Pieces	3.3 oz	250	14
Homestyle Fish, 3 Pieces	5 oz	380	21
Hushpuppies	1	70	2
Long John's Homestyle Fish, 3 Pieces w/ Fryes & Slaw	13.1 oz	830	39
Long John's Homestyle Fish, 4 Pieces w/ Fryes & Slaw	14.8 oz	960	46
Ocean Chef Salad	8.2 oz	234	5
Rice Pilaf	5 oz	142	2
Sandwich, Baked Chicken	6.4 oz	310	8
Sandwich, Batter Dipped Chicken, 2 Pieces	6.5 oz	440	17
Sandwich, Batter Dipped Fish, 1 Piece	5.6 oz	380	16
Seafood Chowder w/ Cod	7 oz	140	6
Seafood Gumbo w/ Cod	7 oz	120	8
Seafood Salad	9.8 oz	230	5
Shrimp Scampi	10.6	610	18
SALAD DRESSINGS AND SAUCES			
Creamy Italian Dressing	1 oz	30	3
Dijon Herb Sauce	.88 oz	90	7
Honey Mustard Sauce	.88 oz	45	tr
Ketchup	⅓ oz	12	0
Malt Vinegar	.4 oz	2	tr
Ranch Dressing	1 oz	90	2

FOOD	PORTION	CALORIES	FAT
Sea Salad Dressing	1 oz	90	4
Seafood Sauce	.88 oz	35	tr
Sweet 'N Sour Sauce	.88 oz	40	tr
Tartar Sauce	.88 oz	70	3

MACHEEZMO MOUSE

FOOD	PORTION	CALORIES	FAT
CHILDREN'S MENU SELECTIONS			
Kid's Plate	7 oz	279	5
Kid's Plate w/ Chicken	9 oz	349	7
MAIN MENU SELECTIONS			
Bean/Cheese Enchilada	12 oz	405	8
Bean/Cheese Enchilada Dinner	22 oz	670	8
Beans	6 oz	214	0
Boss Sauce	1 oz	30	0
Cheese	1 oz	81	5
Cheese Quesadilla	5 oz	337	13
Chicken	3 oz	105	3
Chicken Burrito	13 oz	543	10
Chicken Burrito Dinner	23 oz	808	10
Chicken Enchilada	10 oz	332	10
Chicken Enchilada Dinner	20 oz	597	10
Chicken Quesadilla	9 oz	407	15
Chicken Majita	18 oz	704	9
Chicken Salad Small	10 oz	324	75
Chicken Salad Large	17 oz	612	15
Chicken Tacos	6 oz	294	8
Chicken Tacos Dinner	16 oz	559	8
Chicken w/ Green Salad	13 oz	377	6
Chili	3 oz	135	3
Chili Tacos	6 oz	314	8

FOOD	PORTION	CALORIES	FAT
Chili Tacos Dinner	16 oz	579	8
Chips	3 oz	394	17
Combo Burrito	14 oz	598	11
Combo Burrito Dinner	24 oz	863	11
Corn Tortilla	2 oz	128	0
Enchilada Sauce	1 oz	6	0
Famouse #5	14 oz	583	5
Flour Tortilla	2 oz	160	2
Guacamole	2 oz	201	5
Mex Cheese	1 oz	100	8
Mini Corn Tortilla	3 oz	160	0
Mixed Greens	4 oz	tr	0
Nacho Grande	8 oz	704	38
Nonfat Yogurt	1 oz	15	0
Rice	6 oz	274	0
Salad w/ Marinated, Small Veggies	5 oz	32	1
Salad w/ Marinated Veggies, Large	8 oz	54	1
Sour Cream Blend	1 oz	27	3
Vegetables	4 oz	43	0
Vegetarian Burrito	14 oz	601	7
Vegetarian Burrito Dinner	24 oz	866	7
Vegetarian Plate	15 oz	531	5
Vegetarian Tacos	6 oz	295	6
Vegetarian Tacos Dinner	16 oz	560	6
Veggie Taco Salad, Small	10 oz	379	8
Veggie Taco Salad, Large	17 oz	647	13
Whole Wheat Tortilla	2 oz	160	2

FOOD	PORTION	CALORIES	FAT

McDONALD'S

BEVERAGES

FOOD	PORTION	CALORIES	FAT
Apple Juice	6 oz	90	0
Coca-Cola Classic	16 oz	190	0
Diet Coke	16 oz	1	0
Grapefruit Juice	6 oz	80	0
Milk, 1%	8 oz	110	2
Milk Shake, Lowfat Chocolate	10.4 oz	320	1
Milk Shake, Lowfat Strawberry	10.4 oz	320	1
Milk Shake, Lowfat Vanilla	10.4 oz	290	1
Orange Drink	16 oz	177	0
Orange Juice	6 oz	80	0
Sprite	16 oz	190	0

BREAKFAST SELECTIONS

FOOD	PORTION	CALORIES	FAT
Biscuit w/ Bacon, Egg & Cheese	1	440	26
Biscuit w/ Sausage	1	420	28
Biscuit w/ Sausage & Egg	1	505	33
Biscuit w/ Spread	1	260	13
Breakfast Burrito	1	280	17
Cheerios	¾ cup	80	1
Egg McMuffin	1	280	11
English Muffin w/ Spread	1	170	4
Fat-Free Apple Bran Muffin	1	180	0
Fat-Free Blueberry Muffin	1	170	0
Hash Brown Potatoes	1 serving	130	7
Hotcakes w/ Margarine & Syrup	1 portion	440	12
Sausage	1	160	15
Sausage McMuffin	1	345	20
Sausage McMuffin w/ Egg	1	430	25

FOOD	PORTION	CALORIES	FAT
Scrambled Eggs	1 portion	140	10
Wheaties	¾ cup	90	1
DESSERTS			
Apple Pie	1 (3 oz)	260	15
Cone, Vanilla Lowfat Frozen Yogurt	1 (3 oz)	105	1
Cookies, Chocolaty Chip	1 pkg (2 oz)	330	15
Cookies, McDonaldland	1 pkg (2 oz)	290	9
Danish, Apple	1	390	17
Danish, Cinnamon Raisin	1	440	13
Danish, Iced Cheese	1	390	21
Danish, Raspberry	1	410	16
Sundae, Lowfat Frozen Yogurt, Hot Caramel	1 (6 oz)	270	3
Sundae, Lowfat Frozen Yogurt, Hot Fudge	1 (6 oz)	240	3
Sundae, Lowfat Frozen Yogurt, Strawberry	1 (6 oz)	210	1
MAIN MENU SELECTIONS			
Big Mac	1	500	26
Cheeseburger	1	305	13
Chicken Fajita	1	185	8
Chicken McNuggets	6	270	15
Filet-O-Fish	1	370	18
French Fries	1 sm	220	12
French Fries	1 med	320	17
French Fries	1 lg	400	22
Hamburger	1	255	9
McChicken	1	415	19
McLean Deluxe	1	320	10
McLean Deluxe w/ Cheese	1	370	14

FOOD	PORTION	CALORIES	FAT
Quarter Pounder	1	410	20
Quarter Pounder w/ Cheese	1	510	28
SALADS, DRESSINGS AND SAUCES			
1000 Island Dressing	1 pkg	225	20
Bacon Bits	.1 oz	15	1
Bleu Cheese Dressing	1 pkg	250	20
Chef Salad	1 serving	170	9
Chunky Chicken Salad	1 serving	150	4
Croutons	.3 oz	50	2
Garden Salad	1	50	2
Lite Vinaigrette Dressing	1 pkg	48	2
McNuggets Sauce, Barbeque	1.12 oz	50	1
McNuggets Sauce, Honey	.5 oz	45	0
McNuggets Sauce, Hot Mustard	1.05 oz	70	4
McNuggets Sauce, Sweet 'N Sour	1.12 oz	60	tr
Ranch Dressing	1 pkg	220	20
Red French Reduced Calorie Dressing	1 pkg	160	8
Side Salad	1 serving	30	4

NATHAN'S

French Fries	1 (7 oz)	550	31
Hot Dog & Roll	1	290	19

PIZZA HUT

HAND TOSSED, MEDIUM			
Cheese	2 slices	518	20
Pepperoni	2 slices	500	23
Super Supreme	2 slices	556	25
Supreme	2 slices	540	26

FOOD	PORTION	CALORIES	FAT
PAN PIZZA, MEDIUM			
Cheese	2 slices	492	18
Pepperoni	2 slices	540	22
Super Supreme	2 slices	563	26
Supreme	2 slices	589	30
PERSONAL PAN PIZZA			
Pepperoni	1 pie	675	29
Supreme	1 pie	647	28
THIN 'N CRISPY, MEDIUM			
Cheese	2 slices	398	17
Pepperoni	2 slices	413	20
Super Supreme	2 slices	463	21
Supreme	2 slices	459	22

PONDEROSA

FOOD	PORTION	CALORIES	FAT
BEVERAGES			
Cherry Coke	6 oz	77	0
Chocolate Milk	8 oz	208	9
Coca-Cola	6 oz	72	0
Coffee, Black	6 oz	2	0
Diet Coke	6 oz	tr	0
Diet Coke, Caffeine-Free	6 oz	tr	0
Diet Sprite	6 oz	2	0
Dr Pepper	6 oz	72	0
Lemonade	6 oz	68	0
Milk	8 oz	159	9
Mr. Pibb	6 oz	71	0
Orange Soda	6 oz	82	0
Root Beer	6 oz	80	0
Sprite	6 oz	72	0

FOOD	PORTION	CALORIES	FAT
Tea	6 oz	2	0
DESSERTS			
Ice Milk, Chocolate	3.5 oz	152	3
Ice Milk, Vanilla	3.5 oz	150	3
Topping, Caramel	1 oz	100	1
Topping, Chocolate	1 oz	89	tr
Topping, Strawberry	1 oz	71	tr
Topping, Whipped	1 oz	80	6
MAIN MENU SELECTIONS			
Bake 'R Broil Fish	1 serving (5.2 oz)	230	13
BBQ Sauce	1 tbsp	25	0
Beans, Baked	1 serving (4 oz)	170	6
Beans, Green	1 serving (3.5 oz)	20	0
Breaded Cauliflower	1 serving (4 oz)	115	1
Breaded Okra	1 serving (4 oz)	124	1
Breaded Onion Rings	1 serving (4 oz)	213	9
Breaded Zucchini	1 serving (4 oz)	102	1
Carrots	1 serving (3.5 oz)	31	tr
Cheese Sauce	2 oz	52	2
Cheese, Herb & Garlic Spread	1 tbsp	100	10
Chicken Breast	1 serving (5.5 oz)	90	2
Chicken Wings	2	213	9
Chopped Steak	4 oz	225	16
Chopped Steak	5.3 oz	296	22
Corn	1 serving (3.5 oz)	90	tr
Fish Fried	1 serving (3.2 oz)	190	9

FOOD	PORTION	CALORIES	FAT
Fish Nuggets	1	31	2
Gravy, Brown	2 oz	25	1
Gravy, Turkey	2 oz	25	tr
Halibut, Broiled	1 serving (6 oz)	170	2
Hot Dog	1	144	13
Italian Breadsticks	1	100	1
Kansas City Strip	5 oz	138	6
Macaroni & Cheese	4 oz	67	2
Margarine, Liquid	1 tbsp	100	11
Meatballs	1	58	2
Mini Shrimp	6	47	tr
New York Strip, Choice	8 oz	314	11
New York Strip, Choice	10 oz	384	15
Pasta Shells, Plain	2 oz	78	tr
Peas	1 serving (3.5 oz)	67	tr
Porterhouse	13 oz	441	30
Porterhouse, Choice	16 oz	640	31
Potato, Baked	1	145	tr
Potato Wedges	1 serving (3.5 oz)	130	6
Potatoes, French Fried	1 serving	120	4
Potatoes, Mashed	1 serving (4 oz)	62	tr
Ribeye	5 oz	219	13
Ribeye, Choice	6 oz	281	14
Rice Pilaf	1 serving (4 oz)	160	4
Roll, Dinner	1	184	3
Roll, Sourdough	1	110	1
Roughy, Broiled	1 serving (5 oz)	139	5
Salmon, Broiled	1 serving (6 oz)	192	3
Sandwich Steak	4 oz	408	11

FOOD	PORTION	CALORIES	FAT
Scrod, Baked	1 serving (7 oz)	120	1
Shrimp, Fried	7 pieces	231	tr
Sirloin, Choice	7 oz	241	11
Sirloin Tips, Choice	5 oz	473	8
Spaghetti, Plain	2 oz	78	tr
Spaghetti Sauce	4 oz	110	4
Steak Kabobs (Meat only)	3 oz	153	5
Stuffing	4 oz	230	11
Sweet & Sour Sauce	1 oz	37	1
Swordfish, Broiled	1 serving (6 oz)	271	9
T-Bone	8 oz	176	9
T-Bone, Choice	10 oz	444	18
Teriyaki Steak	5 oz	174	3
Tortilla Chips	1 oz	150	8
Trout, Broiled	1 serving (5 oz)	228	4
Winter Mix	1 serving (3.5 oz)	25	0
SALAD BAR			
Alfalfa Sprouts	1 oz	10	0
Apple	1	80	1
Apples, Canned	4 oz	90	0
Applesauce	4 oz	80	0
Banana	1	87	tr
Banana Chips	.2 oz	25	1
Banana Pudding	1 oz	52	2
Bean Sprouts	1 oz	10	tr
Beets, Diced	4 oz	55	tr
Broccoli	1 oz	9	1
Cabbage, Green	1 oz	9	0
Cabbage, Red	1 oz	1	0

FOOD	PORTION	CALORIES	FAT
Cantaloupe	1 wedge	13	0
Carrots	1 oz	12	tr
Cauliflower	1 oz	8	tr
Celery	1 oz	4	0
Cheese, Imitation, Shredded	1 oz	90	7
Cheese Spread	1 oz	98	7
Cherry Peppers	2 pieces	7	tr
Chicken Salad	3.5 oz	212	15
Chow Mein Noodles	.2 oz	25	1
Cocktail Sauce	1 oz	34	1
Coconut, Shredded	.2 oz	25	2
Cottage Cheese	4 oz	120	5
Croutons	1 oz	115	4
Cucumber	1 oz	4	0
Eggs, Diced	2 oz	94	7
Fruit Cocktail	4 oz	97	tr
Garbanzo Beans	1 oz	102	0
Gelatin, Plain	4 oz	71	0
Granola	.2 oz	24	1
Grapes	10	34	tr
Green Pepper	1 oz	6	tr
Green Onion	1	7	tr
Ham, Diced	2 oz	120	10
Honeydew	1 wedge	24	tr
Lemon	1 wedge	3	tr
Lettuce	1 oz	5	0
Macaroni Salad	3.5 oz	335	12
Margarine, Whipped	1 tbsp	34	1
Meal Mates Sesame Crackers	2	45	2
Melba Snacks	2	18	0

FOOD	PORTION	CALORIES	FAT
Mousse, Chocolate	1 oz	78	4
Mousse, Strawberry	1 oz	74	5
Mushrooms	1 oz	8	tr
Olives, Black	1	4	tr
Olives, Green	1	3	tr
Onions, Red & Yellow	1 oz	11	0
Orange	1	45	tr
Pasta Salad	3.5 oz	269	12
Peaches, Canned	4 oz	70	0
Peanuts, Chopped	.2 oz	30	2
Pears, Canned	4 oz	98	tr
Pickles, Dill Spears	.14 oz	tr	0
Pickles, Sweet Chips	.14 oz	4	0
Pineapple, Fresh	1 wedge	11	tr
Pineapple Tidbits	4 oz	95	tr
Potato Salad	3.5 oz	126	6
Radishes	1 oz	4	0
Ritz Crackers	2	40	2
Saltine Crackers	2	25	tr
Sesame Breadsticks	2	35	0
Spiced Apple Rings	4 oz	100	0
Spinach	1 oz	7	tr
Strawberries	2 oz	14	tr
Strawberry Glaze	1 oz	37	0
Tartar Sauce	1 oz	85	11
Tomatoes	1 oz	6	tr
Turkey & Ham Salad	3.5 oz	186	13
Turkey Julienne	1 oz	29	tr
Vanilla Wafer	2	35	1
Watermelon	1 wedge	111	1

FOOD	PORTION	CALORIES	FAT
Yogurt, Fruit	4 oz	115	1
Yogurt, Vanilla	4 oz	110	2
Zucchini	1 oz	5	0
SALAD DRESSINGS			
Blue Cheese	1 oz	130	13
Cole Slaw	1 oz	150	14
Creamy Italian	1 oz	103	10
Cucumber Reduced Calorie	1 oz	69	6
Italian Reduced Calorie	1 oz	31	3
Parmesan Pepper	1 oz	150	15
Ranch	1 oz	147	15
Salad Oil	1 tbsp	120	14
Sour Cream	1 tbsp	26	3
Sweet-N-Tangy	1 oz	122	9
Thousand Island	1 oz	113	10

QUINCY'S FAMILY STEAKHOUSE

MAIN MENU SELECTIONS			
Catfish Filets	2	309	12
Chicken Strips	4	318	15
Chili Cheeseburger	1	919	54
Chopped Steak	6 oz	466	34
Country Style Steak w/ Mushroom Sauce	6 oz	288	19
Hamburger, ¼-lb	1	403	19
Hamburger w/ Cheese	1	451	23
Luncheon Chopped Steak	4 oz	350	25
Ribeye Steak	7 oz	665	60
Shrimp	7	248	12
Sirloin Club	5 oz	283	10

FOOD	PORTION	CALORIES	FAT
Sirloin Petite	4 oz	446	37
Sirloin Regular	6 oz	649	54
Sirloin Tips	4 oz	236	9
Steak, Filet, Extra-Thick	6 oz	331	12
Steak, Ribeye, Extra-Thick	9 oz	865	78
Steak, Sirloin, Extra-Thick	8 oz	898	73
Steak, T-Bone, Extra-Thick	13 oz	1612	159
T-Bone Steak	8 oz	1045	95
SIDE DISHES			
Baked Potato w/o Butter	1	181	tr
Barbecue Beans	1 portion	296	13
Cole Slaw	1 portion	60	5
Corn Bread	1 piece	178	6
Country Style Roll	1	70	1
Green Beans	1 portion	40	1
Mushroom Sauce	2 oz	27	tr
Peppers & Onions	1 portion	80	5
Steak Fries	1 portion	426	21
Texas Toast w/o Butter	1 portion	73	tr
SOUPS			
Chili w/ Beans	9 oz	346	16
Clam Chowder	9 oz	198	14
Vegetable Beef	9 oz	78	2

RAX

BEVERAGES AND DESSERTS			
Chocolate Chip Cookie	1	262	12
Chocolate Shake	11 oz	445	12
Coca-Cola	16 oz	205	0
Diet Coke	16 oz	1	0

FOOD	PORTION	CALORIES	FAT
MAIN MENU SELECTIONS			
Bacon	1 slice	14	1
Baked Potato	1	264	0
Baked Potato w/ 1 tbsp Margarine	1	364	11
Barbecue Sauce	1 pkg	11	0
Beef, Bacon 'N Cheddar	1	523	32
Cheddar Cheese Sauce	1 oz	29	tr
Country Fried Chicken Breast Sandwich	1	618	29
Deluxe Roast Beef	1	498	30
French Dressing	2 oz	275	22
French Fries	1 reg	282	14
Gourmet Garden Salad w/ French Dressing	1	409	29
Gourmet Garden Salad w/ Lite Italian Dressing	1	305	10
Gourmet Garden Salad w/o Dressing	1	134	6
Grilled Chicken Breast Sandwich	1	402	23
Grilled Chicken Garden Salad w/ French Dressing	1	477	31
Grilled Chicken Garden Salad w/ Lite Italian Dressing	1	264	12
Grilled Chicken Salad w/o Dressing	1	202	9
Lite Italian Dressing	2 oz	63	3
Mushroom Sauce	1 oz	16	tr
Philly Melt	1	396	16
Regular Rax	1	262	10
Swiss Slice	1 slice	42	3

RED LOBSTER

FOOD	PORTION	CALORIES	FAT
Atlantic Cod	1 lunch serving	100	1
Atlantic Ocean Perch	1 lunch serving	130	4

FOOD	PORTION	CALORIES	FAT
Blacktip Shark	1 lunch serving	150	1
Calamari, Breaded & Fried	1 lunch serving	360	21
Calico Scallops	1 lunch serving	180	2
Catfish	1 lunch serving	170	10
Chicken Breast, Skinless	4 oz	140	3
Deep Sea Scallops	1 lunch serving	130	2
Filet Mignon	8 oz	350	16
Flounder	1 lunch serving	100	1
Grouper	1 lunch serving	110	1
Haddock	1 lunch serving	110	1
Halibut	1 lunch serving	110	1
Hamburger	5 oz	410	28
King Crab Legs	1 lb	170	2
Langostino	1 lunch serving	120	1
Lemon Sole	1 lunch serving	120	1
Mackerel	1 lunch serving	190	12
Maine Lobster	18 oz	240	8
Mako Shark	1 lunch serving	140	1
Monkfish	1 lunch serving	110	1
Norwegian Salmon	1 lunch serving	230	12
Pollack	1 lunch serving	120	1
Rainbow Trout	1 lunch serving	170	9
Red Rockfish	1 lunch serving	90	1
Red Snapper	1 lunch serving	110	1
Ribeye Steak	12 oz	980	82
Rock Lobster	1 tail (13 oz)	230	3
Shrimp	8–12 pieces (7 oz)	120	2
Sirloin Steak	8 oz	350	15
Snow Crab Legs	1 lb	150	2

FOOD	PORTION	CALORIES	FAT
Sockeye Salmon	1 lunch serving	160	4
Strip Steak	9 oz	560	40
Swordfish	1 lunch serving	100	4
Tilefish	1 lunch serving	100	2
Yellowfin Tuna	1 lunch serving	180	6

ROY ROGERS

FOOD	PORTION	CALORIES	FAT
BEVERAGES			
Coca-Cola	12 oz	145	0
Coffee, Black	1 reg	0	0
Diet Coke	12 oz	1	0
Hot Chocolate	6 oz	123	2
Ice Tea	1 reg	0	0
Milk, Whole	8 oz	150	8
Orange Juice	7 oz	99	tr
Orange Juice	10 oz	136	tr
Shake, Chocolate	1	358	10
Shake, Strawberry	1	315	10
Shake, Vanilla	1	306	11
BREAKFAST SELECTIONS			
Breakfast Crescent Sandwich	1	401	27
Breakfast Crescent Sandwich w/ Bacon	1	431	30
Breakfast Crescent Sandwich w/ Ham	1	442	29
Breakfast Crescent Sandwich w/ Sausage	1	449	29
Breakfast Crescent Sandwich w/ Sausage	1 lg	608	30
Pancake Platter w/ syrup & butter	1	452	15
Pancake Platter w/ syrup, butter & bacon	1	493	18

FOOD	PORTION	CALORIES	FAT
Pancake Platter w/ syrup, butter & ham	1	506	17
Pancake Platter w/ syrup, butter & sausage	1	608	30
DESSERTS			
Brownie	1	264	11
Danish, Apple	1	249	12
Danish, Cheese	1	254	12
Danish, Cherry	1	271	14
Strawberry Shortcake	1	447	19
Sundae, Caramel	1	293	9
Sundae, Hot Fudge	1	337	13
Sundae, Strawberry	1	216	7
MAIN MENU SELECTIONS			
Bacon Cheeseburger	1	581	39
Biscuit	1	231	12
Cheeseburger	1	563	37
Chicken Breast	4.8 oz	412	24
Chicken Breast & Wing	6.5 oz	604	37
Chicken Leg	1.8 oz	140	8
Chicken Nuggets	6	267	17
Chicken Thigh	3.2 oz	296	20
Chicken Thigh & Leg	5 oz	436	28
Chicken Wing	1.7 oz	192	13
Cole Slaw	1 reg	110	7
French Fries	1 reg	268	14
French Fries	1 lg	357	18
Hamburger	1	456	28
Hot Topped Potato, Plain	1	211	2
Hot Topped Potato w/ Bacon 'N Cheese	1	397	22

FOOD	PORTION	CALORIES	FAT
Hot Topped Potato w/ Broccoli 'N Cheese	1	376	18
Hot Topped Potato w/ Oleo	1	274	7
Hot Topped Potato w/ Sour Cream 'N Chives	1	408	21
Hot Topped Potato w/ Taco Beef 'N Cheese	1	463	22
Large Roast Beef Sandwich	1	360	12
Large Roast Beef Sandwich w/ Cheese	1	467	21
Macaroni Salad	1 reg	186	11
Potato Salad	1 reg	107	6
Roast Beef Sandwich	1	317	10
Roast Beef Sandwich w/ Cheese	1	424	19
RR Bar Burger	1	611	39
SALAD BAR			
Bacon Bits	1 tbsp	33	1
Beets, Sliced	¼ cup	16	0
Broccoli	½ cup	20	0
Carrots, Shredded	¼ cup	42	0
Cheddar Cheese	¼ cup	112	9
Chinese Noodles	¼ cup	55	3
Chopped Egg	2 tbsp	55	4
Croutons	2 tbsp	70	0
Cucumbers	5–6 slices	4	0
Green Peas	¼ cup	7	0
Green Peppers	2 tbsp	4	0
Lettuce	1 cup	10	0
Mushrooms	¼ cup	5	0
Sunflower Seeds	2 tbsp	157	9
Tomatoes	3 slices	20	0

FOOD	PORTION	CALORIES	FAT
SALAD DRESSINGS			
1000 Island	2 tbsp	160	16
Bacon 'N Tomato	2 tbsp	136	12
Blue Cheese	2 tbsp	150	16
Lo-cal Italian	2 tbsp	70	6
Ranch	2 tbsp	155	14

SHONEY'S

FOOD	PORTION	CALORIES	FAT
BEVERAGES			
Clear Soda	1 sm	52	0
Clear Soda	1 lg	105	0
Coffee, Regular & Decaf	1 cup	8	0
Cola	1 sm	69	0
Cola	1 lg	139	0
Creamer	⅜ oz	14	1
Hot Chocolate	1 cup	110	2
Milk, 2%	1 cup	121	5
Orange Juice	4 oz	54	tr
Sugar	1 pkg	13	0
Tea	1 cup	0	0
BREAKFAST SELECTIONS			
100% Natural	½ cup	244	11
Ambrosia Salad	¼ cup	75	3
Apple	1	81	1
Apple Butter	1 tbsp	37	tr
Apple Grape Surprise	¼ cup	19	0
Apple Ring	1	15	0
Apple, Sliced	1 slice	13	tr
Bacon	1 strip	36	3
Beef Stick	1	43	1

FOOD	PORTION	CALORIES	FAT
Biscuit	1	170	8
Blueberries	¼ cup	21	tr
Blueberry Muffin	1	107	4
Bread Pudding	1 sq	305	11
Breakfast Ham	1 slice	26	1
Brunch Cake, Apple	1 sq	160	8
Brunch Cake, Banana	1 sq	152	7
Brunch Cake, Carrot	1 sq	150	7
Brunch Cake, Pineapple	1 sq	147	7
Brunch Cake, Sour Cream	1 sq	160	8
Buttered Toast	2 slices	163	5
Cantaloupe, Diced	½ cup	28	tr
Cantaloupe, Sliced	1 slice	8	tr
Captain Crunch Berry	½ cup	73	2
Cheese Sauce	1 ladle	26	2
Chicken Pieces	1 piece	40	2
Chocolate Pudding	¼ cup	81	2
Cinnamon Honey Bun	1	344	12
Cottage Cheese	1 tbsp	12	tr
Cottage Fries	¼ cup	62	2
Country Gravy	¼ cup	82	7
Croissant	1	260	16
DoughNugget	1	157	10
Egg, Fried	1	159	15
Egg, Scrambled	¼ cup	95	7
English Muffin w/ Margarine	1	140	2
Fluff	¼ cup	16	0
French Toast	1 slice	69	3
Fruit Delight	¼ cup	54	2
Fruit Topping, All Flavors	1 tbsp	24	0

FOOD	PORTION	CALORIES	FAT
Glaced Fruit	¼ cup	51	tr
Golden Pound Cake	1 slice	134	5
Grape Jelly	1 tbsp	60	0
Grapefruit, Canned	¼ cup	24	tr
Grapes	25	57	1
Grits	¼ cup	57	3
Hash Browns	¼ cup	43	2
Home Fries	¼ cup	53	2
Honey Bun	1	265	14
Honeydew, Sliced	1 slice	13	0
Jelly Packet	1	40	0
Jr. Bun, Chocolate	1	141	5
Jr. Bun, Honey	1	141	5
Jr. Bun, Maple	1	141	5
Kiwi, Sliced	1 slice	11	tr
Marble Cake w/ Icing	1 slice	136	5
Mini Cinnamon Donut	1	56	3
Mixed Fruit	¼ cup	37	tr
Mushroom Topping	1 oz	25	2
Oleo, Whipped	1 tbsp	70	8
Omelette Topping	1 spoonful	23	2
Orange	1 med	65	tr
Orange Sections	1 section	7	0
Oriental Salad	¼ cup	79	3
Pancake	1	41	tr
Pear	1	98	1
Pineapple Bits	1 tbsp	9	0
Pineapple, Fresh, Sliced	1 slice	10	tr
Pistachio Pineapple Salad	¼ cup	98	0
Powder Sugar Donut	1	56	3

FOOD	PORTION	CALORIES	FAT
Prunes	1 tbsp	19	0
Raisin Bran	½ cup	87	1
Raisin English Muffin w/ Margarine	1	158	4
Sausage Link	1	91	9
Sausage Patty	1	136	13
Sausage Rice	¼ cup	110	6
Shortcake	1	60	2
Sirloin Steak, Charbroiled	6 oz	357	25
Smoked Sausage	1	103	10
Snow Salad	¼ cup	72	4
Strawberries	5	23	tr
Syrup, Light	1 ladle	60	0
Syrup, Low-Cal	2.2 oz	98	0
Tangerine	1	37	tr
Trix	½ cup	54	tr
Waldorf Salad	¼ cup	81	5
Watermelon, Diced	½ cup	50	1
Watermelon, Sliced	1 slice	9	tr
Whipped Topping	1 scoop	10	1

CHILDREN'S MENU SELECTIONS

Jr. Burger All-American	1 serving	234	11
Kid's Fried Chicken Dinner	1 serving	244	13
Kid's Fish N' Chips (includes fries)	1 serving	337	17
Kid's Fried Shrimp	1 serving	194	12
Kid's Spaghetti	1 serving	247	8

DESSERTS

Apple Pie a la Mode	1 slice	492	23
Carrot Cake	1 slice	500	26
Hot Fudge Cake	1 slice	522	20
Hot Fudge Sundae	1	451	22

FOOD	PORTION	CALORIES	FAT
Strawberry Sundae	1	380	19
Strawberry Pie	1 slice	332	17
Walnut Brownie a la Mode	1	576	34
MAIN MENU SELECTIONS			
All-American Burger	1	501	33
Bacon Burger	1	591	40
Baked Fish	1 serving	170	1
Baked Ham Sandwich	1	290	10
Baked Potato	10 oz	264	tr
BBQ Sauce	1 souffle cup	41	1
Bite-Size Shrimp	1 serving	387	25
Broiled Shrimp	1 serving	93	18
Charbroiled Chicken	1 serving	239	7
Charbroiled Chicken Sandwich	1	451	17
Charbroiled Shrimp	1 serving	138	3
Chicken Fillet Sandwich	1	464	21
Chicken Tenders	1 serving	388	20
Cocktail Sauce	1 souffle cup	36	tr
Country Fried Sandwich	1	588	29
Country Fried Steak	1 serving	449	27
Fish N' Chips (includes fries)	1 serving	639	35
Fish N' Shrimp	1 serving	487	26
Fish Sandwich	1	323	13
French Fries	3 oz	189	8
French Fries	4 oz	252	10
Grecian Bread	1 slice	80	2
Grilled Bacon & Cheese Sandwich	1	440	28
Grilled Cheese Sandwich	1	302	17
Half O'Pound	1 serving	435	34
Ham Club on Whole Wheat	1	642	36

FOOD	PORTION	CALORIES	FAT
Hawaiian Chicken	1 serving	262	7
Italian Feast	1 serving	500	20
Large Shrimper's Feast	1 serving	575	33
Lasagna	1 serving	297	10
Light Baked Fish	1 serving	170	1
Light Beef Patty	1 serving	289	23
Light Fried Fish	1 serving	297	14
Liver N' Onions	1 serving	411	23
Mushroom Swiss Burger	1	616	42
Old-Fashioned Burger	1	470	28
Onion Rings	1	52	3
Patty Melt	1	640	42
Philly Steak Sandwich	1	673	44
Reuben Sandwich	1	596	35
Ribeye	6 oz	605	51
Rice	3.5 oz	137	4
Sautéed Mushrooms	3 oz	75	7
Sautéed Onions	2.5 oz	37	2
Seafood Platter	1 serving	566	28
Shoney Burger	1	498	36
Shrimp Sampler	1 serving	412	23
Shrimper's Feast	1 serving	383	22
Sirloin	6 oz	357	25
Slim Jim Sandwich	1	484	24
Spaghetti	1 serving	496	16
Steak N' Shrimp (charbroiled shrimp)	1 serving	361	23
Steak N' Shrimp (fried shrimp)	1 serving	507	33
Sweet N' Sour Sauce	1 souffle cup	58	0
Tartar Sauce	1 souffle cup	84	8

FOOD	PORTION	CALORIES	FAT
Turkey Club on Whole Wheat	1	635	33
SALAD BAR			
Ambrosia Salad	¼ cup	75	3
Apple Grape Surprise	¼ cup	19	0
Apple Ring	1	15	0
Bacon Bits	1 spoonful	15	1
Beet Onion Salad	¼ cup	25	1
Black Olives	2	10	1
Broccoli	¼ cup	4	tr
Broccoli, Cauliflower, Carrot Salad	¼ cup	53	4
Broccoli & Cauliflower	¼ cup	98	9
Broccoli & Cauliflower Ranch	¼ cup	65	6
Carrot	¼ cup	10	tr
Carrot Apple Salad	¼ cup	99	9
Cauliflower	¼ cup	8	tr
Celery	1 tbsp	5	0
Chocolate Pudding	¼ cup	81	2
Chow Mein Noodles	1 spoonful	13	1
Cole Slaw	¼ cup	69	5
Cottage Cheese	1 tbsp	12	tr
Croutons	1 spoonful	13	tr
Cucumber	1 tbsp	1	0
Cucumber Lite	¼ cup	12	tr
Diced Egg	1 tbsp	15	1
Don's Pasta	¼ cup	82	5
Fruit Delight	¼ cup	54	2
Fruit Topping, All Flavors	¼ cup	64	tr
Glaced Fruit	¼ cup	51	tr
Granola	1 spoonful	25	1
Grapefruit	¼ cup	24	tr

FOOD	PORTION	CALORIES	FAT
Green Olives	2	8	1
Green Pepper	1 tbsp	1	0
Italian Vegetable	¼ cup	11	tr
Jell-O	¼ cup	40	0
Jell-O Fluff	¼ cup	16	tr
Kidney Bean Salad	¼ cup	55	2
Lettuce	1.8 oz	7	tr
Macaroni Salad	¼ cup	207	14
Melba Toast	2	20	0
Mixed Fruit Salad	¼ cup	37	tr
Mixed Squash	¼ cup	49	4
Mushrooms	1 tbsp	1	0
Oil	1 tsp	45	5
Oriental Salad	¼ cup	79	3
Pea Salad	¼ cup	73	6
Pepperoni	1 tbsp	30	3
Pickle Chips	1 slice	5	0
Pickle Spear	1 spear	2	0
Pineapple Bits	1 tbsp	11	0
Pistachio Pineapple Salad	¼ cup	98	3
Prunes	1 tbsp	19	0
Radish	1 tbsp	1	0
Raisins	1 spoonful	26	0
Rotelli Pasta	¼ cup	78	4
Seign Salad	¼ cup	72	4
Shredded Cheese	1 tbsp	21	2
Sliced Onion	1 tbsp	1	0
Snow Delight	¼ cup	72	4
Spaghetti Salad	¼ cup	81	5
Spinach	¼ cup	1	0

FOOD	PORTION	CALORIES	FAT
Spring Pasta	¼ cup	38	3
Summer Salad	¼ cup	114	12
Sunflower Seeds	1 spoonful	40	3
Three Bean Salad	¼ cup	96	5
Trail Mix	1 spoonful	30	0
Turkey Ham	1 tbsp	12	1
Waldorf	¼ cup	81	5
Wheat Bread	1 slice	71	1
Whipped Margarine	1 tsp	23	3
SALADS DRESSINGS			
Biscayne Lo-Cal	2 tbsp	62	1
Blue Cheese	2 tbsp	113	13
Creamy Italian	2 tbsp	135	15
French	2 tbsp	124	12
Golden Italian	2 tbsp	141	15
Honey Mustard	2 tbsp	165	17
Ranch	2 tbsp	95	10
Rue French	2 tbsp	122	10
Thousand Island	2 tbsp	130	13
W.W. Italian	2 tbsp	10	0
SOUP			
Bean	6 oz	63	1
Beef Cabbage	6 oz	86	3
Broccoli Cauliflower	6 oz	124	9
Cheddar Chowder	6 oz	91	2
Cheese Florentine Ham	6 oz	110	8
Chicken Gumbo	6 oz	60	2
Chicken Noodle	6 oz	62	1
Chicken Rice	6 oz	72	1
Clam Chowder	6 oz	94	5

FOOD	PORTION	CALORIES	FAT
Corn Chowder	6 oz	148	5
Cream of Broccoli	6 oz	75	5
Cream of Chicken	6 oz	136	9
Cream of Chicken Vegetable	6 oz	79	1
Onion	6 oz	29	2
Potato	6 oz	102	3
Tomato Florentine	6 oz	63	1
Tomato Vegetable	6 oz	46	tr
Vegetable Beef	6 oz	82	2

TACO BELL

FOOD	PORTION	CALORIES	FAT
Burrito Bean	1	447	14
Burrito Beef	1	493	21
Burrito Chicken	1	334	12
Burrito Combo	1	407	16
Burrito Fiesta Bean	1	226	9
Burrito Supreme	1	503	22
Chilito	1	383	18
Cinnamon Twists	1 order	171	8
Enchirito	1	382	20
Green Sauce	1 oz	4	0
Guacamole	⅔ oz	34	2
Jalapeno Peppers	3.5 oz	20	0
MexiMelt Beef	1	266	15
MexiMelt Chicken	1	257	15
Mexican Pizza	1	575	37
Nacho Cheese Sauce	2 oz	105	8
Nachos	1	346	18
Nachos Bellgrande	1	649	35
Nachos Supreme	1	367	27

FOOD	PORTION	CALORIES	FAT
Pico De Gallo	1	8	0
Pintos 'N Cheese	1	190	9
Ranch Dressing	2.5 oz	236	25
Red Sauce	1 oz	10	0
Salsa	⅓ oz	18	0
Sour Cream	⅔ oz	46	4
Taco	1	183	11
Taco Bellgrande	1	335	23
Taco Fiesta	1	127	7
Taco Salad	1	905	61
Taco Salad w/o Shell	1	484	31
Taco Sauce	1 pkg	2	0
Taco Sauce, Hot	1 pkg	3	0
Taco, Soft	1	225	12
Taco, Soft, Chicken	1	213	10
Taco, Soft, Fiesta	1	147	7
Taco, Soft, Steak	1	218	11
Taco, Soft, Supreme	1	272	16
Taco Supreme	1	230	15
Tostada	1	243	11
Tostada Fiesta	1	167	7

TACO JOHN'S

FOOD	PORTION	CALORIES	FAT
Bean Burrito	1	197	6
Beef Burrito	1	303	18
Chicken Burrito w/ Green Chili	1	344	16
Chicken Super Taco Salad w/ Dressing	1	507	27
Chicken Super Taco Salad w/o Dressing	1	377	15
Chimichanga	1	464	21

FOOD	PORTION	CALORIES	FAT
Chimichanga w/ Chicken	1 serving	441	19
Combo Burrito	1	250	12
Mexican Rice	1 serving	340	8
Nachos	1 serving	468	25
Potato Olé	1 lg	414	6
Smothered Burrito w/ Green Chili	1	367	18
Smothered Burrito w/ Texas Chili	1	455	23
Softshell	1	140	224
Softshell w/ Chicken	1	180	8
Super Burrito	1	389	16
Super Burrito w/ Chicken	1	366	14
Super Nachos	1 serving	669	39
Super Taco Bravo	1	361	19
Super Taco Salad w/ 2 oz Dressing	1	558	32
Super Taco Salad w/o Dressing	1	428	20
Taco	1	178	13
Taco Bravo	1	319	14
Taco Burger	1	281	14
Taco Salad w/ 2 oz Dressing	1	359	24
Taco Salad w/o Dressing	1	228	13

TCBY

FOOD	PORTION	CALORIES	FAT
Nonfat, All Flavors	1 kiddie size	88	tr
Nonfat, All Flavors	1 sm	162	tr
Nonfat, All Flavors	1 reg	226	tr
Nonfat, All Flavors	1 lg	289	tr
Nonfat, All Flavors	1 super	418	tr
Nonfat, All Flavors	1 giant	869	tr
Regular, All Flavors	1 kiddie size	104	2
Regular, All Flavors	1 sm	192	4

FOOD	PORTION	CALORIES	FAT
Regular, All Flavors	1 lg	341	8
Regular, All Flavors	1 super	494	11
Regular, All Flavors	1 giant	1027	24
Sugar Free, All Flavors	1 kiddie size	64	tr
Sugar Free, All Flavors	1 sm	118	tr
Sugar Free, All Flavors	1 reg	164	tr
Sugar Free, All Flavors	1 lg	210	tr
Sugar Free, All Flavors	1 super	304	tr
Sugar Free, All Flavors	1 giant	632	tr

T. J. CINNAMONS

FOOD	PORTION	CALORIES	FAT
Doughnuts, Cake	2	454	22
Doughnuts, Raised	2	352	22
Mini-Cinn, Plain	1	75	5
Mini-Cinn w/ Icing	1	80	5
Original Gourmet Cinnamon Roll, Plain	1	630	34
Original Gourmet Cinnamon Roll w/ Icing	1	686	34
Petite Cinnamon Roll, Plain	1	185	10
Petite Cinnamon Roll w/ Icing	1	202	10
Sticky Bun, Cinnamon Pecan	1	607	35
Sticky Bun, Petite Cinnamon Pecan	1	255	15
Triple Chocolate Classic Roll, Plain	1	412	28
Triple Chocolate Classic Roll w/ Icing	1	462	31

WENDY'S

FOOD	PORTION	CALORIES	FAT
BEVERAGES			
Coffee, Black	6 oz	2	0
Coffee, Decaffeinated Black	6 oz	2	0
Cola	8 oz	100	0

FOOD	PORTION	CALORIES	FAT
Diet Cola	8 oz	1	0
Hot Chocolate	6 oz	110	1
Lemonade	8 oz	90	0
Lemon-Lime	8 oz	100	0
Milk, 2%	8 oz	110	4
Milk, Chocolate	8 oz	160	5
Tea, Hot	6 oz	1	0
Tea, Iced	12 oz	2	0

CHILDREN'S MENU SELECTIONS

FOOD	PORTION	CALORIES	FAT
Kid's Meal Cheeseburger	1	300	13
Kid's Meal Hamburger	1	260	33

DESSERTS

FOOD	PORTION	CALORIES	FAT
Chocolate Chip Cookie	1	275	13
Frosty Dairy Dessert	1 sm	340	10

MAIN MENU SELECTIONS

FOOD	PORTION	CALORIES	FAT
¼-lb Hamburger Patty (no bun)	1	180	12
American Cheese	1 slice	70	6
Bacon	1 strip	30	3
Big Classic	1	570	33
Cheddar Cheese, Shredded	1 oz	110	10
Chicken Breast Fillet	1	220	10
Chicken Club Sandwich	1	506	25
Chicken Sandwich	1	440	19
Chili	1 reg	220	7
Country Fried Steak Sandwich	1	440	25
Crispy Chicken Nuggets	6	280	20
Fish Fillet Sandwich	1	460	25
French Fries	1 sm order	240	12
Grilled Chicken Fillet	1	100	3
Grilled Chicken Sandwich	1	340	13

FOOD	PORTION	CALORIES	FAT
Honey Mustard	1 tbsp	71	6
Hot Stuffed Potato, Bacon & Cheese	1	520	18
Hot Stuffed Potato, Broccoli & Cheese	1	400	16
Hot Stuffed Potato, Cheese	1	420	15
Hot Stuffed Potato, Chili & Cheese	1	500	18
Hot Stuffed Potato, Plain	1	250	tr
Hot Stuffed Potato, Sour Cream & Chives	1	500	23
Jr. Bacon Cheeseburger	1	430	25
Jr. Cheeseburger	1	310	13
Jr. Hamburger	1	260	9
Jr. Swiss Deluxe	1	360	18
Kaiser Bun	1	200	3
Ketchup	1 tbsp	17	tr
Lettuce	1 leaf	1	0
Mayonnaise	1 tbsp	90	10
Mustard	1 tsp	4	tr
Nuggets Sauce, Barbecue	1 pkg	50	tr
Nuggets Sauce, Honey	1 pkg	45	tr
Nuggets Sauce, Sweet & Sour	1 pkg	45	tr
Nuggets Sauce, Sweet Mustard	1 pkg	50	1
Onion	6 rings	4	tr
Pickles	½ oz	2	tr
Plain Single	1	340	15
Sandwich Bun	1	160	3
Single w/ Everything	1	420	21
Sour Cream	1 oz	60	6
Tartar Sauce	⅔ oz	120	14
Tomatoes	2 slices	4	tr

FOOD	PORTION	CALORIES	FAT
SALAD SUPER BAR			
Alfalfa Sprouts	1 oz	8	0
Alfredo Sauce	2 oz	36	1
Applesauce, Chunky	1 oz	22	tr
Bacon Bits	1 tbsp	40	2
Bananas	1 oz	26	tr
Blue Cheese Dressing	1 tbsp	90	10
Breadsticks	2	30	1
Broccoli	½ cup	12	0
Cantaloupe	2 oz	20	0
Carrots	¼ cup	12	0
Cauliflower	½ cup	14	0
Celery Seed Dressing	1 tbsp	70	6
Cheddar Chips	1 oz	160	12
Cheese Ravioli in Spaghetti Sauce	2 oz	45	1
Cheese Sauce	2 oz	39	2
Cheese, Shredded, Imitation	1 oz	80	6
Cheese Tortellini in Spaghetti Sauce	2 oz	60	1
Chef Salad	1 (9 oz)	130	5
Chicken Salad	2 oz	120	8
Chives	1 oz	71	1
Chow Mein Noodles	½ oz	64	4
Cole Slaw	2 oz	70	5
Cottage Cheese	½ cup	108	4
Croutons	½ oz	60	3
Cucumbers	4 slices	2	0
Eggs, Hard Cooked, Chopped	1 tbsp	30	2
Fettuccini	2 oz	190	39
Flour Tortilla	1	110	3
French Style Dressing	1 tbsp	60	6

FOOD	PORTION	CALORIES	FAT
French Sweet Red Dressing	1 tbsp	70	6
Garbanzo Beans	1 oz	46	1
Garden Salad	1 (8 oz)	70	2
Garlic Toast	1	70	3
Green Peas	1 oz	21	0
Green Peppers	¼ cup	10	0
Hidden Valley Ranch Dressing	1 tbsp	50	6
Honeydew Melon	2 oz	20	0
Italian Caesar Dressing	1 tbsp	80	9
Italian Golden Dressing	1 tbsp	45	4
Jalapeno Peppers	1 tbsp	2	0
Lettuce, Iceberg	1 cup	8	0
Lettuce, Romaine	1 cup	9	0
Mushrooms	¼ cup	4	0
Oil	2 tbsp	250	28
Olives, Black	1 oz	35	3
Oranges	2 oz	26	0
Parmesan Cheese	1 oz	130	9
Parmesan Cheese, Imitation	1 oz	80	3
Pasta Medley	2 oz	60	2
Pasta Salad	¼ cup	35	tr
Peaches	2 pieces	31	0
Pepperoni, Sliced	1 oz	140	12
Picante Sauce	2 oz	18	tr
Pineapple Chunks	3 oz	60	0
Potato Salad	2 oz	125	11
Pudding, Butterscotch	2 oz	90	4
Pudding, Chocolate	2 oz	90	4
Red Onions	3 rings	2	0

FOOD	PORTION	CALORIES	FAT
Reduced Calorie Bacon & Tomato Dressing	1 tbsp	45	4
Reduced Calorie Italian Dressing	1 tbsp	25	2
Refried Beans	2 oz	70	3
Rotini	2 oz	90	2
Seafood Salad	2 oz	110	7
Sour Topping	1 oz	58	5
Spaghetti Meat Sauce	2 oz	60	2
Spaghetti Sauce	2 oz	28	tr
Spanish Rice	2 oz	70	1
Strawberries	2 oz	17	0
Sunflower Seeds & Raisins	1 oz	140	10
Taco Chips	1.33 oz	260	10
Taco Meat	2 oz	110	7
Taco Salad	1 (17 oz)	530	23
Taco Sauce	1 oz	16	tr
Taco Shell	1	45	3
Thousand Island Dressing	1 tbsp	70	7
Three Bean Salad	2 oz	60	tr
Tomatoes	1 oz	6	0
Tuna Salad	2 oz	100	6
Turkey Ham	1 oz	35	1
Watermelon	2 oz	18	0
Wine Vinegar	1 tbsp	2	0

WHITE CASTLE

FOOD	PORTION	CALORIES	FAT
Bun	1	74	tr
Cheese	3 oz	31	2
Cheeseburger	1	200	11

FOOD	PORTION	CALORIES	FAT
Chicken Sandwich	1	186	7
Fish Sandwich w/o Tartar	1	155	5
French Fries	1 reg	301	15
Hamburger	1	161	8
Onion Rings	1 reg order	245	13
Sausage Sandwich	1	196	12
Sausage & Egg Sandwich	1	322	22

WINCHELL'S DONUTS

FOOD	PORTION	CALORIES	FAT
Apple Fritter	1	580	37
Cinnamon Crumb	1	240	11
Cinnamon Roll	1	360	21
Glazed Jelly	1	300	13
Glazed Round	1	210	12
Glazed Twist	1	210	11
Iced Chocolate Bar	1	220	11
Iced Chocolate Cake	1	230	10
Iced Chocolate Devil's	1	240	12
Iced Chocolate French	1	220	13
Iced Chocolate Raised	1	210	10
Plain	1	200	11
Plain Donut Hole	1	50	3